Experimentation with Human Subjects

THE DAEDALUS LIBRARY

Experimentation with Human Subjects

Edited by
PAUL A. FREUND

GEORGE BRAZILLER
NEW YORK

For information address the publisher:
George Braziller, Inc.
One Park Avenue, New York 10016

Standard Book Number: 0-8076-0542-5, cloth; 0-8076-0541-7, paper

Library of Congress Catalog Card Number: 70–107776

With the exception of "Protection and Compensation for Injury in Human Studies" by Irving Ladimer, "The Clinical Moratorium" by Judith P. Swazey and Renée C. Fox, and Comments by Arthur J. Dyck, Walsh McDermott, and Donald Fleming, the essays in this book appeared in the Spring 1969 issue of *Daedalus*, the Journal of the American Academy of Arts and Sciences. "Philosophical Reflections in Human Experimentation" by Hans Jonas, which appeared in the same issue, has been extensively revised.

FIRST PRINTING

Printed in the United States of America

Jacket photograph: George Tames, *New York Times*

CONTENTS

CONTENTS

Preface

TODAY, WHEN the news media are filled with reports of efforts to prolong life through new surgical techniques involving human organ transplants, there is no dearth of interest in the matters raised in this book. The transplant development alone, particularly as it relates to heart surgery, would have been sufficient to create a substantial concern about the ethics of experimentation with human subjects had such an interest not already existed. The Academy's involvement in the matter, in fact, antedates by several years the inauguration of these novel surgical techniques. This is another way of saying that our concern transcends the present situation, and is based on the premise that experimentation with human subjects is an integral part of modern scientific research—and not only in the medical field—and that it behooves us to consider carefully the many ethical issues raised by such research.

While it would be impossible to set a date when systematic study of the matters discussed in this volume first received wide attention, some would say that substantial inquiry began to be made soon after World War II. The reasons are obvious: Given what had transpired during the years of Nazi terror, it was altogether reasonable that jurists and physicians—and many others as well—should wish to reflect on that experience and seek to establish codes that would make such bestial activity impossible. It would be difficult to overstate the impetus this uniquely tragic European experience gave to studies of the ethics of human experimentation. Out of a concern with the violence done to human beings came an interest in defining precisely the conditions under which human experimentation might take place.

There were, however, additional reasons for considering such matters, and these had to do more with what seemed to be impending in the sphere of research than with anything that had already taken place. By the late 1950's, particularly in the United States, public funds for medical research had increased many times, and experimentation involving human subjects was proceeding on an unprecedented scale throughout the country. In such circumstances, an articulate demand inevitably developed for assurance that the experimentation for which these public monies were being used would bear public screening. The problem, obviously, was to develop a more rational basis for judging experimental performance.

There were many interests involved: those of the subject, obviously, but also those of the investigator, as well as the scientific team with which he was often associated; and finally and very importantly, also those of the larger society that in one way or other sanctioned such experiments. How can each of these interests be defined, protected, and controlled? The "regulation" of research, particularly that significant segment involving human subjects, has become a matter of the greatest moment. The issues are at once ethical and scientific, but also social and legal. It can even be argued that they have, at least potentially, a certain political importance. They are clearly not the kinds of issues that can be deliberated on and resolved by a group representing only a single profession or interest. Given the American Academy's extensive experience with interdisciplinary inquiry, it is entirely reasonable that it should have sought to foster discussions in such an area.

The Academy showed its concern early in 1966 when its President, Paul A. Freund, appointed a small Working Party to consult on the matter. The Working Party met through 1966 and 1967 in a sort of "continuing seminar" on the subject. While it was generally accepted that the issue of experimentation with human subjects has relevance for many fields other than medicine, it was deemed advisable for the group to concentrate its attention on medical experimentation. The need for an analogous inquiry, particularly in those social sciences that make abundant use of human subjects, would be generally admitted. This may well prove to be an area that the American Academy will shortly wish to explore. There is reason to believe that ethical issues will increasingly preoccupy social scientists, and not only because of a growing resistance to their research proposals. The school and the ghetto are two of the more obvious sites for experimentation with human subjects, and their inhabitants may need to be "protected" in very much the same way that hospital patients and experimental subjects in medical research now are. Alternatives will have to be weighed so that the needs of society are taken into account while the rights of the individual are not neglected. The medical paradigm—with its emphasis on consent, professional competence, review mechanisms, adequacy of research design, legal liability, protection of privacy, governmental regulation, and the like—may prove to have more than a little relevance to the kinds of psychological and educational experimentation that will be countenanced in the future.

If the Working Party chose to concentrate on medical experimentation, it did so in a context that made ample use of the insights of men and women coming from many disciplines and from very different professions, as will be obvious from the list of names given at the back of the volume. We are indebted to those who helped. They participated—sometimes as witnesses, always as collaborators—in sessions of the Working Party; many attended one or both of the larger conferences convened to deliberate on memoranda and papers. In November 1967, the first of these larger meetings was held. Memoranda prepared for the occasion were discussed and criticized. The meeting provided the opportunity for members to become aware of certain of the dimensions of the problem as they had been defined by the Working Party. The meeting stimulated an expansion of the Working Party's original plans. A second conference, held in September 1968, provided the occasion for a study of the drafts of many of the essays printed here.

A number of additional essays, commissioned since the publication of the *Dædalus* issue in which many of these essays initially appeared, are presented here for the first time. They include a number of critical comments on several of the original essays. In short, this book presents evidence of a continuing dialogue.

It is difficult to know whether justice has been done to a theme of such obvious complexity. What may be said with no fear of contradiction is that the product, as presently offered, bears only a slight resemblance to what was said (or written) when the study was initiated. This is only to suggest that the "continuing seminar" has been a unique learning experience for those who participated in it, and that the group hopes to learn much from the responses of the larger audience that it now seeks to reach.

A great debt is owed to Dr. James A. Shannon of the National Institutes of Health for his original support of the Academy's endeavors in this area. A grant from the National Institutes of Health, number 1 RO1 HE11000-01, permitted the Academy to embark on this venture. The papers published here could not have been written in many instances but for the continued criticism they received through the conference procedures described above. It is a pleasant duty to acknowledge the help provided by this grant.

It is impossible to speak too highly of the assistance given by those who have so generously shared their time with us. All would wish to join in expressing our particular appreciation to Professor Freund. To be part of a study group that he chairs is a pleasure difficult to describe, but earnestly to be recommended to anyone who has not already experienced it. We feel deep gratitude to him.

S.R.G.

Experimentation with Human Subjects

PAUL A. FREUND

Introduction

Two CENTURIES ago it was said by a court of law that a physician experiments at his peril; if he departs from the accepted method of treatment, he is responsible for any untoward consequence to the patient. Today we are more likely to say that all serious therapy is experimental. The deepened knowledge of complex biological processes, the proliferation of powerful and sensitive drugs and therapies, the range of options in treatment, and the idiosyncrasies of patients' reactions, all make it inevitable that sound medical practice be experimental in a sense that does not contradict the nineteenth-century admonition, but renders it much less meaningful and serviceable as a guide to professional conduct.

There is another sense in which medical practice has become increasingly experimental—namely, in the interrelation between therapy and scientific investigation of a systematic kind. The embodiment of this kind of medical practice is, of course, the modern teaching hospital.

In casting about for models from other fields that might illuminate the ethical issues involved, members of different professions see different patterns and parallels. Partly this divergence of choice reflects what is most familiar in actuality, and partly, I surmise, it reflects what is thought to be most needed or desirable as a corrective to prevailing distortions. However that may be, it is true that sociologists and lawyers, for example, have turned to different models for ethical analysis.

The sociological model, focusing on the teaching hospital, is the professional collegium, like a university, which underscores the communal aspect of the endeavor, the reciprocity of rights and duties, the positive values to be pursued, encouraged, and facilitated, as well as the hazards, limitations, and safeguards. On the premise that the teaching hospital, oriented toward both research and immediate healing, is the institution best prepared to give the best of medical care, the patient's duty to cooperate in the research function is no less than the physicians' duty to use their best efforts to alleviate the patient's disease. Participation by the patient is a more apt concept, in this view, than legal consent to what would otherwise be assault and battery by the physician. Not many, however, seemed ready to agree with one member of the symposium who maintained that the duty to participate in an experiment on a measured basis (the hazard not being disproportionate to the potential social benefit) is as firm as the duty to submit to vaccination, on the ground that the danger of preventable contagion is no more deadly than the menace of avoidable ignorance.

The lawyers, on the other hand, tended to find models in fiduciary relationships, where a trustee, because of his superior competence and the trust and reliance placed in him, owes a duty of undivided loyalty and devotion to his client, the more so when the fiduciary, like a lawyer or doctor, enjoys as a class certain exclusive privileges to carry on his calling. This model underscores the obligation of full disclosure and explanation and the limitations of consent. At the same time, the lawyers recognized a wide area of consent whereby individuals capable of choosing may engage in hazardous undertakings that have a definite statistical morbidity, but are of approved social value, like driving automobiles at certain speeds or mining coal. Here the problem becomes one of compensation, and the analogy has been drawn between medical experimentation and industrial accidents, where the law has replaced the principle of compensation for injuries caused by the employer's negligence with the concept of compensation for injuries as an inherent cost of the enterprise, regardless of the allocation of fault. The analogy is a suggestive one, and its side effects will have to be considered. What would be the effect of compulsory accident insurance on the standard of prudence followed in experimentation? Would the elimination of inquiry into fault lead to irresponsibility? In the case of automobile accidents, the self-interest of the operator is a check on his behavior; perhaps the reputation of the experimenter and the hospital would be a comparable inner check. In the case of industrial accidents, the surveillance carried out by the insurance companies produces an acceptable level of safety. Who would serve as the insurers for medical experimentation? And would we wish to vest in them, as it were, responsibility for achieving the right balance between conservatism and innovation, between contentment and risk, that is the necessary calculus of experimentation?

These are all suggestive frameworks for viewing the ethical issues, and each gains something by the corrective of another. Although they furnish valuable points of view, they do not come to grips with the concrete judgments that have to be made. For such judgments, standards have to be evolved, influenced but not determined by a general point of view. Standards, in turn, can be of a greater or lesser degree of particularity, somewhere between the Golden Rule, which is inadequate (a masochist might be justified in employing sadistic measures), and a detailed code, which would be impractical. Guidelines, of a middle order of generality, have been developed around the world by various medical groups following the drafting of the so-called Nuremberg Code stimulated by the revulsion over the Nazi practices. These guidelines have been valuable in clarifying the ethical issues, but they are not free of ambiguities and questionable formulas.

Certainly consent should be sought in all such cases, but consent alone is not enough to warrant an experimental procedure. A bad experimental design, one that is incapable of yielding significant data, is itself unethical and cannot be immunized by procuring patients' consent. Similarly, in view of the fiduciary obligation of the physician, an experiment that entails a high degree of serious risk and is not for the direct benefit of the patient ought not to be put to the patient for consent. (The use of so-called normal volunteers will be considered separately.) Some possibility might be suggested of using dying patients in highly hazardous trials, with their consent or that of their family if they are incapable. But for a variety of reasons practical and emotional (results may be clouded by the deterioration of the patient; a dying person should be left to take his leave in peace), members of this group have not been regarded as proper subjects for perilous experimentation.

So far we have considered substantive questions. These are closely bound up with procedures for arriving at judgments and putting them into effect. Because of the potential conflict of roles of the physician-investigator, some outside judgment is called for. This is coming to be found in hospital committees on research (established partly under the stimulus of the NIH as a condition of its research grants), which consider all protocols for research involving human subjects in the institution, and which should include members not of the same department as the prospective experimenters. In addition, the chief of service, or the patient's private physician if he has one, should be required to approve the patient's participation. The protocol should include a statement of how the procedure will be explained to the subjects in seeking their informed consent. We need to know more about how these committees are actually functioning. An open question is whether non-medical representation should be included on the committee. Perhaps the very naïveté of a question put by a lawyer or theologian may open up an avenue of thought that had not occurred to the professional medical mind. Alternatively, such representation could be had on a review committee that makes a kind of audit of the work of the staff committee, through review of abstracts for approval or remand to the committee for clarification or modification. In time, a record of abstracts and action taken might provide a reservoir of source material, a kind of common law of the subject, that might be circulated to other institutions and could furnish material for medical school education in the ethics of experimentation. If medical students resemble law students in this respect—and there is good reason to believe they do—there would be a lively interest in exploring the ethical problems of their profession.

One simple procedural rule that is coming to be adopted is that papers submitted for publication must include a statement of how consent of the subjects was obtained and how approval was secured. A more drastic sanction—rejection by an editor of any paper based on an unethically conducted experiment—raises some question of censorship, especially in view of the indeterminate nature of certain of the ethical judgments in the field. Actual exposure of the methods employed for consent and approval may be an effective control. Sunlight, said Mr. Justice Brandeis, is the most effective of all disinfectants. Whether this is or ever was scientifically accurate, it makes a valid point about disclosure.

Much of the discussion of the patient as experimental subject is applicable to the so-called normal volunteer: the necessity for sound experimental design, for informed consent, for review procedures. The absence of a conflict of roles on the part of the investigator mitigates certain ethical problems, but since there is no physician as protector, the element of informed consent becomes all the more important, including as it does the question as to how severe a risk the normal volunteer should be allowed to assume. In an age of discovery, which bestows its highest accolade on courage in the service of new frontiers of knowledge, there seems little reason to be extremely finicky about accepting daring volunteers, provided the design is sound, the explanations candid, the objectives important, and the will not overborne. While experimental volunteers are probably motivated rather specially as a group, the question of motivation is so subtle and pervasive in so many aspects of life that it seems inappropriate to plumb this factor with special penetration in screening for medical experimentation. A study of attitudes toward volunteering indicated a spectrum from the most willing among menial workers to the least willing among professional people, suggesting at least that escape from boredom or monotony is a cardinal incentive and not an unworthy one, if not the highest possible.

The special problems arise with classes that are under some disability or constraint—children and prisoners. If the experiment may be of direct benefit to the child, the consent of the parent or guardian should be enough. If no direct benefit is indicated, may the parent consent (together with the child if he is at an age of understanding)? The subject is far from clear, but an absolute disqualification would eliminate much useful investigation. A more moderate rule is indicated, one that would permit children to serve as subjects where they are peculiarly suitable and there is no discernible hazard to them.

Prisoners (aside from prisoners of war, who are ineligible) present another controversial group. The basic standard ought to be that their will shall not be overborne either by threats of punishment or by promises of reward. Within those limits, although some investigators rule out prisoners as subjects, there seems to be no good reason for depriving this group of the satisfactions of participation on an informed basis, satisfactions that to them are often great indeed, bolstering their self-esteem and furnishing links to the general community and its values.

In all of our discussions, informed consent has loomed large. The concept has been derided as unreal, a cover for the will of the experimenter, and yet it serves purposes that should not lightly be dismissed. It bears repeating that consent will not protect a badly designed or negligently conducted experiment. Consent serves at the least a symbolic function, recalling the respect for individual integrity that should inform the quest for knowledge. More than that, it serves to force the experimenter to think through and articulate his project in terms of design, risks, and objectives, and thus it has a valuable reflexive effect on the enterprise itself, like the practice of a judge in writing an opinion rendering judgment (sometimes it "won't write").

Finally, a few words may be said on a very large subject: the allocation of scarce resources. In 1943 penicillin was in short supply among our Armed Forces in North Africa. Competitors for its use were two groups of soldiers suffering from infections that would respond to it: victims of venereal disease and victims of battle wounds. The Chief Surgical Consultant advised that priority be given to the wounded; the Theatre Medical Commander directed that priority be given to the other victims. How does one account for this apparently immoral judgment? For one thing, venereal disease sufferers could be restored to fighting trim more rapidly; and secondly, if untreated, they were a threat of infection spreading to others. It was a highly pragmatic judgment, in accord with the morality of social utility in a situation where objectives were closely defined—maximum fighting power as rapidly as possible. For better or worse, life is rarely so circumscribed in its goals.

Consider the allocation of the limited and costly renal dialysis machines among sufferers from otherwise untreatable kidney disease. A first screening can be made on medical grounds: capacity to benefit from the treatment and not succumb to complicating ailments. Beyond this preliminary selection, how should the candidates be assigned? In Seattle, a panel of eminent laymen makes the selection on the basis of worth to the community. This was the subject of considerable debate at the conferences. My own submission was that in a matter of choosing for life or death, not involving specific wrongdoing, no one should assume the responsibility of judging comparative worthiness to live on the basis of unfocused criteria of virtue or social usefulness, and that either priority in time, or a lottery, or a mechanical selection on the basis of age should be followed. One of the symposiasts retorted that it was quite feasible to measure the relevant qualities, but when it was pointed out that the Seattle group considered as a relevant factor attendance at church, he threw up his hands.

The more nearly total is the estimate to be made of an individual, and the more nearly the consequence determines life and death, the more unfit the judgment becomes for human reckoning—or so I suggest. Randomness as a moral principle deserves serious study. A generation ago a French biologist said that science has taught us how to become gods before we have learned to be men. But not even science has taught us how to act as gods on the Day of Judgment.

HANS JONAS

Philosophical Reflections on Experimenting with Human Subjects

EXPERIMENTING with human subjects is going on in many fields of scientific and technological progress. It is designed to replace the over-all instruction by natural, occasional experience with the selective information from artificial, systematic experiment which physical science has found so effective in dealing with inanimate nature. Of the new experimentation with man, medical is surely the most legitimate; psychological, the most dubious; biological (still to come), the most dangerous. I have chosen here to deal with the first only, where the case *for* it is strongest and the task of adjudicating conflicting claims hardest. When I was first asked[1] to comment "philosophically" on it, I had all the hesitation natural to a layman in the face of matters on which experts of the highest competence have had their say and still carry on their dialogue. As I familiarized myself with the material,[2] any initial feeling of moral rectitude that might have facilitated my task quickly dissipated before the awesome complexity of the problem, and a state of great humility took its place. The awareness of the problem in all its shadings and ramifications speaks out with such authority, perception, and sophistication in the published discussions of the researchers themselves that it would be foolish of me to hope that I, an onlooker on the sidelines, could tell those battling in the arena anything they have not pondered themselves. Still, since the matter is obscure by its nature and involves very fundamental, transtechnical issues, anyone's attempt at clarification can be of use, even without novelty. And even if the philosophical reflection should in the end achieve no more than the realization that in the dialectics of this area we must sin and fall into guilt, this insight may not be without its own gains.

1

I. The Peculiarity of Human Experimentation

Experimentation was originally sanctioned by natural science. There it is performed on inanimate objects, and this raises no moral problems. But as soon as animate, feeling beings become the subjects of experiment, as they do in the life sciences and especially in medical research, this innocence of the search for knowledge is lost and questions of conscience arise. The depth to which moral and religious sensibilities can become aroused over these questions is shown by the vivisection issue. Human experimentation must sharpen the issue as it involves ultimate questions of personal dignity and sacrosanctity. One profound difference between the human experiment and the physical (beside that between animate and inanimate, feeling and unfeeling nature) is this: The physical experiment employs small-scale, artificially devised substitutes for that about which knowledge is to be obtained, and the experimenter extrapolates from these models and simulated conditions to nature at large. Something deputizes for the "real thing"—balls rolling down an inclined plane for sun and planets, electric discharges from a condenser for real lightning, and so on. For the most part, no such substitution is possible in the biological sphere. We must operate on the original itself, the real thing in the fullest sense, and perhaps affect it irreversibly. No simulacrum can take its place. Especially in the human sphere, experimentation loses entirely the advantage of the clear division between vicarious model and true object. Up to a point, animals may fulfill the proxy role of the classical physical experiment. But in the end man himself must furnish knowledge about himself, and the comfortable separation of noncommittal experiment and definitive action vanishes. An experiment in education affects the lives of its subjects, perhaps a whole generation of schoolchildren. Human experimentation for whatever purpose is always *also* a responsible, nonexperimental, definitive dealing with the subject himself. And not even the noblest purpose abrogates the obligations this involves.

This is the root of the problem with which we are faced: Can both that purpose and this obligation be satisfied? If not, what would be a just compromise? Which side should give way to the other? The question is inherently philosophical as it concerns not merely pragmatic difficulties and their arbitration, but a genuine conflict of values involving principles of a high order. May I put the conflict in these terms. On principle, it is felt, human beings *ought not* to be dealt with in that way (the "guinea pig" protest); on the other hand, such dealings are increasingly urged on us by considerations, in turn appealing to principle, that claim to override those objections. Such a claim must be carefully assessed, especially when it is swept along by a mighty tide. Putting the matter thus, we have already made one important assumption rooted in our "Western" cultural tradition: The prohibitive rule is, to that way of thinking, the primary and axiomatic one; the permissive counter-rule, as qualifying the first, is secondary and stands in need of justification. We must justify the infringement of a primary inviolability, which needs no justification itself; and the justification of its infringement must be by values and needs of a dignity commensurate with those to be sacrificed.

Before going any further, we should give some more articulate voice to the resistance we feel against a merely utilitarian view of the matter. It has to do with a peculiarity of human experimentation quite independent of the question of possible injury to the subject. What is wrong with making a person an experimental subject is not so much that we make him thereby a means (which happens in social contexts of all kinds), as that we make him a thing—a passive thing merely to be acted on, and passive not even for real action, but for token action whose token object he is. His being is reduced to that of a mere token or "sample." This is different from even the most exploitative situations of social life: there the business is real, not fictitious. The subject, however much abused, remains an agent and thus a "subject" in the other sense of the word. The soldier's case is instructive: Subject to most unilateral discipline, forced to risk mutilation and death, conscripted without, perhaps against, his will—he is still conscripted with his capacities to act, to hold his own or fail in situations, to meet real challenges for real stakes. Though a mere "number" to the High Command, he is not a token and not a thing. (Imagine what he would say if it turned out that the war was a game staged to sample observations on his endurance, courage, or cowardice.)

These compensations of personhood are denied to the subject of experimentation, who is acted upon for an extraneous end without being engaged in a real relation where he would be the counterpoint to the other or to circumstance. Mere "consent" (mostly amounting to no more than permission) does not right this reification. Only

3

genuine authenticity of volunteering can possibly redeem the condition of "thinghood" to which the subject submits. Of this we shall speak later. Let us now look at the nature of the conflict, and especially at the nature of the claims countering in this matter those on behalf of personal sacrosanctity.

II. "Individual Versus Society" as the Conceptual Framework

The setting for the conflict most consistently invoked in the literature is the polarity of individual versus society—the possible tension between the individual good and the common good, between private and public welfare. Thus, W. Wolfensberger speaks of "the tension between the long-range interests of society, science, and progress, on one hand, and the rights of the individual on the other."[3] Walsh McDermott says: "In essence, this is a problem of the rights of the individual versus the rights of society."[4] Somewhere I found the "social contract" invoked in support of claims that science may make on individuals in the matter of experimentation. I have grave doubts about the adequacy of this frame of reference, but I will go along with it part of the way. It does apply to some extent, and it has the advantage of being familiar. We concede, as a matter of course, to the common good some pragmatically determined measure of precedence over the individual good. In terms of rights, we let some of the basic rights of the individual be overruled by the acknowledged rights of society—as a matter of right and moral justness and not of mere force or dire necessity (much as such necessity may be adduced in defense of that right). But in making that concession, we require a careful clarification of what the needs, interests, and rights of society are, for society—as distinct from any plurality of individuals—is an abstract and, as such, is subject to our definition, while the individual is the primary concrete, prior to all definition, and his basic good is more or less known. Thus the unknown in our problem is the so-called common or public good and its potentially superior claims, to which the individual good must or might sometimes be sacrificed, in circumstances that in turn must also be counted among the unknowns of our question. Note that in putting the matter in this way—that is, in asking about the right of society to individual sacrifice—the consent of the sacrificial subject is no necessary part of the *basic* question.

4

"Consent," however, is the other most consistently emphasized and examined concept in discussions of this issue. This attention betrays a feeling that the "social" angle is not fully satisfactory. If society has a right, its exercise is not contingent on volunteering. On the other hand, if volunteering is fully genuine, no public right to the volunteered act need be construed. There is a difference between the moral or emotional appeal of a cause that elicits volunteering and a right that demands compliance—for example, with particular reference to the social sphere, between the *moral claim* of a common good and society's *right* to that good and to the means of its realization. A moral claim cannot be met without consent; a right can do without it. Where consent is present anyway, the distinction may become immaterial. But the awareness of the many ambiguities besetting the "consent" actually available and used in medical research[5] prompts recourse to the idea of a public right conceived independently of (and valid prior to) consent; and, vice versa, the awareness of the problematic nature of such a right makes even its advocates still insist on the idea of consent with all its ambiguities: an uneasy situation either way.

Nor does it help much to replace the language of "rights" by that of "interests" and then argue the sheer cumulative weight of the interest of the many over against those of the few or the single individual. "Interests" range all the way from the most marginal and optional to the most vital and imperative, and only those sanctioned by particular importance and merit will be admitted to count in such a calculus—which simply brings us back to the question of right or moral claim. Moreover, the appeal to numbers is dangerous. Is the number of those afflicted with a particular disease great enough to warrant violating the interests of the non-afflicted? Since the number of the latter is usually so much greater, the argument can actually turn around to the contention that the cumulative weight of interest is on *their* side. Finally, it may well be the case that the individual's interest in his own inviolability is itself a public interest, such that its publicly condoned violation, irrespective of numbers, violates the interest of all. In that case, its protection in *each* instance would be a paramount interest, and the comparison of numbers will not avail.

These are some of the difficulties hidden in the conceptual framework indicated by the terms "society-individual," "interest," and "rights." But we also spoke of a moral call, and this points to another dimension—not indeed divorced from the social sphere,

5

but transcending it. And there is something even beyond that: true sacrifice from highest devotion, for which there are no laws or rules except that it must be absolutely free. "No one has the right to choose martyrs for science" was a statement repeatedly quoted in the November, 1967, *Dædalus* conference. But no scientist can be prevented from making himself a martyr for his science. At all times, dedicated explorers, thinkers, and artists have immolated themselves on the altar of their vocation, and creative genius most often pays the price of happiness, health, and life for its own consummation. But no one, not even society, has the shred of a right to expect and ask these things in the normal course of events. They come to the rest of us as a *gratia gratis data*.

III. The Sacrificial Theme

Yet we must face the somber truth that the *ultima ratio* of communal life is and has always been the compulsory, vicarious sacrifice of individual lives. The primordial sacrificial situation is that of outright human sacrifices in early communities. These were not acts of blood-lust or gleeful savagery; they were the solemn execution of a supreme, sacral necessity. One of the fellowship of men had to die so that all could live, the earth be fertile, the cycle of nature renewed. The victim often was not a captured enemy, but a select member of the group: "The king must die." If there was cruelty here, it was not that of men, but that of the gods, or rather of the stern order of things, which was believed to exact that price for the bounty of life. To assure it for the community, and to assure it ever again, the awesome *quid pro quo* had to be paid over again.

Far should it be from us to belittle, from the height of our enlightened knowledge, the majesty of the underlying conception. The particular *causal* views that prompted our ancestors have long since been relegated to the realm of superstition. But in moments of national danger we still send the flower of our young manhood to offer their lives for the continued life of the community, and if it is a just war, we see them go forth as consecrated and strangely ennobled by a sacrificial role. Nor do we make their going forth depend on their own will and consent, much as we may desire and foster these. We conscript them according to law. We conscript the best and feel morally disturbed if the draft, either by design or in effect, works so that mainly the disadvantaged, socially less useful, more expendable, make up those whose lives are to buy ours. No rational persuasion of the pragmatic necessity here at work can do away with the feeling, a mixture of gratitude and guilt, that the sphere of the sacred is touched with the vicarious offering of life for life. Quite apart from these dramatic occasions, there is, it appears, a persistent and constitutive aspect òf human immolation to the very being and prospering of human society—an immolation in terms of life and happiness, imposed or voluntary, of few for many. What Goethe has said of the rise of Christianity may well apply to the nature of civilization in general: *"Opfer fallen hier, / Weder Lamm noch Stier, / Aber Menschenopfer unerhoert."*[6] We can never rest comfortably in the belief that the soil from which our satisfactions sprout is not watered with the blood of martyrs. But a troubled conscience compels us, the undeserving beneficiaries, to ask: Who is to be martyred? in the service of what cause and by whose choice?

Not for a moment do I wish to suggest that medical experimentation on human subjects, sick or healthy, is to be likened to primeval human sacrifices. Yet something sacrificial is involved in the selective abrogation of personal inviolability and the ritualized exposure to gratuitous risk of health and life, justified by a presumed greater, social good. My examples from the sphere of stark sacrifice were intended to sharpen the issues implied in that context and to set them off clearly from the kinds of obligations and constraints imposed on the citizen in the normal course of things or generally demanded of the individual in exchange for the advantages of civil society.

IV. The "Social Contract" Theme

The first thing to say in such a setting-off is that the sacrificial area is not covered by what is called the "social contract." This fiction of political theory, premised on the primacy of the individual, was designed to supply a rationale for the *limitation* of individual freedom and power required for the existence of the body politic, whose existence in turn is for the benefit of the individuals. The principle of these limitations is that their *general* observance profits all, and that therefore the individual observer, assuring this general observance for his part, profits by it himself. I observe property rights because their general observance assures my own; I observe traffic rules because their general observance assures my own safety; and so on. The obligations here are mutual and general; no one is singled out for special sacrifice. Moreover, for the most part, *qua* limitations of my liberty, the laws thus deducible from the hypothetical "social contract" enjoin me from certain actions rather than obligate me to positive actions (as did the laws of feudal society). Even where the latter is the case, as in the duty to pay taxes, the rationale is that I am myself a beneficiary of the services financed through these payments. Even the contributions levied by the welfare state, though not originally contemplated in the liberal version of the social contract theory, can be interpreted as a personal insurance policy of one sort or another—be it against the contingency of my own indigence, be it against the dangers of disaffection from the laws in consequence of widespread unrelieved destitution, be it even against the disadvantages of a diminished consumer market. Thus, by some stretch, such contributions can still be subsumed under the principle of enlightened self-interest. But no complete abrogation of self-interest at any time is in the terms of the social contract, and so pure sacrifice falls outside it. Under the putative terms of the contract alone, I cannot be required to die for the public good. (Thomas Hobbes made this forcibly clear.) Even short of this extreme, we like to think that nobody is entirely and one-sidedly the victim in any of the renunciations exacted under normal circumstances by society "in the general interest"—that is, for the benefit of others. "Under normal circumstances," as we shall see, is a necessary qualification. Moreover, the "contract" can legitimitize claims only on our overt, public actions and not on our invisible private being. Our powers, not our persons, are beholden to the common weal. In one important respect, it is true, public interest and control do extend to the private sphere by general consent: in the compulsory education of our children. Even there, the assumption is that the learning and what is learned, apart from all future social usefulness, are also for the benefit of the individual in his own being. We would not tolerate education to degenerate into the conditioning of useful robots for the social machine.

Both restrictions of public claim in behalf of the "common good"—that concerning one-sided sacrifice and that concerning the private sphere—are valid only, let us remember, on the premise of the primacy of the individual, upon which the whole idea of the "social contract" rests. This primacy is itself a metaphysical axiom or option peculiar to our Western tradition, and the whittling away of its force would threaten the tradition's whole foundation. In passing, I may remark that systems adopting the alternative primacy of the community as their axiom are naturally less bound by the restrictions we postulate. Whereas we reject the idea of "expendables" and regard those not useful or even recalcitrant to the social purpose as a burden that society must carry (since their individual claim to existence is as absolute as that of the most useful), a truly totalitarian regime, Communist or other, may deem it right for the collective to rid itself of such encumbrances or to make them forcibly serve some social end by conscripting their persons (and there are effective combinations of both). We do not normally—that is, in nonemergency conditions—give the state the right to conscript labor, while we do give it the right to "conscript" money, for money is detachable from the person as labor is not. Even less than forced labor do we countenance forced risk, injury, and indignity.

But in time of war our society itself supersedes the nice balance of the social contract with an almost absolute precedence of public necessities over individual rights. In this and similar emergencies, the sacrosanctity of the individual is abrogated, and what for all practical purposes amounts to a near-totalitarian, quasi-communist state of affairs is *temporarily* permitted to prevail. In such situations, the community is conceded the right to make calls on its members, or certain of its members, entirely different in magnitude and kind from the calls normally allowed. It is deemed right that a part of the population bears a disproportionate burden of risk of a disproportionate gravity; and it is deemed right that the rest of the community accepts this sacrifice, whether voluntary or enforced, and reaps its benefits—difficult as we find it to justify this acceptance and this benefit by any normal ethical categories. We justify it transethically, as it were, by the supreme collective emergency, formalized, for example, by the declaration of a state of war.

Medical experimentation on human subjects falls somewhere between this overpowering case and the normal transactions of the social contract. On the one hand, no comparable extreme issue of social survival is (by and large) at stake. And no comparable extreme sacrifice or foreseeable risk is (by and large) asked. On the other hand, what is asked goes decidedly beyond, even runs counter to, what it is otherwise deemed fair to let the individual sign over of his person to the benefit of the "common good." Indeed, our sensitivity to the kind of intrusion and use involved is such that only an end of transcendent value or overriding urgency can make it arguable and possibly acceptable in our eyes.

V. Health as a Public Good

The cause invoked is health and, in its more critical aspect, life itself—clearly superlative goods that the physician serves directly by curing and the researcher indirectly by the knowledge gained through his experiments. There is no question about the good served nor about the evil fought—disease and premature death. But a good to whom and an evil to whom? Here the issue tends to become somewhat clouded. In the attempt to give experimentation the proper dignity (on the problematic view that a value becomes greater by being "social" instead of merely individual), the health in question or the disease in question is somehow predicated on the social whole, as if it were society that, in the persons of its members, enjoyed the one and suffered the other. For the purposes of our problem, public interest can then be pitted against private interest, the common good against the individual good. Indeed, I have found health called a national resource, which of course it is, but surely not in the first place.

In trying to resolve some of the complexities and ambiguities lurking in these conceptualizations, I have pondered a particular statement, made in the form of a question, which I found in the *Proceedings* of the earlier *Dædalus* conference: "Can society afford to discard the tissues and organs of the hopelessly unconscious patient when they could be used to restore the otherwise hopelessly ill, but still salvageable individual?" And somewhat later: "A strong case can be made that society can ill afford to discard the tissues and organs of the hopelessly unconscious patient; they are greatly needed for study and experimental trial to help those who can be salvaged."[7] I hasten to add that any suspicion of callousness that the "commodity" language of these statements may suggest is immediately dispelled by the name of the speaker, Dr. Henry K. Beecher, for whose humanity and moral sensibility there can be nothing but admiration. But the use, in all innocence, of this language gives food for thought. Let me, for a moment, take the question literally. "Discarding" implies proprietary rights—nobody can discard what does not belong to him in the first place. Does society then own my body? "Salvaging" implies the same and, moreover, a use-value to the owner. Is the life-extension of certain individuals then a public interest? "Affording" implies a critically vital level of such an interest—that is, of the loss or gain involved. And "society" itself—what is it? When does a need, an aim, an obligation become social? Let us reflect on some of these terms.

VI. What Society Can Afford

"Can Society afford . . . ?" Afford what? To let people die intact, thereby withholding something from other people who desperately need it, who in consequence will have to die too? These other, unfortunate people indeed cannot afford not to have a kidney, heart, or other organ of the dying patient, on which they depend for an extension of their lease on life; but does that give them a right to it? And does it oblige society to procure it for them? What is it that *society* can or cannot afford—leaving aside for the moment the question of what it has a *right* to? It surely can afford to lose members through death; more than that, it is built on the balance of death and birth decreed by the order of life. This is too general, of course, for our question, but perhaps it is well to remember. The specific question seems to be whether society can afford to let some people die whose death might be deferred by particular means if these were authorized by society. Again, if it is merely a question of what society can or cannot afford, rather than of what it ought or ought not to do, the answer must be: Of course, it can. If cancer, heart disease, and other organic, non-contagious ills, especially those tending to strike the old more than the young, continue to exact their toll at the normal rate of incidence (including the toll of private anguish and misery), society can go on flourishing in every way.

Here, by contrast, are some examples of what, in sober truth, society cannot afford. It cannot afford to let an epidemic rage unchecked; a persistent excess of deaths over births, but neither—we must add—too great an excess of births over deaths; too low an average life expectancy even if demographically balanced by fertility, but neither too great a longevity with the necessitated correlative dearth of youth in the social body; a debilitating state of general health; and things of this kind. These are plain cases where the whole condition of society is critically affected, and the public interest can make its imperative claims. The Black

11

Death of the Middle Ages was a *public* calamity of the acute kind; the life-sapping ravages of endemic malaria or sleeping sickness in certain areas are a public calamity of the chronic kind. Such situations a society as a whole can truly not "afford," and they may call for extraordinary remedies, including, perhaps, the invasion of private sacrosanctities.

This is not entirely a matter of numbers and numerical ratios. Society, in a subtler sense, cannot "afford" a single miscarriage of justice, a single inequity in the dispensation of its laws, the violation of the rights of even the tiniest minority, because these undermine the moral basis on which society's existence rests. Nor can it, for a similar reason, afford the absence or atrophy in its midst of compassion and of the effort to alleviate suffering—be it widespread or rare—one form of which is the effort to conquer disease of any kind, whether "socially" significant (by reason of number) or not. And in short, society cannot afford the absence among its members of *virtue* with its readiness for sacrifice beyond defined duty. Since its presence—that is to say, that of personal idealism— is a matter of grace and not of decree, we have the paradox that society depends for its existence on intangibles of nothing less than a religious order, for which it can hope, but which it cannot enforce. All the more must it protect this most precious capital from abuse.

For what objectives connected with the medico-biological sphere should this reserve be drawn upon—for example, in the form of accepting, soliciting, perhaps even imposing the submission of human subjects to experimentation? We postulate that this must be not just a worthy cause, as any promotion of the health of anybody doubtlessly is, but a cause qualifying for transcendent social sanction. Here one thinks first of those cases critically affecting the whole condition, present and future, of the community we have illustrated. Something equivalent to what in the political sphere is called "clear and present danger" may be invoked and a state of emergency proclaimed, thereby suspending certain otherwise inviolable prohibitions and taboos. We may observe that averting a disaster always carries greater weight than promoting a good. Extraordinary danger excuses extraordinary means. This covers human experimentation, which we would like to count, as far as possible, among the extraordinary rather than the ordinary means of serving the common good under public auspices. Naturally, since foresight and responsibility for the future are of the essence of institutional society, averting disaster extends into long-term prevention, although the lesser urgency will warrant less sweeping licenses.

VII. Society and the Cause of Progress

Much weaker is the case where it is a matter not of saving but of improving society. Much of medical research falls into this category. As stated before, a permanent death rate from heart failure or cancer does not threaten society. So long as certain statistical ratios are maintained, the incidence of disease and of disease-induced mortality is not (in the strict sense) a "social" misfortune. I hasten to add that it is not therefore less of a human misfortune, and the call for relief issuing with silent eloquence from each victim and all potential victims is of no lesser dignity. But it is misleading to equate the fundamentally human response to it with what is owed to society: it is owed by man to man—and it is thereby owed by society to the individuals as soon as the adequate ministering to these concerns outgrows (as it progressively does) the scope of private spontaneity and is made a public mandate. It is thus that society assumes responsibility for medical care, research, old age, and innumerable other things not originally of the public realm (in the original "social contract"), and they become duties toward "society" (rather than directly toward one's fellow man) by the fact that they are socially operated.

Indeed, we expect from organized society no longer mere protection against harm and the securing of the conditions of our preservation, but active and constant improvement in all the domains of life: the waging of the battle against nature, the enhancement of the human estate—in short, the promotion of progress. This is an expansive goal, one far surpassing the disaster norm of our previous reflections. It lacks the urgency of the latter, but has the nobility of the free, forward thrust. It surely is worth sacrifices. It is not at all a question of what society can afford, but of what it is committed to, beyond all necessity, by our mandate. Its trusteeship has become an established, ongoing, institutionalized business of the body politic. As eager beneficiaries of its gains, we now owe to "society," as its chief agent, our individual contributions toward its *continued pursuit*. I emphasize "continued pursuit." Maintaining

13

the existing level requires no more than the orthodox means of taxation and enforcement of professional standards that raise no problems. The more optional goal of pushing forward is also more exacting. We have this syndrome: Progress is by our choosing an acknowledged interest of society, in which we have a stake in various degrees; science is a necessary instrument of progress; research is a necessary instrument of science; and in medical science experimentation on human subjects is a necessary instrument of research. Therefore, human experimentation has come to be a societal interest.

The destination of research is essentially melioristic. It does not serve the preservation of the existing good from which I profit myself and to which I am obligated. Unless the present state is intolerable, the melioristic goal is in a sense gratuitous, and this not only from the vantage point of the present. Our descendants have a right to be left an unplundered planet; they do not have a right to new miracle cures. We have sinned against them, if by our doing we have destroyed their inheritance—which we are doing at full blast; we have not sinned against them, if by the time they come around arthritis has not yet been conquered (unless by sheer neglect). And generally, in the matter of progress, as humanity had no claim on a Newton, a Michelangelo, or a St. Francis to appear, and no right to the blessings of their unscheduled deeds, so progress, with all our methodical labor for it, cannot be budgeted in advance and its fruits received as a due. Its coming-about at all and its turning out for good (of which we can never be sure) must rather be regarded as something akin to grace.

VIII. The Melioristic Goal, Medical Research, and Individual Duty

Nowhere is the melioristic goal more inherent than in medicine. To the physician, it is not gratuitous. He is committed to curing and thus to improving the power to cure. Gratuitous we called it (outside disaster conditions) as a *social* goal, but noble at the same time. Both the nobility and the gratuitousness must influence the manner in which self-sacrifice for it is elicited, and even its free offer accepted. Freedom is certainly the first condition to be observed here. The surrender of one's body to medical experimentation is entirely outside the enforceable "social contract."

Or can it be construed to fall within its terms—namely, as repayment for benefits from past experimentation that I have enjoyed myself? But I am indebted for these benefits not to society, but to the past "martyrs," to whom society is indebted itself, and society has no right to call in my personal debt by way of adding new to its own. Moreover, gratitude is not an enforceable social obligation; it anyway does not mean that I must emulate the deed. Most of all, if it was wrong to exact such sacrifice in the first place, it does not become right to exact it again with the plea of the profit it has brought me. If, however, it was not exacted, but entirely free, as it ought to have been, then it should remain so, and its precedence must not be used as a social pressure on others for doing the same under the sign of duty.

Indeed, we must look outside the sphere of the social contract, outside the whole realm of public rights and duties, for the motivations and norms by which we can expect ever again the upwelling of a will to give what nobody—neither society, nor fellow man, nor posterity—is entitled to. There are such dimensions in man with trans-social wellsprings of conduct, and I have already pointed to the paradox, or mystery, that society cannot prosper without them, that it must draw on them, but cannot command them.

What about the moral law as such a transcendent motivation of conduct? It goes considerably beyond the public law of the social contract. The latter, we saw, is founded on the rule of enlightened self-interest: *Do ut des*— I give so that I be given to. The law of individual conscience asks more. Under the Golden Rule, for example, I am required to give as I wish to be given to under like circumstances, but not in order that I be given to and not in expectation of return. Reciprocity, essential to the social law, is not a condition of the moral law. One subtle "expectation" and "self-interest," but of the moral order itself, may even then be in my mind: I prefer the environment of a moral society and can expect to contribute to the general morality by my own example. But even if I should always be the dupe, the Golden Rule holds. (If the social law breaks faith with me, I am released from its claim.)

IX. Moral Law and Transmoral Dedication

Can I, then, be called upon to offer myself for medical experimentation in the name of the moral law? *Prima facie*, the Golden Rule seems to apply. I should wish, were I dying of a disease, that enough volunteers in the past had provided enough knowledge through the gift of their bodies that I could now be saved. I should wish, were I desperately in need of a transplant, that the dying patient next door had agreed to a definition of death by which his organs would become available to me in the freshest possible condition. I surely should also wish, were I drowning, that somebody would risk his life, even sacrifice his life, for mine.

But the last example reminds us that only the negative form of the Golden Rule ("Do not do unto others what you do not want done unto yourself") is fully prescriptive. The positive form (Do unto others as you would wish them to do unto you"), in whose compass our issue falls, points into an infinite, open horizon where prescriptive force soon ceases. We may well say of somebody that he ought to have come to the succor of B, to have shared with him in his need, and the like. But we may not say that he ought to have given his life for him. To have done so would be praiseworthy; not to have done so is not blameworthy. It cannot be asked of him; if he fails to do so, he reneges on no duty. But *he* may say of himself, and only he, that he ought to have given his life. *This* "ought" is strictly between him and himself, or between him and God; no outside party—fellow man or society—can appropriate its voice. It can humbly receive the supererogatory gifts from the free enactment of it.

We must, in other words, distinguish between moral obligation and the much larger sphere of moral value. (This, incidentally, shows up the error in the widely held view of value theory that the higher a value, the stronger its claim and the greater the duty to realize it. The highest are in a region beyond duty and claim.) The ethical dimension far exceeds that of the moral law and reaches into the sublime solitude of dedication and ultimate commitment, away from all reckoning and rule—in short, into the sphere of the *holy*. From there alone can the offer of self-sacrifice genuinely spring, and this—its source—must be honored religiously. How? The first duty here falling on the research community, when it enlists and uses this source, is the safeguarding of true authenticity and spontaneity.

X. The "Conscription" of Consent

But here we must realize that the mere issuing of the appeal, the calling for volunteers, with the moral and social pressures it inevitably generates, amounts even under the most meticulous rules of consent to a sort of *conscripting*. And some soliciting is necessarily involved. This was in part meant by the earlier remark that in this area sin and guilt can perhaps not be wholly avoided. And this is why "consent," surely a non-negotiable minimum requirement, is not the full answer to the problem. Granting then that soliciting and therefore some degree of conscripting are part of the situation, who may conscript and who may be conscripted? Or less harshly expressed: Who should issue appeals and to whom?

The naturally qualified issuer of the appeal is the research scientist himself, collectively the main carrier of the impulse and the only one with the technical competence to judge. But his being very much an interested party (with vested interests, indeed, not purely in the public good, but in the scientific enterprise as such, in "his" project, and even in his career) makes him also suspect. The ineradicable dialectic of this situation—a delicate incompatibility problem—calls for particular controls by the research community and by public authority that we need not discuss. They can mitigate, but not eliminate the problem. We have to live with the ambiguity, the treacherous impurity of everything human.

XI. Self-Recruitment of the Community

To whom should the appeal be addressed? The natural issuer of the call is also the first natural addressee: the physician-researcher himself and the scientific confraternity at large. With such a coincidence—indeed, the noble tradition with which the whole business of human experimentation started—almost all of the associated legal, ethical, and metaphysical problems vanish. If it is full, autonomous identification of the subject with the purpose that is required for the dignifying of his serving as a subject—here it is; if strongest motivation—here it is; if fullest understanding—here it is; if freest decision—here it is; if greatest integration with the person's total, chosen pursuit—here it is. With the fact of self-solicitation the issue of consent in all its insoluble equivocality is bypassed *per se*. Not even the condition that the particular purpose be truly important and the project reasonably promising, which must hold in any solicitation of others, need be satisfied here. By himself, the scientist is free to obey his obsession, to play his hunch, to wager on chance, to follow the lure of ambition. It is all part of the "divine madness" that somehow animates the ceaseless pressing against frontiers. For the rest of society, which has a deep-seated disposition to look with reverence and awe upon the guardians of the mysteries of life, the profession assumes with this proof of its devotion the role of a self-chosen, consecrated fraternity, not unlike the monastic orders of the past, and this would come nearest to the actual, religious origins of the art of healing.

It would be the ideal, but is not a real solution, to keep the issue of human experimentation within the research community itself. Neither in numbers nor in variety of material would its potential suffice for the many-pronged, systematic, continual attack on disease into which the lonely exploits of the early investigators have grown. Statistical requirements alone make their voracious demands; and were it not for what I have called the essentially "gratuitous" nature of the whole enterprise of progress, as against the mandatory respect for invasion-proof selfhood, the simplest answer would be to keep the whole population enrolled, and let the lot, or an equivalent of draft boards, decide which of each category will at any one time be called up for "service." It is not difficult to picture societies with whose philosophy this would be consonant. We are agreed that ours is not one such and should not become one. The specter of it is indeed among the threatening utopias on our own horizon from which we should recoil, and of whose advent by imperceptible steps we must beware. How then can our mandatory faith be honored when the recruitment for experimentation goes outside the scientific community, as it must in honoring another commitment of no mean dignity? We simply repeat the former question: To whom should the call be addressed?

XII. "Identification" as the Principle of Recruitment in General

If the properties we adduced as the particular qualifications of the members of the scientific fraternity itself are taken as general criteria of selection, then one should look for additional subjects where a maximum of identification, understanding, and spontaneity can be expected—that is, among the most highly motivated, the most highly educated, and the least "captive" members of the community. From this naturally scarce resource, a descending order of permissibility leads to greater abundance and ease of supply, whose use should become proportionately more hesitant as the exculpating criteria are relaxed. An inversion of normal "market" behavior is demanded here—namely, to accept the lowest quotation last (and excused only by the greatest pressure of need); to pay the highest price first.

The ruling principle in our considerations is that the "wrong" of reification can only be made "right" by such authentic identification with the cause that it is the subject's as well as the researcher's cause—whereby his role in its service is not just permitted by him, but *willed*. That sovereign will of his which embraces the end as his own restores his personhood to the otherwise depersonalizing context. To be valid it must be autonomous and informed. The latter condition can, outside the research community, only be fulfilled by degrees; but the higher the degree of the understanding regarding the purpose and the technique, the more valid becomes the endorsement of the will. A margin of mere trust inevitably remains. Ultimately, the appeal for volunteers should seek this free and generous endorsement, the appropriation of the research purpose into the person's own scheme of ends. Thus, the appeal is in truth addressed to the one, mysterious, and sacred source of any such generosity of the will—"devotion," whose forms and objects of commitment are various and may invest different motivations in different individuals. The following, for instance, may be responsive to the "call" we are discussing: compassion with human suffering, zeal for humanity, reverence for the Golden Rule, enthusiasm for progress, homage to the cause of knowledge, even longing for sacrificial justification (do not call that "masochism," please). On all these, I say, it is defensible and right to draw when the research objective is worthy enough; and it is a prime duty of the research community (especially in view of what we called the "margin of trust") to see that this sacred source is never abused for frivolous ends. For a less than adequate cause, not even the freest, unsolicited offer should be accepted.

XIII. The Rule of the "Descending Order" and Its Counter-Utility Sense

We have laid down what must seem to be a forbidding rule to the number-hungry research industry. Having faith in the transcendent potential of man, I do not fear that the "source" will ever fail a society that does not destroy it—and only such a one is worthy of the blessings of progress. But "elitistic" the rule is (as is

19

the enterprise of progress itself), and elites are by nature small. The combined attribute of motivation and information, plus the absence of external pressures, tends to be socially so circumscribed that strict adherence to the rule might numerically starve the research process. This is why I spoke of a descending order of permissibility, which is itself permissive, but where the realization that it is a *descending* order is not without pragmatic import. Departing from the august norm, the appeal must needs shift from idealism to docility, from high-mindedness to compliance, from judgment to trust. Consent spreads over the whole spectrum. I will not go into the casuistics of this penumbral area. I merely indicate the principle of the order of preference: The poorer in knowledge, motivation, and freedom of decision (and that, alas, means the more readily available in terms of numbers and possible manipulation), the more sparingly and indeed reluctantly should the reservoir be used, and the more compelling must therefore become the countervailing justification.

Let us note that this is the opposite of a social utility standard, the reverse of the order by "availability and expendability": The most valuable and scarcest, the least expendable elements of the social organism, are to be the first candidates for risk and sacrifice. It is the standard of *noblesse oblige;* and with all its counter-utility and seeming "wastefulness," we feel a rightness about it and perhaps even a higher "utility," for the soul of the community lives by this spirit.[8] It is also the opposite of what the day-to-day interests of research clamor for, and for the scientific community to honor it will mean that it will have to fight a strong temptation to go by routine to the readiest sources of supply—the suggestible, the ignorant, the dependent, the "captive" in various senses.[9] I do not believe that heightened resistance here must cripple research, which cannot be permitted; but it may indeed slow it down by the smaller numbers fed into experimentation in consequence. This price—a possibly slower rate of progress—may have to be paid for the preservation of the most precious capital of higher communal life.

XIV. Experimentation on Patients

So far we have been speaking on the tacit assumption that the subjects of experimentation are recruited from among the healthy.

Philosophical Reflections on Human Experimentation

To the question "Who is conscriptable?" the spontaneous answer is: Least and last of all the sick—the most available of all as they are under treatment and observation anyway. That the afflicted should not be called upon to bear additional burden and risk, that they are society's special trust and the physician's trust in particular—these are elementary responses of our moral sense. Yet the very destination of medical research, the conquest of disease, requires at the crucial stage trial and verification on precisely the sufferers from the disease, and their total exemption would defeat the purpose itself. In acknowledging this inescapable necessity, we enter the most sensitive area of the whole complex, the one most keenly felt and most searchingly discussed by the practitioners themselves. No wonder, it touches the heart of the doctor-patient relation, putting its most solemn obligations to the test. There is nothing new in what I have to say about the ethics of the doctor-patient relation, but for the purpose of confronting it with the issue of experimentation some of the oldest verities must be recalled.

A. THE FUNDAMENTAL PRIVILEGE OF THE SICK

In the course of treatment, the physician is obligated to the patient and to no one else. He is not the agent of society, nor of the interests of medical science, nor of the patient's family, nor of his co-sufferers, or future sufferers from the same disease. The patient alone counts when he is under the physician's care. By the simple law of bilateral contract (analogous, for example, to the relation of lawyer to client and its "conflict of interest" rule), the physician is bound not to let any other interest interfere with that of the patient in being cured. But manifestly more sublime norms than contractual ones are involved. We may speak of a sacred trust; strictly by its terms, the doctor is, as it were, alone with his patient and God.

There is one normal exception to this—that is, to the doctor's not being the agent of society vis-à-vis the patient, but the trustee of his interests alone: the quarantining of the contagious sick. This is plainly not for the patient's interest, but for that of others threatened by him. (In vaccination, we have a combination of both: protection of the individual and others.) But preventing the patient from causing harm to others is not the same as exploiting him for the advantage of others. And there is, of course, the abnormal exception of collective catastrophe, the analogue to a state of war.

21

The physician who desperately battles a raging epidemic is under a unique dispensation that suspends in a nonspecifiable way some of the strictures of normal practice, including possibly those against experimental liberties with his patients. No rules can be devised for the waiving of rules in extremities. And as with the famous shipwreck examples of ethical theory, the less said about it the better. But what is allowable there and may later be passed over in forgiving silence cannot serve as a precedent. We are concerned with non-extreme, non-emergency conditions where the voice of principle can be heard and claims can be adjudicated free from duress. We have conceded that there are such claims, and that if there is to be medical advance at all, not even the superlative privilege of the suffering and the sick can be kept wholly intact from the intrusion of its needs. About this least palatable, most disquieting part of our subject, I have to offer only groping, inconclusive remarks.

B. THE PRINCIPLE OF "IDENTIFICATION" APPLIED TO PATIENTS

On the whole, the same principles would seem to hold here as are found to hold with "normal subjects": motivation, identification, understanding on the part of the subject. But it is clear that these conditions are peculiarly difficult to satisfy with regard to a patient. His physical state, psychic preoccupation, dependent relation to the doctor, the submissive attitude induced by treatment—everything connected with his condition and situation makes the sick person inherently less of a sovereign person than the healthy one. Spontaneity of self-offering has almost to be ruled out; consent is marred by lower resistance or captive circumstance, and so on. In fact, all the factors that make the patient, as a category, particularly accessible and welcome for experimentation at the same time compromise the quality of the responding affirmation that must morally redeem the making use of them. This, in addition to the primacy of the physician's duty, puts a heightened onus on the physician-researcher to limit his undue power to the most important and defensible research objectives and, of course, to keep persuasion at a minimum.

Still, with all the disabilities noted, there is scope among patients for observing the rule of the "descending order of permissibility" that we have laid down for normal subjects, in vexing inversion of the utility order of quantitative abundance and qualitative "expendability." By the principle of this order, those patients who most identify with and are cognizant of the cause of research—members of the medical profession (who after all are sometimes patients themselves)—come first; the highly motivated and educated, also least dependent, among the lay patients come next; and so on down the line. An added consideration here is seriousness of condition, which again operates in inverse proportion. Here the profession must fight the tempting sophistry that the hopeless case is expendable (because in prospect already expended) and therefore especially usable; and generally the attitude that the poorer the chances of the patient the more justifiable his recruitment for experimentation (other than for his own benefit). The opposite is true.

C. NONDISCLOSURE AS A BORDERLINE CASE

Then there is the case where ignorance of the subject, sometimes even of the experimenter, is of the essence of the experiment (the "double blind"-control group-placebo syndrome). It is said to be a necessary element of the scientific process. Whatever may be said about its ethics in regard to normal subjects, especially volunteers, it is an outright betrayal of trust in regard to the patient who believes that he is receiving treatment. Only supreme importance of the objective can exonerate it, without making it less of a transgression. The patient is definitely wronged even when not harmed. And ethics apart, the practice of such deception holds the danger of undermining the faith in the *bona fides* of treatment, the beneficial intent of the physician—the very basis of the doctor-patient relationship. In every respect, it follows that concealed experiment on patients—that is, experiment under the guise of treatment— should be the rarest exception, at best, if it cannot be wholly avoided.

This has still the merit of a borderline problem. The same is not true of the other case of necessary ignorance of the subject— that of the unconscious patient. Drafting him for nontherapeutic experiments is simply and unqualifiedly impermissible; progress or not, he must never be used, on the inflexible principle that utter helplessness demands utter protection.

When preparing this paper, I filled pages with a casuistics of this harrowing field, but then scrapped most of it, realizing my dilettante status. The shadings are endless, and only the physician-researcher can discern them properly as the cases arise. Into his lap the decision is thrown. The philosophical rule, once it has admitted into itself the idea of a sliding scale, cannot really specify its own application. It can only impress on the practitioner a general maxim or attitude for the exercise of his judgment and conscience in the concrete occasions of his work. In our case, I am afraid, it means making life more difficult for him.

It will also be noted that, somewhat at variance with the emphasis in the literature, I have not dwelt on the element of "risk" and very little on that of "consent." Discussion of the first is beyond the layman's competence; the emphasis on the second has been lessened because of its equivocal character. It is a truism to say that one should strive to minimize the risk and to maximize the consent. The more demanding concept of "identification," which I have used, includes "consent" in its maximal or authentic form, and the assumption of risk is its privilege.

XV. No Experiments on Patients Unrelated to Their Own Disease

Although my ponderings have, on the whole, yielded points of view rather than definite prescriptions, premises rather than conclusions, they have led me to a few unequivocal yeses and noes. The first is the emphatic rule that patients should be experimented upon, if at all, *only* with reference to *their disease*. Never should there be added to the gratuitousness of the experiment as such the gratuitousness of service to an unrelated cause. This follows simply from what we have found to be the *only* excuse for infracting the special exemption of the sick at all—namely, that the scientific war on disease cannot accomplish its goal without drawing the sufferers from disease into the investigative process. If under this excuse they become subjects of experiment, they do so *because,* and only because, of *their* disease.

This is the fundamental and self-sufficient consideration. That the patient cannot possibly benefit from the unrelated experiment therapeutically, while he might from experiment related to his condition, is also true, but lies beyond the problem area of pure experiment. I am in any case discussing nontherapeutic experimentation only, where *ex hypothesi* the patient does not benefit. Experiment as part of therapy—that is, directed toward helping the subject himself—is a different matter altogether and raises its own problems, but hardly philosophical ones. As long as a doctor can say, even if only in his own thought: "There is no known cure for your condition (or: You have responded to none); but there is promise in a new treatment still under investigation, not quite tested yet as to effectiveness and safety; you will be taking a chance, but all things considered, I judge it in your best interest to let me try it on you"—as long as he can speak thus, he speaks as the patient's physician and may err, but does not transform the patient into a subject of experimentation. Introduction of an untried therapy into the treatment where the tried ones have failed is not "experimentation on the patient."

Generally, and almost needless to say, with all the rules of the book, there is something "experimental" (because tentative) about every individual treatment, beginning with the diagnosis itself; and he would be a poor doctor who would not learn from every case for the benefit of future cases, and a poor member of the profession who would not make any new insights gained from his treatments available to the profession at large. Thus, knowledge may be advanced in the treatment of any patient, and the interest of the medical art and all sufferers from the same affliction as well as the patient himself may be served if something happens to be learned from his case. But this gain to knowledge and future therapy is incidental to the *bona fide* service to the present patient. He has the right to expect that the doctor does nothing to him just in order to learn.

In that case, the doctor's imaginary speech would run, for instance, like this: "There is nothing more I can do for you. But you can do something for me. Speaking no longer as your physician but on behalf of medical science, we could learn a great deal about future cases of this kind if you would permit me to perform certain experiments on you. It is understood that you yourself would not benefit from any knowledge we might gain; but future patients would." This statement would express the purely experimental situation, assumedly here with the subject's concurrence and with all cards on the table. In Alexander Bickel's words: "It is a different situation when the doctor is no longer trying to make [the patient] well, but is trying to find out how to make others well in the future."[10]

But even in the second case, that of the nontherapeutic experiment where the patient does not benefit, at least the patient's

25

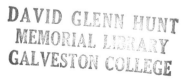

own disease is enlisted in the cause of fighting that disease, even if only in others. It is yet another thing to say or think: "Since you are here—in the hospital with its facilities—anyway, under our care and observation anyway, away from your job (or, perhaps, doomed) anyway, we wish to profit from your being available for some other research of great interest we are presently engaged in." From the standpoint of merely medical ethics, which has only to consider risk, consent, and the worth of the objective, there may be no cardinal difference between this case and the last one. I hope that the medical reader will not think I am making too fine a point when I say that from the standpoint of the subject and his dignity there is a cardinal difference that crosses the line between the permissible and the impermissible, and this by the same principle of "identification" I have been invoking all along. Whatever the rights and wrongs of any experimentation on any patient—in the one case, at least that residue of identification is left him that it is his own affliction by which he can contribute to the conquest of that affliction, his own kind of suffering which he helps to alleviate in others; and so in a sense it is his own cause. It is totally indefensible to rob the unfortunate of this intimacy with the purpose and make his misfortune a convenience for the furtherance of alien concerns. The observance of this rule is essential, I think, to at least attenuate the wrong that nontherapeutic experimenting on patients commits in any case.

XVI. On the Redefinition of Death

My other emphatic verdict concerns the question of the redefinition of death—that is, acknowledging "irreversible coma as a new definition for death."[11] I wish not to be misunderstood. As long as it is merely a question of when it is permitted to cease the artificial prolongation of certain functions (like heartbeat) traditionally regarded as signs of life, I do not see anything ominous in the notion of "brain death." Indeed, a new definition of death is not even necessary to legitimize the same result if one adopts the position of the Roman Catholic Church, which here at least is eminently reasonable—namely that "when deep unconsciousness is judged to be permanent, extraordinary means to maintain life are not obligatory. They can be terminated and the patient allowed to die."[12] Given a clearly defined negative condition of the brain, the physician is allowed to allow the patient to die his own death by *any* definition, which of itself will lead through the gamut of all possible definitions. But a disquietingly contradictory purpose is combined with this purpose in the quest for a new definition of death —that is, in the will to *advance* the moment of declaring him dead: Permission not to turn off the respirator, but, on the contrary, to keep it on and thereby maintain the body in a state of what would have been "life" by the older definition (but is only a "simulacrum" of life by the new)—so as to get at his organs and tissues under the ideal conditions of what would previously have been "vivisection."[13]

Now this, whether done for research or transplant purposes, seems to me to overstep what the definition can warrant. Surely it is one thing when to cease delaying death, another when to start doing violence to the body; one thing when to desist from protracting the process of dying, another when to regard that process as complete and thereby the body as a cadaver free for inflicting on it what would be torture and death to any living body. For the first purpose, we need not know the exact borderline between life and death—we leave it to nature to cross it wherever it is, or to traverse the whole spectrum if there is not just one line. All we need to know is that coma is irreversible. For the second purpose we must know the borderline with absolute certainty; and to use any definition short of the maximal for perpetrating on a *possibly* penultimate state what only the ultimate state can permit is to arrogate a knowledge which, I think, we cannot possibly have. *Since we do not know the exact borderline between life and death,* nothing less than the maximum definition of death will do—brain death plus heart death plus any other indication that may be pertinent—before final violence is allowed to be done.

It would follow then, for this layman at least, that the use of the definition should itself be defined, and this in a restrictive sense. When only permanent coma can be gained with the artificial sustaining of functions, by all means turn off the respirator, the stimulator, any sustaining artifice, and let the patient die; but let him die all the way. Do not, instead, arrest the process and start using him as a mine while, with your own help and cunning, he is still kept this side of what may in truth be the final line. Who is to say that a shock, a final trauma, is not administered to a sensitivity diffusely situated elsewhere than in the brain and still vulnerable to suffering a sensitivity that we ourselves have been keeping alive. No fiat of definition can settle this question.[14] But

27

I wish to emphasize that the question of possible suffering (easily brushed aside by a sufficient show of reassuring expert consensus) is merely a subsidiary and not the real point of my argument; this, to reiterate, turns on the indeterminacy of the boundaries between *life and death*, not between sensitivity and insensitivity, and bids us to lean toward a maximal rather than a minimal determination of death in an area of basic uncertainty.

There is also this to consider: The patient must be absolutely sure that his doctor does not become his executioner, and that no definition authorizes him ever to become one. His right to this certainty is absolute, and so is his right to his own body with all its organs. Absolute respect for these rights violates no one else's rights, for no one has a right to another's body. Speaking in still another, religious vein: The expiring moments should be watched over with piety and be safe from exploitation.

I strongly feel, therefore, that it should be made quite clear that the proposed new definition of death is to authorize *only* the one and *not* the other of the two opposing things: only to break off a sustaining intervention and let things take their course, not to keep up the sustaining intervention for a final intervention of the most destructive kind.

XVII. Conclusion

There would now have to be said something about nonmedical experiments on human subjects, notably psychological and genetic, of which I have not lost sight. But I must leave this for another occasion. I wish only to say in conclusion that if some of the practical implications of my reasonings are felt to work out toward a slower rate of progress, this should not cause too great dismay. Let us not forget that progress is an optional goal, not an unconditional commitment, and that its tempo in particular, compulsive as it may become, has nothing sacred about it. Let us also remember that a slower progress in the conquest of disease would not threaten society, grievous as it is to those who have to deplore that their particular disease be not yet conquered, but that society would indeed be threatened by the erosion of those moral values whose loss, possibly caused by too ruthless a pursuit of scientific progress, would make its most dazzling triumphs not worth having. Let us finally remember that it cannot be the aim of progress to abolish the lot of mortality. Of some ill or other, each of us will die. Our mortal condition is upon us with its harshness but also its wisdom—because without it there would not be the eternally renewed promise of the freshness, immediacy, and eagerness of youth; nor would there be for any of us the incentive to number our days and make them count. With all our striving to wrest from our mortality what we can, we should bear its burden with patience and dignity.

REFERENCES

1. In preparation for the Conference from which this volume originated.

2. G. E. W. Wolstenholme and Maeve O'Connor (editors), *CIBA Foundation Symposium, Ethics in Medical Progress: With Special Reference to Transplantation* (Boston, 1966); "The Changing Mores of Biomedical Research," *Annals of Internal Medicine* (Supplement 7), Vol. 67, No. 3 (Philadelphia, September, 1967); *Proceedings of the Conference on the Ethical Aspects of Experimentation on Human Subjects,* November 3–4, 1967 (Boston, Massachusetts; hereafter called *Proceedings*); H. K. Beecher, "Some Guiding Principles for Clinical Investigation," *Journal of the American Medical Association,* Vol. 195 (March 28, 1966), pp. 1135–36; H. K. Beecher, "Consent in Clinical Experimentation: Myth and Reality," *Journal of the American Medical Association,* Vol. 195 (January 3, 1966), pp. 34–35; P. A. Freund, "Ethical Problems in Human Experimentation," *New England Journal of Medicine,* Vol. 273 (September 23, 1965), pp. 687–92; P. A. Freund, "Is the Law Ready for Human Experimentation?," *American Psychologist,* Vol. 22 (1967), pp. 394–99; W. Wolfensberger, "Ethical Issues in Research with Human Subjects," *World Science,* Vol. 155 (January 6, 1967), pp. 47–51; See also a series of five articles by Drs. Schoen, McGrath, and Kennedy, "Principles of Medical Ethics," which appeared from August to December in Volume 23 of *Arizona Medicine.* The most recent entry in the growing literature is E. Fuller Torrey (editor), *Ethical Issues in Medicine* (New York, 1968), in which the chapter "Ethical Problems in Human Experimentation" by Otto E. Guttentag should be especially noted.

3. Wolfensberger, "Ethical Issues in Research with Human Subjects," p. 48.

4. *Proceedings,* p. 29.

5. Cf. M. H. Pappworth, "Ethical Issues in Experimental Medicine" in D. R. Cutler (editor), *Updating Life and Death* (Boston, 1969), pp. 64–69.

6. *Die Braut von Korinth:* "Victims do fall here, /Neither lamb nor steer, / Nay, but human offerings untold."

7. *Proceedings,* pp. 50–51.

8. Socially, everyone is expendable relatively—that is, in different degrees; religiously, no one is expendable absolutely: The "image of God" is in all. If it can be enhanced, then not by anyone being expended, but by someone expending himself.

9. This refers to captives of circumstance, not of justice. Prison inmates are, with respect to our problem, in a special class. If we hold to some idea of guilt, and to the supposition that our judicial system is not entirely at fault, they may be held to stand in a special debt to society, and their offer to serve—from whatever motive—may be accepted with a minimum of qualms as a means of reparation.

10. *Proceedings*, p. 33. To spell out the difference between the two cases: In the first case, the patient himself is meant to be the beneficiary of the experiment, and directly so; the "subject" of the experiment is at the same time its object, its end. It is performed not for gaining knowledge, but for helping him—and helping him in the *act* of performing it, even if by its results it also contributes to a broader testing process currently under way. It is in fact part of the treatment itself and an "experiment" only in the loose sense of being untried and highly tentative. But whatever the degree of uncertainty, the motivating anticipation (the wager, if you like) is for success, and success here means the subject's own good. To a pure experiment, by contrast, undertaken to gain knowledge, the difference of success and failure is not germane, only that of conclusiveness and inconclusiveness. The "negative" result has as much to teach as the "positive." Also, the true experiment is an act distinct from the uses later made of the findings. And, most important, the subject experimented on is distinct from the eventual beneficiaries of those findings: He lets himself be used as a means toward an end external to himself (even if he should at some later time happen to be among the beneficiaries himself). With respect to his own present needs and his own good, the act is gratuitous.

11. "A Definition of Irreversible Coma," Report of the *Ad Hoc* Committee of Harvard Medical School to Examine the Definition of Brain Death, *Journal of the American Medical Association*, Vol. 205, No. 6 (August 5, 1968), pp. 337–40.

12. As rendered by Dr. Beecher in *Proceedings*, p. 50.

13. The Report of the *Ad Hoc* Committee no more than indicates this possibility with the second of the "two reasons why there is need for a definition": "(2) Obsolete criteria for the definition of death can lead to controversy in obtaining organs for transplantation." The first reason is relief from the burden of indefinitely drawn out coma. The report wisely confines its recommendations on application to what falls under this first reason—namely, turning off the respirator—and remains silent on the possible use of the definition under the second reason. But when "the patient is declared dead on the basis of these criteria," the road to the other use has theoretically been opened and will be taken (if I remember rightly, it has even been taken once, in a much debated case in England), unless it is

blocked by a special barrier in good time. The above is my feeble attempt to help doing so.

14. Only a Cartesian view of the "animal machine," which I somehow see lingering here, could set the mind at rest, as in historical fact it did at its time in the matter of vivisection: But its truth is surely not established by definition.

ARTHUR J. DYCK

Comment on "Philosophical Reflections on Experimenting with Human Subjects"

FOR MANY reasons, our century has tended to be hostile to philosophical reflections on social issues. Indeed, we are currently living in a time when our intellectual sensibilities are all too frequently besieged by numerous forms of relatively mindless activism, whether of the establishment or anti-establishment variety. Our souls rejoice, therefore, to be able to feed on the solid intellectual fare so amply provided in the essay by Hans Jonas. Like Socrates of old, he nourishes our enthusiasm for the examined life and restores our respect for disciplined thought upon the most vital human problems.

In his invaluable essay, Professor Jonas has provided us with many insights into the proper goals and limits of scientific experimentation. Hence, this commentary, though mainly critical in import and in detail, is fundamentally a sympathetic attempt to amplify and, in some measure, to refine the major issues he has delineated. We shall consider the nature of human experimentation, the relation of the individual to society, and the problem of consent.

The Nature of Human Experimentation

Although the title of his essay suggested that Professor Jonas would reflect upon human experimentation generally, we find that he has confined his discussion to medical experimentation. Furthermore, the kind of medical experimentation that most concerns Professor Jonas is research with patients or healthy persons where this involves risks, but where no direct benefits accrue to the experimental subjects. It is not surprising, therefore, that he tends to picture the experimental subject as one who is somehow put upon, violated, or victimized. Professor Jonas finds it necessary and

32

illuminating to discuss the way in which human sacrifice has entered into the calculations and purposes of various societies.

Now, I think it is helpful to recognize that experimentation with humans may, in varying degrees, call for sacrifices. Furthermore, Professor Jonas is quite right to affirm the inviolable rights of human beings to be spared from involuntary subjection to the kind of manipulation that has characterized scientific experimentation with inanimate objects. But the scientific quest for knowledge about human beings does not, as such, require this kind of direct assault upon the inviolable rights of individual persons. As Margaret Mead has indicated in her excellent essay in this volume,[1] a great deal of scientific research has been a cooperative venture entered upon in a situation of open trust, confidence, and voluntary participation. In their articles, Professors Parsons and Freund[2] have also stressed this collegial and associational aspect of the scientist's quest for information about human beings. Scientific observation and research, therefore, can take the form of a social venture that enlists and engages some of the highest moral aspirations both of the observer and of the observed. Nevertheless, as Hans Jonas rightly discerns, and he is not alone in this, there are situations in which this relationship of mutual trust and cooperation does not obtain, and there are experimental situations in which the design of the experiment would appear to preclude this form of association, as in the so-called double-blind experiment.[3] It is important, therefore, to identify the outer limits that should be placed upon victimization and manipulation, and this is something that Professor Jonas has done rather well.

The Individual's Relation to Society

If we justify experimentation with humans by considering it a right of society, Professor Jonas quite rightly notes that we are exposing individuals to the risk of being recruited to make sacrifices for the general good. In such a context, the fact that consent is given by these individuals can be relatively meaningless. Furthermore, it does not help to move from the language of rights to the language of interests, because it is not difficult to show that the interests of society at large far outweigh the interests of single individuals or small groups. There is no way to avoid the consideration of the worth of those interests. It will not do simply to decide that they are for the good of society, for even once we have decided that a given social interest or goal is extremely valuable, any risks by individuals on behalf of such a goal must be voluntary and taken with the consent of those individuals. Hence, we find that Professor Jonas is very protective here of the rights and inviolability of the individual against the so-called rights of society.

But throughout his essay, Professor Jonas continues to think of the individual as one whose interests conflict with those of his society. This way of thinking, of course, is inconsistent with his general model of experimentation as a set of demands that society makes of its individual members. There are instances, however, where Professor Jonas does suggest a framework that would go beyond this polar relationship between the individual and his society, and the resulting tensions of that polarity. Thus, he says, for example, that "it may well be the case that the individual's interest in his own inviolability is itself a public interest, such that its publicly condoned violation, irrespective of numbers, violates the interest of all. In that case, its protection in *each* instance would be a paramount interest, and the comparison of numbers will not avail."[4] Or as he says in another passage, "Society, in a subtler sense, cannot 'afford' a single miscarriage of justice, a single inequity in the dispensation of its laws, the violation of the rights of even the tiniest minority, because these undermine the moral basis on which society's existence rests."[5] Or again he speaks of "the erosion of those moral values whose loss, possibly caused by too ruthless a pursuit of scientific progress, would make its most dazzling triumphs not worth having."[6] In these passages, we see a tendency to speak about certain kinds of values that must be honored by society as a whole, if the society is to sustain itself and have value for its members.

Here Professor Jonas has his hand on a vital point that needs to be further clarified and refined. The developmental psychologist Jean Piaget has distinguished between what he calls "constructive rules" and "constituted rules."[7] "Constitutive rules" are those that are necessary for drawing up rules at all. "Constituted rules" are the results of the various deliberative processes by means of which rules are conceptualized, administered, and enforced. Although Piaget did not identify these constitutive rules, Dyck and Richardson[8] have tried to isolate precisely those norms that are structurally required by a society in the sense that society would no longer be viable unless such norms were to some extent embodied in its constituted rules and institutional practices. Dyck and Richardson have argued that it is in the interest both of society and of its individual members to maximize the extent to which the practices surrounding experimentation with human beings are consistent with the requirements of justice, freedom, and veracity. The major ethical problem facing the investigator and the society in which his investigations take place is to find and to develop the practices that will facilitate and satisfy these norms. The failure to get voluntary and informed consent for participation in an experiment not only constitutes an assault on a given individual, but also undermines the basic necessity in society to maximize freedom and to maintain the trust that emanates from fidelity to truth and to mutually agreed upon contractual relations. In any calculation of the relative harms and benefits for society of a given experiment, it is not possible to bargain away any precedent-setting violation of these norms. It is only the utmost emergency that would allow one even to contemplate an exceptional violation of one of these norms.

But violations of these norms even within emergencies, however extreme, must also be carefully limited. Professor Jonas notes that war is one of those emergencies that does lead a society to require involuntary sacrifices on the part of its individual members. This discussion of conscription for the purposes of waging war gives one the impression that there are not limits to the demands made for sacrifice in war. It is important to bear in mind, however, that in any war, whether just or unjust, we have come, at least in the Western world, to exempt from combatant services those whose conscience will not permit them to go to war at all. Indeed, our sensitivity to the generally unjust nature of war is increasingly leading us to think about broadening these exemptions.[9] To take cognizance of these limits upon the violation of conscience even in the extremities of modern warfare is very much in the spirit of his essay and surely Professor Jonas would wish to do so.

The Problem of Consent

Professor Jonas has given a sensitive account of the role of voluntary consent in human experimentation. On the one hand, he explicitly recognizes the violation of human rights that would occur were experimentation to take place without the voluntary consent of the participants. He is aware that the requirement of consent, as an institutionalized guideline governing experimental procedure, is requisite for honoring and perpetuating the moral basis of man's life in community. On the other hand, Professor Jonas clearly discerns that obtaining voluntary consent will not by itself justify a given experimental use of humans. Two additional considerations must be taken into account in the justification of an experiment with humans: identification as the principle of recruitment and the adequacy of the cause.

Using identification as the principle of recruitment, Professor Jonas has evolved a set of helpful criteria for assuring some measure of informed and voluntary consent: subjects are to be recruited from the most highly motivated persons, from those whose experiences are most relevant to the knowledge that is being sought, and from those who are otherwise intellectually most capable of grasping the purposes and procedures of the experiment. These criteria provide working guidelines for approximating the collegial relationship that should, according to Mead and Parsons, generally characterize experimentation with human beings. In this way, Professor Jonas is providing important concrete means by which the violation of human rights can more readily be avoided, and he is also recognizing some of the nobler motives that can lead both the investigator and the experimental subject to participate in research.

His discussion of an adequate cause for the experiment is considerably less helpful. Professor Jonas certainly agrees that what we have called constitutive rules should not be violated by any of the practices guiding research with humans, and his guidelines for consent help dramatize this. But what guidelines are there for moral reasoning regarding the adequacy of the ends sought in an experiment where some partial violation of the usual guidelines is to be considered justifiable? Here Professor Jonas has little to suggest although he does sound a general warning against simply seeking the good of society and does recognize that grave threats to mankind are a more likely source of justifications for violating human rights.

Professor Jonas has not, therefore, explicitly ruled out a crass utilitarian calculus of the adequacy of our goals. Although he has mentioned the Golden Rule, he does not see its potential connection to the moral calculus of a benefit/harm ratio. The Golden Rule, however, can assist us in assigning relative weights to the possible benefits and harms of a given act. When in our calculus of relative benefits and harms we try to satisfy the Golden Rule in the form of love for our neighbor, we will put considerably heavier weight upon the more immediate and tangible consequences of our actions rather than the more remote and intangible ones.[10] We are not likely, for example, to sanction the napalming of our "neighbors" in order to strengthen our position against Communism in the Pacific or to make the world safe for democracy. Much more immediate and tangible threats to us or our loved ones are needed before we will expose someone we love to the risks of napalm bombs. Love for others, in the form of the sensitivity that we learn to have for the welfare of the members of our own family, serves as a practical moral restraint against a utilitarian calculus that would rationalize a callous disregard of our fellows in the name of a noble cause.

Some Concluding Remarks

It would take a considerably longer commentary to reflect upon the sensitive treatment Professor Jonas has given to the issue of redefining death. Suffice it to say that any discussion of this question should grapple with his distinction between defining death for the purposes of deciding when to break off sustaining intervention, and defining death in order to keep up the sustaining intervention for the purposes of organ transplantation.

The major theme that underlies and shapes the philosophical reflections of Hans Jonas on human experimentation is that the progress that may or may not come from scientific research is not automatically worthy of our efforts or our approbation. As Professor Jonas himself so eloquently observes, there are moral values "whose loss, possibly caused by too ruthless a pursuit of scientific progress, would make its most dazzling triumphs not worth having." This note of warning merits serious continual discussion; we have endeavored, however briefly, to augment that discussion.

REFERENCES

1. Pp. 152–177.

2. Pp. 105–115 and pp. 116–151.

3. As Margaret Mead has noted, even in a double-blind experiment the persons who are being asked to participate in it can and should be told that

it is an experiment of that kind and what this would imply for them should they volunteer their services.

4. P. 5.

5. P. 12.

6. P. 28.

7. Jean Piaget, *The Moral Judgment of the Child* (1932).

8. Arthur J. Dyck and Herbert W. Richardson, "The Moral Justification for Research Using Human Subjects," *Use of Human Subjects in Safety Evaluation of Food Chemicals,* National Academy of Sciences-National Research Council (1967).

9. See, for example, Ralph Potter, "Conscientious Objection to Particular Wars," in Donald A. Giannella, editor, *Religion and the Public Order Number Four* (1968). Recently, Federal District Judge Charles Wyzanski handed down a decision that would extend the class of those who would qualify as conscientious objectors in the direction indicated in Ralph Potter's article.

10. For a discussion of some of the difficulties inherent in traditional utilitarian modes of reasoning and for a detailed account of the way in which the principle of neighbor love can exert a corrective influence upon moral reasoning, see Arthur J. Dyck, "Referent-Models of Loving," *Harvard Theological Review,* Vol. 61 (1968), pp. 525–45.

HERRMAN L. BLUMGART

The Medical Framework for Viewing the Problem of Human Experimentation

THE PHYSICIAN'S view of the ethics of human experimentation inevitably reflects his life experience and his sense of the interactions between his profession and society. For him, the doctor-patient relationship ought to be the central focus. When so much can be accomplished medically for those who are ill, it would be tragic if the patient could not be completely confident that his welfare was the physician's only concern. In a world frequently indifferent and sometimes hostile, the patient often cherishes his relationship with the physician as his main refuge and comfort. This relationship must remain inviolate. Everyone recognizes the importance of acquiring new knowledge regarding disease and its treatment. This does not, however, necessitate the violation of the patient's traditional trust and its acceptance by the physician. Furthermore, a similar concern must govern the investigator in his relation to the experimental subject.

The doctor-patient relationship has the welfare of the patient as its prime objective and may be characterized as a therapeutic alliance. The experimenter-subject relationship, on the other hand, has the discovery of new knowledge as its primary objective and may be termed a scientific alliance. Each of these categories will be discussed separately with comment on some of their similarities and differences.

The Nature of the Doctor-Patient Relationship

The care of the patient encompasses both the science and the art of medicine.[1] The science of medicine embraces the entire stockpile of knowledge accumulated about man as a biological entity. The art of medicine consists of the skillful application of this knowledge to a particular individual for the maintenance of health or the amelioration of disease. In his usual relationship to patients, the doctor is wholly concerned with therapy, not experimentation, although both he and his patient are the beneficiaries of experimentation.

In recent years, one has heard repeated outcries that the science of medicine has so engulfed physicians that they are no longer interested in the patient as a person. The patient, it is said, knows how he feels, but does not know what he has got, while the doctor knows what the patient has got, but does not know how he feels. Fascination with the disease, it is contended, has excluded compassionate regard for the patient who is suffering. The milk of human kindness has been curdled by molecular biology; a robot generation of milliequivalent practitioners is being produced.

In defense of molecular biology and, indeed, of the broad scientific approach to medicine, one must recall that the recent great advances in science have revolutionized our way of life. Average life expectancy has increased from sixty-three to seventy-one years in the past twenty years, a change due not to the dawn of greater compassion but to scientific progress.[2] Nevertheless, it has become increasingly difficult to combine the science and the art of medicine at the bedside—to weigh the evidence and decide wisely.

The Necessity for Specialization

As science progresses, the interests of the investigators get narrower and narrower, whereas the scope of the clinicians must become broader and broader. For example, no single person on the forty-member editorial board of a journal of cardiovascular disease could claim sufficient knowledge to pass on all the papers submitted in this field. Indeed, most of the editors claimed expertness in only three to five of the thirty or forty particular aspects of cardiovascular disease. All of which confirms Ralph Barton Perry's remark that "it is comparatively easy to get educated; it is hard to stay educated."

The knowledge possessed by each physician today runs deeper than it did in the past, although it is often limited to a more restricted area. The necessity of gradually knowing more and more about less and less is an inevitable consequence of expanding frontiers and a fixed cerebral capacity. As specialization becomes increasingly imperative, the perplexed patient searches avidly for the broad-visioned physician who is learned in one circumscribed segment of medicine, but who can nevertheless analyze the clinical problem, identify the area of knowledge applicable to the patient's disability, and refer him to the appropriate consultant when that is indicated. Never before has it been so crucial that each physician be equally clear both about what he knows and what he does *not* know. Even more than formerly, the physician does not meet his patient on equal terms of scientific medical sophistication. He is sought because of his special knowledge and experience by patients who cannot have an informed or valid judgment regarding his skill or the diagnosis and treatment he proposes. The patient's safety depends on the physician's ability and integrity, the collective conscience of the medical profession as embodied in its code of conduct, the right of the patient for consultative opinion, and the patient's evaluation of the doctor as a person.[3]

As a result of specialization and the need for specialists, the continuity of the doctor-patient relationship has become fragmented. More physicians have become involved in the treatment of complicated conditions, but the number of doctors has not increased proportionately. The overworked physician finds it ever more difficult to spend the time necessary to know his patient as a person. Any realistic discussion of therapeutic trials and their scientific evaluation within the doctor-patient or the investigator-subject relationship must take into account the uncertainties due to the swiftly moving context in which these problems occur; the theories of today become the diagnosis and treatment of tomorrow. A newly graduated physician probably could be legally and certainly ethically guilty of malpractice within ten years if he did not constantly replenish his scientific armamentarium.

The Physician's Communication System

To enable the physician to maintain his competence, a vast communications network is available. Thousands of scientific journals reporting specialized information and general reviews are at hand. National as well as state and local medical societies offer well-organized educational programs utilizing bulletins, postgraduate seminars, television, and radio. Free interchange of information and discussion among the staff of a hospital—with their many specialized interests—afford extraordinary educational opportunities. If, in addition, the hospital participates in undergraduate or postgraduate medical education, the physician will be the recipient of the finest learning experience—namely, his own teaching activities. Certain operational aspects of hospitals also exert important educational influences. Every detail of treatment is observed by the resident staff, who weigh and discuss the advantages and disadvantages. If surgery is performed, the members of the operating team similarly evaluate each detail. A pathologist studies any tissue that is removed, such as the appendix, thereby substantiating or disproving the preoperative diagnosis. The consolidated hospital experience in the diagnosis and treatment of various diseased states is the subject of reports and discussions at staff meetings. The practicing physician's participation in the advance of knowledge and its intelligent application benefits both patient and doctor.

Diagnostic and Therapeutic Procedures Within the Doctor-Patient Relationship

Accumulated clinical experience, wisely and imaginatively interpreted, has been a valuable source of the medical profession's contribution to the care of the patient. Many of the greatest discoveries in the prevention and treatment of disease have resulted from such human "experimentation."

Example 1: Edward Jenner was a general practitioner in England in the latter part of the eighteenth century. He noted that even during epidemics milkmaids never contracted smallpox, although they always had sores on their fingers from infected udders. He therefore surmised that infection of cowpox on the fingers probably conferred protection from smallpox. Experimental inoculations with cowpox material carried no appreciable risk and possibly considerable gain and led to the discovery of vaccination against smallpox.

Example 2: William Withering, a physician and notable botanical scholar, observed about 1780 that an old woman in Shropshire frequently cured patients of the dropsy when the illustrious practitioners had failed. Withering states: "This medicine was composed of twenty or more different herbs, but it was not very difficult for one conversant in these subjects to perceive that the active herb could be no other than the foxglove." The use of foxglove—digitalis—required further study to determine the indications and the proper dosage, but in each instance the observations were with therapeutic intent and within the doctor-patient relationship.

In the clinical management of the patient entrusted to his care, the physician must be certain that the expected benefit of a particular procedure outweighs the estimated risk. At one end of the spectrum is the increasing number of investigations that confer little or no conceivable benefit to the subject undergoing hazardous examination. Specifically, I refer to such studies as the catheterization of the urinary tract of healthy female babies in a foundling home to establish the identity of normal bacterial flora, the cardiac catheterization and coronary angiography of patients without heart disease with inadvertent production of myocardial infarction, and the production of unconsciousness and convulsions by a combination of Valsalva maneuver and forced hyperventilation to study the CO_2 tension and electroencephalogram. Such studies are to be considered a violation of the doctor-patient relationship and are fortunately in the minority. They are experimentation within, but nevertheless contrary to, the ethics of the doctor-patient relationship because the motive is indirect benefit to society, not benefit to the patient.[4]

The tendency of medical science to consider its mission solely the increase of knowledge, regardless of the use to which it is put, has been implicit in certain scientific articles that are fortunately in the minority. Science pursued for its own sake has yielded rich rewards, but these must be viewed in the context of humanistic criteria. Otherwise, one would deal only with a world of computers and automation in which efficiency would be God and human welfare and ethical values would be wholly submerged and forgotten. The thesis that science itself contains within its domain social values and social responsibilities requires reaffirmation.

The Ethical Principles of the Doctor-Patient Relationship in the Testing and Use of Drugs

The use of drugs by physicians is illustrative of experimental therapeutics within the doctor-patient relationship devoted wholly to the welfare of the patient. With the scientific advances discussed above, one possesses a power, heretofore unknown in medicine, to manipulate the chemical composition of the intracellular and extracellular environment. Never has the responsibility in the use of drugs been so great. Physicians, despite their vigilance, are inevitably ignorant of all the potentialities of drugs for good and evil, often because knowledge regarding these agents is incomplete. The recent past illustrates how illness and even death may be inflicted inadvertently. The grim tragedy of Thalidomide and phocomelia, chloromycetin and aplastic anemia, and yellow fever vaccine with its thousands of cases of hepatitis (although this misfortune in turn opened up new vistas in our understanding of the latter disease) are but a few examples. With approximately five hundred new drugs entering the market each year, the problems confronting physician and patient grow apace.

Every time a physician administers a drug to a patient, he is in a sense performing an experiment. It is done, however, with therapeutic intent and within the doctor-patient relationship since it involves a judgment that the expected benefit outweighs the risk. Even the most commonly used agents—such as quinidine, digitalis, the thiazides, and the hormonal agents (thyroid, insulin, steroids and progestins)—involve risk. We can standardize drugs, but we cannot standardize patients; medical care of the patient demands adjusting the drug to the individual's unique characteristics. Several studies have vividly portrayed the prevalence of untoward effects in everyday practice. In one of the leading teaching hospitals, major toxic reactions and accidents were encountered in 5 per cent of the patients. A particularly well-documented study by Robert H. Moser is aptly entitled "Diseases of Medical Progress."[5]

The initial studies and subsequent therapeutic trials of a new drug usually follow a well-regulated series of steps outlined and controlled by the Food and Drug Administration of the United States Department of Health, Education and Welfare. A substance is suspected of possible therapeutic value because of its chemical similarity to a potent, previously known therapeutic agent or because it is already present in a minute or similar form within the body. Its chemical and biological qualities are studied extensively in the test tube, in plants, in animals, or in other biological experiments. The drug's physiologic and possible therapeutic attributes as well as its possible adverse effects are extensively studied in animals before its release for clinical studies, but man must be the final experimental test site. Such studies in man are undertaken on an experimental basis by physicians only with the express approval of the Food and Drug Administration and only when the physicians are aware of the already known effects and have clinical and laboratory facilities for a careful clinical evaluation of the drug's pharmacological actions. The latter, designated as Phase I, include observations of human toxicity and safe dosage range. Initial trials on a limited number of patients, Phase II, are then conducted cautiously for specific control of disease to evaluate the therapeutic value and any undesirable side effects. In these clinical studies of Phase II as well as in the wider clinical trials and when the drug is marketed for use by the general medical profession, the physician is not principally an investigator; he is using the drug primarily for therapeutic purposes, rendering a value judgment that the expected benefit outweighs the calculated risk. In Phases I, II, and III when knowledge of the drug action is necessarily incomplete, the Food and Drug Administration has stipulated that the physician must inform his patient of the experimental status of the drug, the possible advantages that have led him to advise its administration, and the possible ill effects.

When the drug is released for general use, adverse effects hitherto unknown may still become apparent. Certain toxic effects may occur only rarely and yet be extremely serious. One may recall that some early batches of poliomyelitis vaccines occasionally caused poliomyelitis when injected in hundreds of cases, although this was not evident in the first cases. Likewise, aplastic anemia following the use of chloromycetin occurs only infrequently and was not recognized during the first years of its use. Similarly, "Mer-29," used for lowering the cholesterol levels of the blood, was employed for several years before its propensity to cause cataracts and loss of hair was recognized. That heroin was initially introduced as a non-addictive substitute for morphine illustrates human fallibility in these matters. While using a drug solely for the benefit of his patient, the physician performs an invaluable service as an investigator of untoward effects, reporting them, when indicated, in medical periodicals or to governmental agencies.

A recent report is illustrative. The feasibility of blood transfusion is an illustrious medical achievement. In relation to acute hemorrhage, anemia, cardiac and other surgery, restoration of blood is life-saving. Roughly 4.5 million transfusions are given in the United States yearly. But transfusions also cause death. It has been estimated that blood transfusions cause about thirty thousand cases of hepatitis each year, of which more than three thousand are fatal. There is no way of entirely obliterating this risk except by abandoning transfusions altogether. The life-saving potential of blood is far too great to advocate such a drastic solution. The National

Research Council has recommended, on the basis of recent studies, that use of whole pooled plasma be discouraged and even discontinued; single donor transfusions are preferable. It also advises that substitutes be used when available—notably serum albumin, derived from plasma. In the meantime, strenuous research continues in an effort to render blood transfusions innocuous.

Communication Between Doctor and Patient

In all the aforementioned matters relating to the patient, the physician must recognize the individual's right to participate in decisions affecting his physical welfare. A few patients resent any explanation of the nature of their illness. And, at times, information must be withheld from the patient in his own interest and transmitted instead to some responsible member of the family. Most patients, however, are comforted when the nature of their illness and its expected course are explained in kindly and considerate terms. No condition is so complex that it cannot be explained in simple, intelligible language. To clothe the illness in unintelligible terminology only increases the patient's anxiety.

All patients or subjects must be convinced that their physician is scientifically competent and wise in his judgments. He must be interested in their disease, but equally concerned with them as persons. When the patient describes his symptoms and problems in detail, he transfers to the physician the material that has been the focus of his anxiety. In a real sense, his anxiety becomes the doctor's problem, rather than his own. Mutual participation by patient and doctor or investigator in all decisions is of the utmost importance. The physician adapts his conduct to the specific needs of the particular person; firmness, deliberateness, kindliness, and encouragement are supports frequently of greater importance than the choice of sedatives. With other patients, particularly those who have been accustomed to authoritative, autocratic parents, a more severe and positive attitude is necessary. Such patients may be disquieted by explanation, misinterpreting this as an indication of weakness and uncertainty on the physician's part.

The Nature of the Investigator-Subject Relationship and a Comparison with the Doctor-Patient Relationship

In the investigator-subject relationship, the primary purpose is to gain knowledge; the direct benefit to the subject may be nil, minor, or even beneficial, but is in any case subsidiary. The investigator may or may not be a physician; the subject may or may not be a patient. But the contrast to the doctor-patient relationship is clear. In the former, the main objective is to secure knowledge; in the latter, the welfare of the patient is the overriding consideration. As stated initially, the former relationship may be characterized as a scientific alliance; the investigator's concern for his subject's welfare should, however, be no less than the physician's for his patient. The conditions of the procedure, the risks, and the possible benefits should be clearly stated to the subject so that he can understand them as fully as possible. As the *Nuremberg Code* states, the subject must know "the nature, duration and purpose of the experiment, the method and means by which it is conducted, all inconveniences and hazards reasonably to be expected, and the effects upon his health or person which may possibly come from his participation in the experiment" so that he can make the most "understanding and enlightened decision."

The issue formulated by the Nuremberg, Helsinki, and other codes is not simple, nor are the concepts absolutes. The meaning of "informed consent" involves subjective judgments that depend on the intellectual acuity, the emotional integrity, and the wisdom of the physician or investigator.[6] To use a person for an experiment without his consent is untenable; the advance of science may be retarded, but more important values are at stake.

Free, full, and informed consent not only is mandatory in the investigator-subject relationship, but is also generally to be observed in the doctor-patient relationship when the risk of the procedure or drug is considerable. The quality of informed consent often depends on the quality of the information the physician imparts. In many decisions involving pain, discomfort, disability, and risk to life in order to obtain benefit, the patient or his representative cannot comprehend the scientific criteria used to evaluate the factors at play. Since a patient can hardly consent to something he does not understand, the physician should not only express his own considered judgment, but also freely permit the patient to seek consultant advice if he so desires. Under these circumstances, informed consent is a goal we strive to attain, but one that is plainly impossible to achieve in any complete sense.

Moreover, physicians with similar intellectual ability, emotional integrity, and wisdom may vary considerably in their decisions. Somewhat analogous situations evidently occur at times in our courts of law. Likewise, investigators vary widely in experience, in maturity of judgment, and in their knowledge of the risks involved in the experimentation. The quality of individual judgment can only be enhanced by the group wisdom of review committees that deal with the ethical as well as the scientific aspects of an investigation. The additional judgment is also beneficial to the investigator since responsibility is shared. Also necessary and complementary are reviews by the granting public and private agencies, rigorous editorial supervision of published reports, and other control mechanisms. All published articles reporting the results of human experimentation, particularly if normal or control subjects are used, should include the author's description of how he obtained informed consent.

The Board of Regents of New York State, in their decision on human experimentation, made an important contribution to this ethical problem. In their capacity as the licensing board for the practice of medicine, they suspended the licenses of two physicians for one year, although the execution of the sentences was stayed. By this act, they affirmed that medical experimentation represents a public interest to be protected by the law.

It had been known that tissue-cultured cancer cells injected subcutaneously into healthy persons were rejected in 4-6 weeks. In patients with advanced cancer, however, the rejection period was much longer, i.e.: from 6 weeks to several months. The possibility of an immunological factor in malignancy raised potential therapeutic possibilities. To learn whether the slower rejection by cancer patients was related to their own cancer and not to general debility, the experiment was next performed on equally debilitated patients with noncancerous conditions. The latter patients were not told clearly that the procedure was unrelated to treatment of their own condition nor were they informed that the substance injected consisted of cancer cells.[7]

Those concerned did not doubt that patients should not be used in experiments unrelated to treatment unless they have given informed consent, but two refinements of that principle were clearly set forth. First, the Regents found that the patient, not the physician, has the right to decide what factors are or are not relevant to his consent, regardless of the rationality of his assessment. Their opinion asserts:

Any fact which might influence the giving or withholding of consent is material. A patient has the right to know he is being asked to volunteer and to refuse to participate in an experiment for any reason, intelligent or otherwise, well-informed or prejudiced. A physician has no right to withhold from a prospective volunteer any fact which he knows may influence the decision. It is the volunteer's decision to make and the physician may not take it away from him by the manner in which he asks the question or explains or fails to explain the circumstances. There is evidenced in the record . . . an attitude on the part of some physicians that they can go ahead and do anything which they conclude is good for the patient, or which is of benefit experimentally or educationally and is not harmful to the patient and that the patient's consent is an empty formality. With this we cannot agree.[8]

The Regents stressed a second principle: that the physician, when he is acting as experimenter, has no claim to the doctor-patient relationship that, in a therapeutic situation, would give him the generally acknowledged right to withhold information if he judged it to be in the patient's best interest. In the absence of a doctor-patient relationship, the Regents said:

There is no basis for the exercise of their usual professional judgment applicable to patient care. . . . No person can be said to have volunteered for an experiment unless he had first understood what he was volunteering for. Any matter which might influence him in giving or withholding his consent is material. Deliberate nondisclosure of the material fact is no different from deliberate misrepresentation of such a fact.[9]

Human experiments of scientific value, but of no therapeutic benefit to the subject embrace a wide variety of circumstances— some that entail no discernible harm to the subject, others that involve pain, and still others that pose hazards to health and well-being. One of the first questions the investigator must face is the scientific validity of the procedure. Faulty design may prevent a study from illuminating the problem at issue. In some instances, the contemplated study may reveal scientific data that does not benefit the subject, but adds materially to our knowledge of vital functions, knowledge that may eventually benefit society and ultimately, perhaps, the subject himself. The subjects may be healthy volunteers motivated by idealism, money payment, or certain other implied or specific rewards, as in the case of convicts.

Example: The question of how long blood can be stored and retain its usefulness for transfusion after venesection is of enormous importance in times of peace as well as war. An experiment undertaken several years ago consisted of transfusing into healthy, normal volunteers blood stored for days, weeks, or months under certain conditions and then observing by appro-

49

priate microscopic study how long the transfused red blood cells survived in the recipient's blood stream. There was no apparent risk to the volunteers. Some of the stored blood became contaminated with bacteria, however, and transfusion of the stored blood resulted in deaths. The design of the experiment was appropriate and the objectives were significant. The importance of rigorous adherence to every safeguard and the element of human fallibility in estimating risk as well as benefit in such matters are apparent.

Studies without therapeutic benefit to the recipient may be undertaken when the major activity is a therapeutic endeavor within the patient-doctor relationship and the additional minor procedure entails no discernible risk or discomfort.

Example: After certain heart operations to correct deformed valves, small silver clips of fine wire were inserted into the heart muscle. Previous experience had shown that no harm would result. Serial photography of the heartbeat revealed changes in contraction of the heart muscle that could be gauged by the narrowing or widening of the space between the silver clips. Differences of opinion have been expressed regarding the ethical validity of such experiments and whether the patients should have been informed of this procedure. The absence of any discernible risk or damage by this additional act and the possible advantageous information made available would seem to validate the propriety of this measure, provided full and informed consent was obtained.

In some studies, observations are made that entail some risk and no immediate benefit to the patient. The increased understanding of the deranged function of the organs may, however, open the way for the use of appropriate drugs or procedures that may eventually redound to the welfare of the patient.

Example: Long rubber catheters were inserted into the arm veins of patients with severe lung and heart disease and passed into their hearts. The risk of injury and even death was definite. This procedure was done in conjunction with chemical studies of cardiac blood withdrawn through these catheters. The experiment produced much valuable information that afforded increased understanding of the disease, but was of little or no immediate benefit to the subjects.

The ethical necessity of securing prior informed and free consent under such circumstances is apparent. The importance of the work itself and its ultimate benefit to mankind was reflected in the award of Nobel Prizes to the investigators.

The necessity of securing informed consent is not negated in a hazardous experiment even if the investigator himself participates. Application of the Golden Rule is obviously not always a sufficient safeguard. A physician's willingness to experiment on himself is not justification for repeating the experiment on a patient.

Example: To facilitate cardiac resuscitation, Werner Forssman, a young surgical intern in Eberswald, Germany, sought to inject drugs directly into the heart through a catheter passed into the heart via the arm veins, rather than by piercing the chest wall and heart muscle with a long needle.[10] He first established the procedure's feasibility in corpses. He then elected to be the first experimental subject, having induced a surgical colleague to insert a lubricated ureteral catheter into an arm vein. Forssman directed the passing of the catheter into his own heart by viewing the fluoroscope on a mirror held by a nurse. Suffering no ill effects, he repeated the procedure several times and suggested in his published report its application to physiological studies. He shared in the Nobel Prize for pioneering and demonstrating the feasibility of this technique.

That opinions may differ widely among equally sophisticated persons is indicated by the following:

Example: A twenty-eight-year-old man of subnormal intelligence was treated in a hospital because of varicose veins. Informed consent was considered to have been obtained, but his subnormal intelligence made this impossible—particularly since he readily misconstrued as part of his treatment for varicose veins an incision in his groin permitting the passage of a catheter to the femoral artery and then to the heart. In passing the catheter into the heart, a coronary artery was blocked, causing collapse and an acute coronary attack—myocardial infarction—in an otherwise normal heart. A board of inquiry consisting of several directors of the hospital, several surgeons, and the hospital's Medical Director decided that the procedure was warranted in order to increase the skill of the surgeons and to bring therapeutic benefit to subsequent patients. The patient's subnormal intelligence prevented informed consent; nor were the family or other responsible persons informed of the procedure's purpose, which was of no possible benefit to the subject.

When the patient or subject is unable—because of subnormal mental intelligence, psychosis, relationship to the physician, or similar reasons—to give free and informed consent, the physician or investigator is beset with further problems. Infants, children, or minors must be represented by their parents or legal guardians, as in the experiments of infectious hepatitis in feeble-minded children in New York State. In some instances, there is divided opinion. The use of convicts in malaria experiments has received approval and disapproval. Some people contend that prisoners are under pressure to consent, lest they be punished by deprivation of food, poor living accommodations, and many other hardships that can be imposed by prison authorities. Others maintain that prisoners are able to feel that they are contributing to the welfare of society by volunteering for experiments for the public good. That there may be an implied willingness to shorten the sentence has been cited as an argument for and against using convicts for experimentation. It would seem, however, that studies of this type have much to commend them if the risks are clearly outlined to the prisoners and they are competent to make a rational decision. In some nutritional investigations, such as the effect of low-fat, low-cholesterol, or high-cholesterol diets, the controlled environment of prisoners is unusually favorable.

Some medical schools hold that participation by the students enhances their understanding of the significance of research, strengthens their sense of responsibility in undertaking investigations, and thereby affords an important educational and emotional experience. At other schools, it is felt that faculty investigators are generally held in such high esteem that the student is likely to consent on the false assumption that no participation would be requested if it involved risk or any untoward results. The Harvard Medical School and others have argued that the school represents, conceptually, the doctor in the doctor-patient relationship and that no research involving students should be undertaken if it entails any risk or any indisposition that might interrupt the student's studies. To assure this at the Harvard Medical School, a detailed protocol must be submitted by each investigator to the Administrative Board, which after careful consideration and consultation with experts may or may not give approval. Some investigations requiring simple with-drawal of blood samples or respiratory measurements may be permitted; rarely is consent given to any research requiring injections of pharmacologically active substances. A somewhat analogous instance of a group physician-patient relationship obtains when a person enters a hospital or clinic because of its excellent reputation rather than as a patient of a particular physician.

Weighing the Balance Between General Welfare and Individual Benefit

The problems of therapeutics and experimentation become difficult when the doctor's role as a physician comes into conflict with his responsibilities as a citizen. There is, for example, no specific statute regarding the physician's legal responsibility for reporting to traffic authorities that a patient suffers from occasional spells of dizziness or unconsciousness or from impaired motor reflexes and judgment. The particular point at which the doctor decides that it would be dangerous for the patient to continue driving and the measures he takes depend on the evaluation of many variables—including the relevant laws and regulations, the degree of impairment, the evaluation of the hazard, and the importance of driving to the patient. In epilepsy, the frequency of attacks, the degree to which they are controllable by medication, the reliability of the patient to take the medicine, the possibility of an aura that would permit the patient to bring the automobile to a standstill, and the likelihood of his so doing are some of the factors that may influence the physician's decision.

Many qualitative judgments also operate in regard to prescribing birth control pills. In Massachusetts it is legally and ethically permissible to prescribe contraceptive pills to unmarried women who have painful, disabling menstrual cramps, but unlawful to prescribe them for contraception. Thus, in many instances the propriety of a prescription depends on the physician's judgment as to the degree of dysmenorrhea and the reliability of the spoken hearsay evidence he gets from the patient.

The particularly complex ethical, religious, and legal problems raised by abortion or sterilization vary from state to state, and from physician to physician insofar as a physician's personal judgments are based on his concept of himself as a physician, as a citizen of his commonwealth, and, perhaps, as a member of a religious group. The physician must define for himself and weigh carefully the legal boundaries that set the limits beyond which his conduct would be unlawful and unethical. These laws prescribe what must be done and may include resuscitation in drowning, tracheotomy in suffocation, or the use of antibiotics in severe infections. They also stipulate what must not be done and may include ill-advised or radical surgery, such as ovariectomy or amputations without prior consent, excessive radiation therapy, or negligence. Having defined the legal boundaries within which he is free to act, the physician must then weigh as best he can the various counterbalancing factors to reach what he considers the wisest possible decision.

The opinion has been advanced that human experimentation for the welfare of society may be necessary and justifiable even though it jeopardizes the welfare of certain individuals. This, I submit, cannot be condoned except in certain special and unusual circumstances, examples of which have been described above. Lapses in ethical practices unnecessarily detrimental to the welfare of individuals represent a small minority of investigations; they can largely be avoided by review committees and, with a modicum of ingenuity, by other more innocuous approaches to the problem. In times of peril, such as war, society invokes for its own welfare legal and medical measures that disregard the welfare of the individual. Vivid examples are the selective service draft in time of war, capital punishment for treason, and the calculation of the number of battle casualties inherent in attaining certain objectives. There are certain medical equivalents, some of which are ugly realities. When only a limited number of wounded can be removed from the battlefield, who is chosen? And who is to be treated when stretchers and medications are in short supply? In the instance of new antibiotics that may be more effective in treatment of infected wounds, the cautious, gradual explorations of efficacy may be abridged or even omitted in the interest of urgency or short supply. In the instance of drugs that may prevent or cure illnesses that lessen military manpower (such as malaria, dysentery, meningitis, or rheumatic fever), deliberate control experiments must be initiated. The control group deprived of effective therapy may sustain serious illness or death. Or they may escape the deleterious, indeed dangerous, side effects of the therapy! But even under such urgent circumstances, epidemiological and other review boards constantly cooperate with the responsible authorities in designing, supervising, controlling, and evaluating these human experimental procedures in the Armed Forces.

In civilian life, perilous therapeutic procedures may be undertaken on an experimental basis when the danger of the procedure or drug, however great, is less than the alternative possibilities. The earliest use of penicillin in the gravely ill and the administration of the first batches of insulin to diabetic patients in acidosis or coma are in this category.

The Physician and the Ethics of Renal Dialysis and Organ Transplantation

With scientific advances, new problems arise because new choices are possible. The current excitement over the development of new techniques and the transplantation of organs—including the kidney, heart, liver, and spleen—has posed many ethical, legal, and social issues for the physician and the general public. Decades of quiet, dedicated research have set the stage.

In patients in whom the excretory function of the kidneys is less than necessary to maintain life, the accumulated poisons are eliminated by inserting needles into an artery and into a vein and circulating the blood through a cellophane membrane with fine pores. These permit the small molecules of toxic material to pass through, but retain the larger life-sustaining molecules of the blood. Dialysis units for treatment at home are now available for patients after their initial hospital evaluation and treatment.

In the United States, approximately six to eight thousand uremic patients could benefit from such treatment, although treatment facilities are available for only a thousand or so. To create a nationwide network of treatment centers would cost $25,000, or more, per case per year for the presently untreated seven thousand patients and would require a large cadre of trained personnel. If one includes the patients with acute kidney disease, the number of people requiring dialysis might reach forty thousand with a cost of $10,000 to $15,000 per patient. To supply sufficient facilities for treatment for all might involve the sacrifice of other social benefits. In our own affluent nation, probably only dispensable luxuries would be affected. This problem is under study by many private and public agencies. The present selection of recipients is necessarily arbitrary, and to an important degree it is based on the ability to pay. The physician, acting alone or as a member of the deciding group, is in the untenable position of playing God. The necessary extension of our present governmental program of medical care to include renal dialysis and similar new techniques would seem imperative. Besides the economic and social problems, there are serious emotional ones as well. The stresses suffered by patients and by spouses who carry out the home dialysis procedures are great. Depression, anxiety, frustration, repressed hostility, and conflict quite frequently produce serious crises and turmoil.[11] These emotional and personality factors are important considerations in selecting recipients.

Kidney transplantations likewise involve tormenting ethical, economic, and social problems for the physician. The success of renal transplantation is greatest the closer the degree of the donor's consanguinity, ranging from identical twins to siblings, parents, relatives, and others wholly unrelated. Concern for the recipient has to be matched by concern for the donor. A donor not only loses the factor of safety and reserve provided by the second kidney, but also undergoes all the consequences of a major abdominal operation. One can conjure the problem of a teenage girl who donates a kidney to her identical twin and at the same time loses the added factor of renal safety before she has passed through periods of life, such as pregnancy, when renal infection or other damage may occur. The physician acting singly or as a member of a group must translate these scientific and ethical problems into readily understandable terms as he serves as counselor for the interested parties.

Certain comparisons between heart and kidney transplantation are of interest. According to animal experimentation, the transplanted heart may be less liable to rejection than the kidney. Rejection of the foreign tissue has been somewhat reduced by the use of antilymphocytic serum, irradiation, tissue typing, steroids, and ancillary drug therapy. Nevertheless, only a small number of survivals of six months or longer have been achieved in probably thousands of heart transplants in dogs, including litter-mates of thoroughbred dogs. Moreover, the availability of one of the paired kidneys of twins, siblings, relatives, and friends is in sharp contrast to the relatively few human hearts that can be made available. After kidney transplantation, the phenomenon of rejection can be evaluated in the recipient by renal needle biopsy and urinary changes; in the event of failure, the recipient may be kept alive for extended periods until another attempt is made. In transplanted hearts, time cannot be purchased by interim dialysis or prolonged artificial heart pumps; the recipient's life cannot be salvaged if the transplanted heart does not function.

The success of renal transplants performed since January 1, 1965, is illustrated by the thirteen- to fifteen-month survi·/al. The Cumulative Probability of Success has been as follows:

Siblings (126)	0.717 C.P.S.
Parents (199)	0.630 C.P.S.
Spouse (58)	0.382 C.P.S.
Cadaver (368)	0.345 C.P.S.

Tissue typing, antilymphocytic serum or globulin, and other advances will improve these results.

Relevant to prior references of "benefit commensurate to risk" is an authoritative opinion regarding the present status of heart transplantation by a pioneer in cardiac surgery, Dr. Dwight E. Harken.

As we estimate a significant death rate from *biologic barriers* (rejection, lymphatic, and neurogenic factors), we must add the immediate surgical mortality which for properly selected recipients, often with poor lungs, livers, and so forth, would be a 20 per cent mortality, perhaps more. Thus, probable mortality rates, biologic barriers, surgery, and other complications rise to a level *precariously close to the probability* of medical prognostic error for the recipient who is to lose the heart that is currently sustaining his life.

The circumstances have not been defined in this perspective. Heart transplantation in an early experimental prototype form is here. Each man who contemplates entry into the field of cardiac transplants must arrive at his own decision by balancing the use of the considerable resources for a few transplants, against his obligation to treat ailing people and extend heart surgery techniques in other ways. So far, I have elected the rehabilitation of a fair number of people while attempting to improve prosthetic valves, coronary circulation, and mechanically assisted circulation. I reserve the right to change tomorrow but today I am proud of our restraint in not performing heart transplantations yesterday.[12]

At this time of writing, sixty-five heart transplants have been undertaken, according to reports in the press. Information regarding these cases is fragmentary and incomplete. The operative mortality and death rate within the first post-operative month are undoubtedly high. The length of time that the recipient can survive is as yet conjectural. The available clinical data pertaining to the pre-operative histories of the recipients and the post-operative course are inadequate. It is hoped that this will be remedied by

57

interchange of information through the organization of a centralized communication network or agency. That transplantation is technically feasible is a bold, important achievement, but its utility to patients with heart disease will require more knowledge of the rejection phenomenon and its prevention. Additional studies in the laboratory on higher mammals are urgently needed on this problem. New, complex legal, moral, ethical, religious, and sociological considerations also require critical exploration to afford confident judgment by responsible physicians.

Only a relatively few donor hearts can be envisaged presently for the many thousands of heart disease patients that may benefit eventually from transplants. The earlier the heart is removed from the donor after death the greater the likelihood of viability in the recipient. There is diversity among medical and lay judgments as to what constitutes death. Is it when the heart stops beating or when the brain stops functioning due to lack of oxygen? Both criteria are erroneous. The heart may suffer from standstill, but may nevertheless be revived for years of life by the newer methods of electrical stimulation or manual massage. Similarly, although the patient's brain may suffer from oxygen deficit, he may survive for years by forced feeding and other artificial supports, albeit with greatly impaired cerebral function.

Declaration of death of the donor is a medical decision that is made legally by the physician in charge except in those instances when the medical examiner has taken jurisdiction. Traditionally, death has been considered to occur when the heart stops beating. Re-examination of the question by a committee chaired by Dr. Henry K. Beecher has contributed valuable concepts to the ongoing discussions.[13] The committee proposed that irreversible coma be the criterion of death in persons with no discernible central nervous system activity. The latter is characterized specifically to include total unawareness to externally applied stimuli and to inner need as well as complete unresponsiveness even to the most intense, painful stimuli. Further requirements consist of no spontaneous muscular movements or spontaneous respiration or response to any external stimuli and complete abolition of central nervous system activity as reflected in no elicitable reflexes. Repeated examinations over a period of twenty-four hours or longer should be required in order to obtain evidence of irreversibility.

The numerous moral, ethical, legal, and religious aspects of the problem are being actively explored by many study groups representing the public and the various professions. Serious emotional problems are also posed particularly for donors and next of kin. Some groups of individuals have been formed who have expressed their wish to be donors in the event of death through accident or under certain other circumstances in which their organs can be used for transplantation. Through death the lives of others may be sustained.

Certain precautions have been outlined by the Board on Medicine of the American National Academy of Sciences that should be followed in a heart transplant procedure.[14] The physician must recognize that cardiac transplantation is not an accepted therapeutic procedure, but an experimental investigation that "must meet the same meticulous scientific standards that obtain in the laboratory." It is of the utmost importance that the responsible physicians prepare a complete protocol of contemplated studies beforehand. They must further ensure that all facilities are available that are necessary for investigating the biological processes that threaten functional survival of the transplant.

Investigators skilled in immunology, including tissue typing and the management of immunosuppressive procedures, should be readily available as collaborators in the transplantation effort. As the procedure is a scientific investigation and not as yet an accepted form of therapy, [the physician's] primary justification for this activity in respect to both the donor and recipient is that from the study will come new knowledge of benefit to others in our society.[15]

The complexity of the many scientific, legal, and ethical problems in cardiac transplantation indicates the necessity of an independent supervisory and consulting peer group of physicians and scientists not directly attached to the transplant team who will render an opinion on the acceptability of the donor and the suitability of the recipient. The group would refer particularly to the evidence of the donor's irreversible bodily damage and imminent death, and the recipient's far-advanced hopeless state despite application of all other forms of reasonably indicated therapy. Qualified scientific judgment must indicate that transplantation offers the patient the only alternative to life. The Board of Medicine of the American National Academy of Sciences concluded that in order to obtain the scientific information necessary for the next phase in this form of organ transplantation only a relatively small number of careful investigations involving cardiac transplantation need be done at this time.

The Dying Patient, Human Experimentation, and the Doctor-Patient Relationship

The propriety of pharmacological and other studies in dying patients has been defended, particularly if patients are unconscious or dying after renal failure or cerebrovascular accidents. But it is difficult to discern any difference in the obligation of the physician to the patient under such circumstances. If, however, the patient experiences no pain or discomfort, observations of scientific value, such as the chemical analyses of blood, are permissible. That dying patients may at times be suitably used for experimentation is indicated by the author's following experience.

Example: The use of radioactive iodine generally in doses of 5 to 10 millicuries for the treatment of hyperthyroidism had been widely accepted. The possibility of secondary adverse effects had been raised, however, but none were observed at this dosage level in patients over thirty years of age. A research was undertaken to learn whether the destruction of the normal thyroid in patients with congestive failure or angina pectoris might be accomplished by radioactive iodine and thereby lead to clinical improvement in otherwise hopeless cardiac patients by lessening the heart's work. The normal thyroid would be much more resistant to radiation and would require much larger doses for its destruction. The possibility of divided doses totaling as much as 100 to 150 millicuries of radioactive iodine was envisaged. Such large doses might lead to untoward effects on the blood, on the kidneys, and possibly on other organs. We were reluctant to use cardiac patients for such studies since their expected span of life might be many months or even several years. It was felt that patients who were in the final stages of widespread malignancy would be more suitable. Comparable doses in animals had previously had no adverse effects. The greatly increased exposure to radiation was unlikely to be deleterious under the circumstances and might, indeed, have a favorable effect on the malignancy. The possible adverse effects on the blood and other organs would not be expected to cause pain or future suffering. This situation was discussed with responsible members of the families of patients with widespread malignancy. The majority of these relatives agreed to the procedure. The patients drank approximately one tablespoon of water containing the radioactive iodine. No untoward effects on organs other than the thyroid were apparent either during life or on post-mortem examination. The safety of the larger doses having been demonstrated, many hundreds of patients with hitherto intractable heart disease have been treated with generally favorable results.

In the presence of almost certain death, the physician is sometimes justified in undertaking therapeutic procedures whose chances of success are small. When desperate therapy involves perpetuation of pain and discomfort and a minimum of hope, however, its justification is dubious. Most physicians would agree that it would be generally reprehensible to administer penicillin to treat pneumonia in a patient dying with painful, widespread malignancy, even though no legal, ethical, or religious precepts dictate such a decision. Similar considerations apply to vigorous attempts of artificial feeding or forcible respiration that only add to the discomfort and prolong the agonal state. As pointed out by Dr. Beecher in this connection, it is incumbent on the physician to take all reasonable, ordinary means of restoring spontaneous vital functions and consciousness and to employ such extraordinary means as are available to him to this end. It is not obligatory, however, to continue to use extraordinary means indefinitely in hopeless cases. It is the Roman Catholic Church's view as expressed by Pope Pius XII that a time comes when resuscitative efforts should stop and death be unopposed.

Certain therapeutic and investigational procedures are not so readily appraisable. Thus, the use of chemotherapeutic agents in incurable malignant lymphoma with a high probability of painful widespread gastrointestinal ulceration is open to question. Certain physicians employ such measures after consultation with the family. Some of these dying patients suffer far more from the trial use of new agents in cancer than from the disease itself. The patient or the responsible members of the family may feel that any novel therapy, however experimental in nature, may be preferable since death is inevitable with all hitherto known measures. But the justification of discomfort and additional agony to the patient is not always apparent. Frequently, dying, not comfortable living, is prolonged.

The question of "telling the truth" to the patient with malignant disease, with hopeless neurological or other incurable disorders, is intimately related to the feasibility of full consent for experimental procedures discussed previously. There is no easy single or uniform reply, but certain considerations afford valuable guidance. The physician should conduct himself so that he supports the specific needs and strengthens the particular defenses of the patient for whom he has accepted responsibility.[16] As Francis Bacon stated, certain patients "Fear death as children fear to go in the dark. And as the natural fear in children is increased with tales, so is the other." Such men protect themselves by denying reality. Not infrequently, they have previously said to members of their family or to their physician: "If I ever have such a condition, I do not want to know it." They may express satisfaction in their fancied improvement even as they waste away. Every physician has observed many such patients who peacefully and calmly pass into eternity, successfully protected from their fear by the barriers that they themselves have constructed. Under such circumstances, the responsible members of the family or closest friends must act as agent for the patient.

The patient's cultural and religious background also influences how the physician deals with him in regard to informed consent. A poignant example was Pope John XXIII, who, as he received extreme unction, said to his confessor: "I have been able to follow the course of my death step by step. Now I am going sweetly to my end. I am on the point of leaving. We are going to the House of the Lord." Indeed, all Catholics look upon death as a brief interlude, and all devout Christians, Jews, Hindus, and Moslems, as well as members of certain other faiths, believe in life after death. For such people, as well as for others, the plain unvarnished truth is, in the words of John Donne: "One short sleep past, we wake eternally. And death shall be no more; death, thou shalt die." Complete candor should also prevail for those who accept death as realistically as life.

In the treatment of fatal illness, such as malignancy, the physician must maintain the comfort of his patient and permit him to endure his final days with dignity. Obviously, neither addiction nor euthanasia is a consideration. Neither the law nor the tenets of any religious faith require postponement of death or continued suffering by adherence to the usual time schedule of the usual doses of sedatives and narcotics. If unusually large doses of narcotics or other agents are necessary to control distress or pain, these should be given even though life may thereby be shortened. There is no need for the dying to envy the dead. A person has a right not only to live in dignity, but also to die in dignity.

To summarize, in the preceding discussion I have attempted to clarify the issues of human experimentation from the physician's viewpoint. Human experimentation is essential for scientific progress and the welfare of man. This does not, however, necessitate the violation of the patient's traditional trust and its acceptance by the physician. Furthermore, a similar concern must govern the investigator in his relation to the experimental subject. The doctor-patient relationship has the welfare of the patient as its prime objective; it may be characterized as a therapeutic alliance. The experimenter-subject relationship has the discovery of new knowledge as its primary objective; it may be termed a scientific alliance.

These two categories possess some similarities and some differences. The governing ethical principles relating to various clinical and research efforts entail the infinite variety of concrete problems and conflicting values encountered by physicians. These preclude the formulation of an exact generalization that can be neatly applied to a specific instance. As Justice Holmes cautioned: "General propositions do not decide concrete cases." The increasing complexity and scope of medical science will undoubtedly only add to the present difficulties. In the future, as in the present, the ultimate guardian is the wise, responsible, and humane physician, acting singly or in concert with others. I believe that certain constructive steps must be taken both to protect the rights of the subject and to ensure human experimentation for the welfare of society. Open discussion of the problems should be encouraged in order to develop an informed public opinion. All reports of investigations on human subjects should contain a validation by the investigator regarding the propriety of his study and his observance of the rights, privacy, and welfare of the subjects. Public and private granting agencies should share responsibility by recognizing the problem and by specifically approving the protocol of any investigation that involves human subjects. Review committees of hospitals, medical societies, or other responsible groups of physicians may be helpful to investigator and patient alike. Publishers and editors in the medical field should also accept responsibility for these general principles of ethical experimentation by insisting that an author state how he obtained informed consent, giving all the pertinent facts that bear on the general ethical problem. Finally, I believe that a discussion of these matters is as germane as factual information in the educational program of the future physician. As medical students learn to prevent disease and promote health, they should also begin to learn how "to exercise those wise restraints that make men free."

REFERENCES

1. F. W. Peabody, "Care of the Patient," *Journal of the American Medical Association,* Vol. 88 (1927), pp. 877-82.

2. H. L. Blumgart, "Caring for the Patient," *New England Journal of Medicine,* Vol. 270 (February 27, 1964), pp. 449-56.

3. R. Ormrod, "Medical Ethics," *British Medical Journal,* Vol. 2, No. 7 (April 6, 1968).

4. H. K. Beecher, "Ethics and Clinical Research," *New England Journal of Medicine,* Vol. 274 (1966), p. 1354.

5. R. H. Moser, *Diseases of Medical Progress: A Contemporary Analysis of Illness Produced by Drugs and Other Therapeutic Procedures* (2d edition; Springfield, Illinois, 1959).

6. M. H. Pappworth, *Human Guinea Pigs: Experimentation on Man* (London, 1967).

7. E. Langer, "Human Experimentation: New York Verdict Affirms Patients' Rights," *Science* (February 11, 1966).

8. *Ibid.*

9. *Ibid.*

10. Werner Forssman, "Die Sondierung des rechten Herzens," *Klinische Wochenschrift,* Vol. 8 (1929), p. 2085.

11. P. W. Shambaugh, C. L. Hampers, G. L. Bailey, D. Snyder, and J. P. Merrill, "Hemodialysis in the Home—Emotional Impact on the Spouse," *Transactions of the American Society on Artificial Internal Organs,* Vol. 13, p. 41.

12. D. E. Harken, Personal Communication.

13. H. K. Beecher (Chairman), R. D. Adams, A. C. Barger, W. J. Curran, D. Denny-Brown, D. L. Farnsworth, J. Folch-Pi, E. I. Mendelsohn, J. P. Merrill, J. Murray, R. Potter, R. Schwab, W. Sweet, Report of an *Ad Hoc* Committee at Harvard Medical School to Examine the Definition of Brain Death, "A Definition of Irreversible Coma," *Journal of the American Medical Association,* Vol. 205 (August 5, 1968), pp. 337-40.

14. Report of the Board on Medicine, National Academy of Sciences (Washington, D. C.; February 28, 1968).

15. *Ibid.*

16. G. L. Bibring, "Psychiatry and Medical Practice in a General Hospital," *New England Journal of Medicine,* Vol. 254 (February 23, 1956), pp. 366.

HENRY K. BEECHER

Scarce Resources and Medical Advancement

THERE IS profit in most fields of human endeavor in taking an appraising look at past and present practices. Such comparison can tell much about the direction we are traveling, whether up or down. In medicine, there are a number of routes that can lead to useful insights. Present concern with human experimentation is a case in point. Within this field one can find various levers useful for prying loose significant information. The attitudes of the past and the present toward scarce resources in medical research are revealing. It is our purpose to examine them in some detail.

Among the recurring problems in the history of medicine, from ancient times to the present, is that of the sound allocation of scarce resources. A fairly comprehensive history of medicine could be written on the subject. But our immediate interest is an attempt to identify and to face up to several grave problems created by existing knowledge and limited resources. Nearly all advances in medicine involve experimentation and, usually, experimentation is hampered by scarce resources in its early period.

Scarce resources in the advancement of medicine are attributable to a variety of causes—some are deliberate, man-made, and some are owing to "natural" scarcities that obtain when a rare and newly discovered drug is found to have great effectiveness, where facilities for its adequate production have to be developed despite almost overwhelming difficulties. Sometimes the difficulty is a costly technique, where the problems are monetary cost and shortages of competent manpower. Sometimes moral and ethical considerations determine shortages. There is reason to believe that these may in some cases be based on outmoded views: The use of children is fraught with many problems and, in England at least, with legal difficulties; this area needs and is getting study. Another area where customs and moral, ethical, and legal problems abound is the definition of brain death with surviving heart beat. Clearly, the first problem is definition, but not to be neglected is the secondary fact that many tissues and organs not now adequately available for transplantation would be were the proposed new definition of irreversible coma accepted. *To do nothing in this area is far more radical than to act as proposed.*

I believe that the understanding of scarce resources and recognition of their causes can do much to alert us to such blocks and to their avoidance or correction in future growth. In the preparation of this manuscript, any early thoughts that the two aspects—availability and allocation—could be neatly divided had to be abandoned; the two are usually inextricably interwoven.

Once availability was assured, even though of limited extent, it was often surprisingly difficult or impossible to discover the *principles* that determined allocation of the new substance or technique to one man while it was withheld from another. Many of those who could have answered questions as to underlying principles of allocation are dead; but firsthand experience with the living does not lead to optimism as to what the dead might have divulged. Some of those who could still give information have failed to reply to requests. Some have said it was "too dangerous" to spell out the principles involved. One is led to the conclusion that in many cases no very extensive, thought-out policies were involved. A first-come-first-served basis seems to have been employed. There are notable exceptions to this. Some have evidently enjoyed the power of allocation and exercised it in a personal but nevertheless usually responsible way. And some—such as Professors Charles H. Best, William Castle, and George Thorn—have been completely helpful in discussing their pioneer work.

Our present concern is for the ethical use of scarce resources in medical experimentation in man. Passing references have been made above to areas where shortages and other difficulties have been encountered. It may be helpful for the purposes of orientation to spell them out a little more fully.

I. *A Few Historical Examples from the Last Three Hundred Years*

THE CHAMBERLEN FORCEPS

A member of the Chamberlen family (probably Peter, Sr.) developed an obstetrical forceps in the seventeenth century.[1] A similar instrument had been suggested by Pierre Franco in 1561. Nonetheless the Chamberlen family kept the secret of their instrument secure for many years.[2] At any rate, no outsider saw it until Hugh Chamberlen decided to sell it, for a high price, first in Paris, to François Mauriçeau, the leading obstetrician of his time. That sale was lost owing to the demonstration's fatal outcome. Eventually Hugh sold the secret in Holland to Roger Roonhuysen and others. Here was limitation on the use of a discovery for private gain.

IGNORANCE AND THE SCURVY

Sometimes ignorance is responsible for the scarcity of essential material. The importance of lemon and orange juice for seafarers had been known by the Dutch and others at least from 1564.[3] Lind published his "Treatise of the Scurvy" in 1753; but it was not until 1796, more than forty years later, that the Admiralty added lime juice to the naval ration, and the dread scurvy vanished from the fleets. The British sailors were referred to contemptuously by the Yankees as limeys. The Yankees took no stock in lemon juice, with the result that our Navy and merchant sailors suffered from scurvy for a century longer than the British, until steam shortened voyages to a safe duration.[4]

ANESTHESIA

During the first public demonstration of anesthesia at the Massachusetts General Hospital on October 16, 1846, William Thomas Green Morton was permitted to keep secret the nature of his "Letheon" and to obscure the fact that the active agent was diethyl ether. But a few days later, despite the resounding success of the first public demonstration, Morton was informed that the "surgeons of the hospital thought it their duty to decline the use of the preparation until informed what it was."[5] Under this pressure, Morton capitulated and revealed the nature of his agent.

He was attacked; some held his attempt at secrecy to be monstrous. Others defended him on the basis that he was not a physician, but a dentist. It was then customary for dentists to patent their devices, and no one thought the worse of them for it. Morton had worked hard, and a great discovery had come from his labors. He claimed that the reason for keeping his preparation secret was that he wished to perfect the method of its use and not come before the world until he was certain of the efficiency of his discovery. The surgeons of the Massachusetts General Hospital believed in Morton's sincerity and maintained their confidence in him.

Whatever Morton's true motivations were, selfish or not, he attempted to maintain his epoch-making material as a scarce resource. He was prevented from doing so by the surgeons of the Massachusetts General Hospital; the pressure of society removed his substance from the limited category and made it available to anyone who could learn to use it.

THE THYROID HORMONE AND MYXOEDEMA

Until the latter part of the nineteenth century, myxoedema was considered to be an incurable disease. Observations in man and experimentation in animals led to the suggestion by Victor Horsley that a sheep's thyroid be transplanted into a patient suffering from myxoedema. This was done in Portugal with immediate improvement of the patient, improvement that was evident the day after operation, far too soon to have been the result of the graft "taking." The reasonable conclusion was made that the benefit came from absorption of the "juice of the healthy thyroid." With this information in mind, G. R. Murray cut up a sheep's thyroid and placed it in a little glycerine and 0.5 per cent solution of carbolic acid.[6] After standing for twenty-four hours, the juice was filtered off and injected into a woman suffering from myxoedema, twice weekly at first and later at two- or three-week intervals. Over three months' time, two and a half sheep's thyroid glands were used. The recovery of the patient was spectacular. The tedious and other unsatisfactory aspects of this procedure led to the isolation by Kendall of thyroxine from the thyroid gland. Its chemical structure was established, and finally it was prepared synthetically. Thus the remedy that had been so successful for one patient became easily available, through physiological and chemical studies, to all who need it.

INSULIN

Ever since von Mehring and Minkowski had produced diabetes by excision of the pancreas in dogs in 1889, a number of attempts had been made to isolate the pancreatic substance that controlled carbohydrate metabolism. Finally this was accomplished by F. G. Banting and Charles H. Best in 1920 (published in 1922). They isolated the secretion of the islands of Langerhans and called it insulin.

Professor Best has recently had this to say:

The general principle involved in the early days of the clinical use of insulin was that only severe cases, who were desperately in need of some better treatment, would receive insulin. Furthermore it was felt that these cases should have had a very careful and thorough study so that any changes ascribed to the new therapy would be, in fact, due to it and not be within the variations encountered in diabetics.

In 1922, six distinguished physicians from the United States were invited to Toronto and fully briefed on the available information concerning insulin, and a revolution in medical care was launched. One of these six was Dr. E. P. Joslin of Boston. Dr. Priscilla White, his junior colleague in those early days, has described how Dr. Joslin's first concern was for those who were beginning to fail, especially children where the mortality was 100 per cent. They got first priority. Other considerations in the use of the scarce insulin were psychological stamina and "people who could take the routine and not break."

PENICILLIN

Investigations of the therapeutic usefulness of penicillin and measures to increase its supply were carried out by the Committee on Medical Research of the Office of Scientific Research and Development, by the Division of Medical Sciences of the National Research Council, and by certain commercial companies. These studies were initiated and continued as a phase of the war effort, *primarily for the benefit of the Armed Forces.*[7]

Although discovered by Fleming in London in 1929, penicillin's unique capabilities were revealed only in 1940-41 by Florey, Chain, and their collaborators at Oxford. Stimulated by Florey's visit to this country in the summer of 1941, some sixteen companies soon (by 1943) became engaged in the production of penicillin.

The first clinical tests of penicillin in this country were reported in 1941. In June of 1942, the Committee on Chemotherapeutic and Other Agents of the National Research Council, under the chairmanship of Dr. Chester S. Keefer, was invited to organize and to supervise clinical investigations in selected hospitals, the records to be coordinated by Dr. Keefer and his Committee.

In April 1943, the Surgeon General of the Army arranged for clinical tests to be made at the Bushnell General Hospital in Utah. There were many soldiers in that hospital who had returned from the Pacific area with unhealed compound fractures, osteomyelitis, and wounds containing long-established infections. The results of treatment with penicillin were so encouraging that within a matter of weeks similar studies were planned in ten General Army Hospitals and venereal studies in six. Plans were made for the Navy to carry on comparable but less extensive studies.

By the time Dr. Richards' report was made (May 22, 1943), more than three hundred patients were being treated with penicillin despite the great production problems. The earlier Oxford studies were confirmed. At the time of his report, Dr. Richards foresaw that the supply for civilian medical needs would be extremely limited.

On August 28, 1943, Dr. Keefer and his Committee reported on five hundred cases of infection treated with penicillin. Twenty-two groups of investigators were involved. Penicillin was then a scarce resource, and the situation urgent. In order to conserve material and time, the use of penicillin was restricted to a limited number of infectious states. After penicillin had been established as effective in treating staphylococcus and streptococcus infections, its use was soon extended to pneumonia and pneumococcal infections. Then it was shown to have an almost miraculous effect on gonorrhea and later a similar effect on syphilis, and a considerable number of other infections.[8] First came the concept, then the availability of the agent. As the material became plentiful, the breadth of its usefulness widened. The Committee saw it as their reponsibility to direct "study toward those infections that are most likely to occur in our armed forces and to those that are resistant to the sulfonamides." A few cases (seventeen at the time of Keefer's 1943 report) of subacute bacterial endocarditis, however, were studied with disappointing results. Owing to the scarcity of penicillin and the lack of extensive experience, inadequate doses were used in those early days. Later, penicillin was found to be very effective in treating subacute bacterial endocarditis. This is an indication of the types of erroneous conclusion one may encounter while materials are scarce and experience limited.

Allocation of penicillin within the Military was not without its troubles: When the first sizable shipment arrived at the North African Theatre of Operations, U.S.A., in 1943, decision had to be made between using it for "sulfa fast" gonorrhea or for infected war wounds. Colonel Edward D. Churchill, Chief Surgical Consultant for that Theatre, opted for use in those wounded in battle. The Theatre Surgeon made the decision to use the available penicillin for those "wounded" in brothels. Before indignation takes over, one must recall the military manpower shortage of those days. In a week or less, those overcrowding the military hospitals with venereal disease could be restored to health and returned to the battle line. Moreover, no one is going to catch osteomyelitis from an associate; venereal disease was a widely disseminated and serious hazard to the individual and to the war effort.

When penicillin became available for civilians, the aim was to widen its spectrum of usefulness and to determine the doses needed for effectiveness. To do this, Chester Keefer, who was in charge of the program, carried out a model project, notwithstanding extreme pressures to accede to the importunities of friends, strangers, even the White House, indirectly.

ADRENOCORTICOTROPIC HORMONE (A.C.T.H.) AND CORTISONE

Dr. John R. Mote, while associated with the Armour Laboratories, had control of the distribution of A.C.T.H. Although the hormone had been isolated in an impure form from the pituitary gland in 1925 by Dr. Herbert Evans, it was not until later that it had been purified enough to permit clinical studies. Mote took the purified A.C.T.H. to university hospitals where trained investigators, especially young ones "who had not yet been trapped by their previous training," were given supplies for study. His "guiding principle was to give A.C.T.H. to any competent individual of any age in an accredited teaching institution [with] the freedom to explore his ideas be they ever so bizarre in the light of previous medical concepts."

Dr. George W. Thorn comments:

I have little to comment regarding ACTH and cortisone since we did have available adrenal cortical extract and DOCA at the time these other agents were first marketed. It was entirely possible to keep patients alive with adrenal cortical extract and DOCA, providing suitable financing was available.

However, I can add a little note to our early days with adrenal cortical extract when this was being made in the Department of Physiology Laboratory at the University of Buffalo. Our total output was limited and it was necessary to discontinue treatment on one patient who had been restored from crisis when another Addisonian patient entered the hospital. We attempted to maintain the life of the first patient with supplementary sodium chloride and glucose. The extract was reserved for acute crises. Namely, the patient next to death was given the limited amount of adrenal extract.[9]

II. The Present

SUBJECTS: THE USE OF CHILDREN

An indispensable resource in human experimentation is suitable subjects; they are almost always in short supply, whether normal or ailing, whether free or "captive," as ward patients, inmates of asylums, prisoners, or children. These matters have been discussed extensively by myself and others.[10] Owing to limitations of space, only one of these problems will be dealt with here—namely, children, inasmuch as they present certain as yet unresolved problems.

Parents have the obligation to inculcate into their children attitudes of unselfish service. This can be extended to include participation in research for the public welfare if judged important and there is no discernible risk. There is, of course, useful legislation to protect children from mistreatment; but society has to depend on the integrity, mental stability, and good faith of the parents for the protection of their children. If the parents fail, the law steps in. Parents are the protectors of their children, not their owners.

THE ENGLISH VIEW

When experimentation in children is for diagnosis or treatment to the direct benefit of the child, the ethical problems are few so long as the consent of the parent or guardian has been obtained. The situation is vastly more complicated when the experimentation is not for the direct benefit of the child. A strict interpretation of English law declares this to be illegal, even with the approval of the parents, according to the Medical Research Council, 1962-63.

The situation in respect of minors and mentally subnormal or mentally disordered persons is of particular difficulty. In the strict view of the [English] law parents and guardians of minors cannot give consent on their behalf to any procedures which are of no particular benefit to them and which may carry some risk of harm. Whilst English law does not fix any arbitrary age in this context, it may safely be assumed that the Courts will not regard a child of 12 years or under (or 14 years or under for boys in Scotland) as having the capacity to consent to any procedure which may involve him in an injury. Above this age the reality of any purported consent which may have been obtained is a question of fact and as with an adult the evidence would, if necessary, have to show that irrespective of age the person concerned fully understood the implications to himself of the procedures to which he was consenting.

In the case of those who are mentally subnormal or mentally disordered the reality of the consent given will fall to be judged by similar criteria to those which apply to the making of a will, contracting a marriage or otherwise taking decisions which have legal force as well as moral and social implications. When true consent in this sense cannot be obtained, procedures which are of no direct benefit and which might carry a risk of harm to the subject should not be undertaken.

Even when true consent has been given by a minor or a mentally subnormal or mentally disordered person, considerations of ethics and prudence still require that, if possible, the assent of parents or guardians or relatives, as the case may be, should be obtained.

Investigations that are of no direct benefit to the individual require, therefore, that his true consent to them shall be explicitly obtained. After adequate explanation, the consent of an adult of sound mind and understanding can be relied upon to be true consent. In the case of children and young persons the question whether purported consent was true consent would in each case depend upon facts such as the age, intelligence, situation and character of the subject and the nature of the investigation. When the subject is below the age of 12 years, information requiring the performance of any procedure involving his body would need to be obtained incidentally to and without altering the nature of a procedure intended for his individual benefit.

THE SILENCE OF AMERICAN LAW

Only two precedents are even remotely relevant: There was the decision of the Supreme Judicial Court of Massachusetts in the case of the identical twins, one with kidney failure, one well.[11] The question was the propriety of permitting the well twin to give his kidney to his ailing brother. The decision evaded the central issue by declaring that the well twin would also profit from the transaction in a negative sense, since he would be permanently injured psychologically if he were not permitted to give his kidney to his ailing brother. The other "precedent" concerned the use of a minor as a donor for skin grafts to his cousin who had been badly burned. The donor's mother was ill and was not informed. The matter was brought to court and the judge *implied* that if the mother had been informed, the grafting would have been acceptable.

Although American law often follows English law, it has so far been silent on this issue, and there are no really relevant precedents. Too many decisions in the field of experimentation are now made in this country by default. In my view, it would be much sounder to achieve *group* agreement and then to assert forthrightly a policy to cover the situation, noting that the law is silent. It is quite possible that such a statement—made by thoughtful and distinguished individuals—would, when a legal test came, powerfully influence judicial decision and lead to the establishment of a valuable legal precedent.

DEFINITION OF A CHILD

Since physical and psychological growth generally reaches a plateau between age sixteen and twenty-one, eighteen has been suggested as a dividing age between the American child and the adult. The law, however, very often takes into account *understanding*. English courts will not regard a child of less than twelve years of age as being capable of consenting to any procedure that may do him harm. In Scotland, it is age fourteen; in America, sixteen or more. If self-supporting, if a high-school graduate, if married, or if in military service, the American child can be considered to be capable of understanding and consenting to experimentation that may entail some risk, but is properly approved by the child's parents and by the investigator's peers. Recent law concerning voluntary commitment to psychiatric institutions in Massachusetts uses age sixteen as the dividing line. The voting age in Georgia is eighteen, as is the draft age in the country. Since a "child" of eighteen may be required to give his life in military service, it seems reasonable to conclude that at such an age he may make independent judgments concerning his welfare. While the above matters may enter into a court's consideration, the *legal* age is still twenty-one years, after which the individual is capable of consent to participation in research if he is mentally sound.

RESEARCH ON NORMAL CHILDREN

I believe that the following statements are tenable and reasonable and propose them as policy.

1. The informed consent of the parents, or the legal guardian, and the child, when this is feasible, shall be required for all subjects under twenty-one years of age. The nature of *informed* consent and the complexities often surrounding its attainment are such that sometimes it becomes only a goal toward which we strive. It would be wrong to suppose, as most so-called codes do, that this goal is easily attainable for the asking. A great advantage to come from striving to get truly informed consent is that the parents and subjects, if at the age of understanding, are then alerted to the fact that they are indeed to be subjects of an experiment. Unfortunately this was not always the case in the past.

2. If the subject is too young to give consent, the consent of the parent or guardian is sufficient when no discernible risk is involved and the safety and value of the proposed study are supported by the investigator's peers. When the child is capable of understanding, he shall never be forced to cooperate in experimentation by over-zealous or unstable parents or guardians.

Discussion with children of sexual attitudes or practices is especially likely to bring down a storm on the heads of those who investigate such matters. Another delicate area is the privacy of the home: Parents often discuss their attitudes quite candidly in the house, but object when an investigator puts relevant questions to the children. In the parents' view this, in effect, puts the child in the position of spying on the parents. There is another troublesome area: When local issues are present on which there are strong feelings, the research worker can get into trouble with the parents, especially if he allows his own bias to be discovered.

3. Many thousands of psychomotor tests and sociological studies have been carried out in children during the child's development and have revealed much information of value. It would be difficult to fault this work, provided anonymity (if desired) is preserved. Sound nutritional studies without risk have been carried out. So also have certain blood studies.

Limitation of research in children to studies directly beneficial to them is not necessary. For example, such a restriction would greatly hamper behavioral studies as well as studies of inborn errors of metabolism. Such work is *potentially*, and sometimes unexpectedly, of direct benefit to the given subject. Much can be carried on without discernible risk.

These and other valuable and essentially risk-free endeavors are jeopardized by studies—such as those at Willowbrook where 250 mentally defective children, many five to eight years old, were deliberately infected with hepatitis virus; studies proving the hepatotoxic effects of "Tri-A" in mentally defective subjects and juvenile delinquents; the thymectomies in infants carried out in a transplant study; or the repeated biopsies of the testicles in normal prisoners less than twenty-one years of age.

4. Parents have the right to decide whether or not their children will participate in experimentation even if not for their direct benefit, provided the studies contemplated have no discernible risk and have been approved by a high-level review committee as being

necessary and valuable for human progress and do not unfairly take advantage of the child.

Some, Geoffrey Edsall for example, hold it to be unwarranted intrusion for an impersonal body, such as "the law," to step in between parent and child and say this cannot be done.[12] He goes on to say: "Laws have a tendency to be unintentionally rigid and short-sighted, and they require extremely careful thought and farsighted planning if they are to be written in such a way that they will really serve their purpose."

It is perhaps rather characteristic of the British that they have a law against the use of children in experimentation when it is not for their direct benefit. Edsall goes on to say: "They [the English] are also distinguished for having the most rigid antivivisection laws in the world—laws which drove Lord Lister to France for his experimental work on sutures, and laws which have handicapped the British in much experimental work ever since. . . . The British have displayed a tendency to be carried away by their emotional reactions in such affairs time and again."

5. Research that entails discernible risk may not be performed on subjects too young to give mature, informed consent, unless it is for their direct benefit.

RESEARCH ON SICK CHILDREN

The child brought to a physician for relief of an ailment has given, in the act of coming, his and his guardian's consent to reasonable efforts to relieve him. This usually requires experimentation. Sometimes it requires going beyond "standard" therapy. In this case, the guardian and the child, if feasible, should be informed and should consent.

If studies other than those required in therapy are to be undertaken, no discernible risk shall be the rule, and, if carried out, they should be widely discussed and approved by the child's parents and guardian as well as a high-level review board. The Golden Rule should be adhered to.

IN CONCLUSION

As long as the law is silent on experimentation in children, as it is in America at present, legal responsibility rests with the parents or guardian. The issues are: 1) no risk, if below the age of understanding; 2) screening and approval of a review board; 3) purposeful, useful goals; 4) no coercion or deception of the parents, but their full understanding and consent. Here, as in other problem cases, an additional safeguard is to be found in the child's physician rather than the physician-experimenter.

INTERMITTENT HEMODIALYSIS

Intermittent hemodialysis is of very limited availability. It does not, of course, involve the transplantation of tissues or organs, but it is often a means of maintaining life while awaiting the availability of a suitable kidney for transplantation.

Hemodialysis is an example of a limited experimental-practical procedure that is enveloped in problems both mundane and ethical. H. E. de Wardener has discussed the ethical and economic problems of keeping people alive with hemodialysis.[13] The main function here, of course, is the adjustment of the electrolyte and water content of the body so that they are kept within constant limits and certain wastes derived from protein metabolism are eliminated. If the kidneys cannot do this, the subject will die; life can be maintained even in the absence of kidney function, however, by circulating the blood through an artificial kidney. This process is called hemodialysis. It requires that the patient be placed on the artificial kidney some twelve to fourteen hours twice weekly. It is customary to carry this out at night in order to interfere as little as possible with normal activities. The patient's liberty is severely curtailed; the site of the arterial and venous connections must be kept absolutely clean and cannot be put into a bath; nor can the subject swim. Vigorous exercise is unwise. The site must be protected from injury. Strict dietary limitations are necessary. In most cases, the procedure much be carried out, at the present time at least, in a hospital.

Correctly carried out the mortality is low. For example, J. P. Pendras and R. V. Erickson at Seattle have treated twenty-three patients for over forty patient-years with three deaths.[14] De Wardener reports that he at Charing Cross and Shaldon at the Royal Free Hospital have treated thirty-five patients for a period of forty-three patient-years with one death owing to a technical accident.[15] Eight of Shaldon's patients are on home dialysis. Combining the data from the three centers gives a total of fifty-eight patients treated for eighty-three patient-years with four deaths.

With these elementary considerations in mind, one can turn to the ethical questions that must be faced, and in this it will be helpful to follow de Wardener's thoughtful comments.

Have we the right to prolong life in this way? Despite the limitations imposed, life can still be pleasant and productive; the answer is an unqualified yes to the general question.

Granted that the procedure is justified, who shall be treated? It has been the practice of the initial center to broaden responsibility by committee action, as at Seattle, where the committee includes both lay and medical members.

De Wardener doubts that the results of spreading responsibility are any better than decisions made by one or two individuals. G. E. Schreiner also argues against committee decision as to which candidate will be placed on dialysis, for a committee decision that involves laymen requires in the end organization and presentation of medical data to the lay group and in this the physicians' biases can be expressed.[16] But many aspects of society must be considered in the decision of who will and who will not be accepted in a dialysis program, aspects where the physician is as incompetent to make decisions as the layman is to decide on medical issues. Pendras seems to be on firm ground. His group considers two bases for selecting patients: the medical-psychological aspect and the social-moral, rehabilitation one. In essence, the Seattle screening is done by two committees in which laymen as well as physicians function.[17] In choosing candidates, they consider "worth to the community." For example, a thirty-two-year-old man with a stable history of employment and responsibility, with a family of six to support, was chosen over a forty-five-year-old widow whose children were grown up and had left home. Pendras is a strong advocate of the group decision.

In de Wardener's program, decision has to be made only when a place becomes available; the first obligation is toward those patients who are already being treated.[18] A new patient is not accepted until the last one has been well launched, for experience has shown that most difficulties occur in the early weeks of treatment. Moreover, a new patient is not accepted when any staff shortages are present. To be chosen, the subject must be showing signs of deterioration notwithstanding a low-protein diet. Since hemodialysis facilities are in short supply, a choice must be made among needy candidates. Usually such a choice is made among those between puberty (below this age, they will not mature if on dialysis) and menopause, subjects who are clear mentally and cooperative, and not suffering from some other disease that dialysis will not control. Often patients who have young children are chosen.

A definition of suitability for dialysis depends on a number of factors, some arbitrary, some empirical. For instance, the subject chosen should have the possibility of a prolonged survival. It seems reasonable during the period of establishment of a new technique to choose in the early years those subjects who will probably do best.

What are the financial consequences? The initial cost of the equipment is $4,200 (1966) per bed in England. When dialysis is carried out for three patients six nights a week, the capital cost per patient, thus, is $1,400. (This does not include the cost of housing.) Maintenance cost, nursing staff, technicians, and disposable items come to $84 per patient per week. De Wardener estimates that 2,230 patients in England in 1962 would have been acceptable and would have profited from dialysis. Aside from initial capital expenditure, the cost of treating this number in a hospital would be $9,800,000 for one year. He also estimates the British need to be ultimately the care of eleven thousand patients where the annual cost would be equivalent to the cost of two 800-bed district hospitals; clearly, dilemmas persist. He provides other interesting estimates of cost over a period of years.

In America, Pendras at Seattle estimates the cost at $5,000 to $10,000 per patient per year.[19] He believes that present facilities can accommodate only about 10 per cent of those in need. He estimates that with a cumulative patient load, after five years, 75 to 250 million dollars would be required for therapy for some fifteen to twenty-five thousand patients. At present, hemodialysis can be offered only on a limited basis owing to the scarcity of dialysis centers and the great cost.

Who ought to pay? Few individuals can afford the cost of dialysis. In some countries, only those who can pay are accepted for hemodialysis; in other countries, the State pays; in still other countries, no hemodialysis is available to anyone.

The cost is such that few can pay for the procedure without reducing their standard of living and without jeopardizing their children's future. Such a patient has to choose between family problems and dying. Some call this a form of suicide, a charge hotly denied by others. The sad fact is that a patient may feel obliged to make such a choice when his judgment may be clouded by disease. Once the treatment has begun, a drastic step is required by the sick man to stop the treatment and spare the family further financial distress. He can do this, for example, by a dietary indiscretion, such as choosing a high potassium diet, or by tearing out the tubes and allowing himself to bleed to death. It is unquestionably true that financial hardship preys on the minds of many confronted with these problems.

In the face of such tragic decisions, it is good to know that the United States is financing programs from both government and charitable funds. These are still in short supply, but the trend is hopeful. In Britain, if the Health Service is to be truly comprehensive, it is the responsibility of the Ministry of Health to provide for intermittent hemodialysis. The Minister of Health accepted this responsibility in 1965.

Is it right for the large sums involved to be directed to the pur poses of hemodialysis? The size of the financial commitment has discouraged some. De Wardener takes the creditable view that this is nothing new because, as Lord Platt has pointed out, in earlier years vast sums were spent on tuberculosis patients without questioning the cost. De Wardener has recently found that the cost per week of sanatorium care of a patient with tuberculosis is the same as maintaining a patient on intermittent hemodialysis in a hospital. Few tuberculosis patients confined to a sanatorium can lead productive lives, whereas those on intermittent hemodialysis can. This is a sound argument in favor of extending the availability of hemodialysis. Others can argue, if they choose, that the placement of the tuberculosis patient in a sanatorium removes a threat to the health of those who might otherwise come into contact with him; that the man with renal failure will not infect those about him, and therefore there is less urgency in treating him—a specious argument.

De Wardener presents interesting comparisons of the cost of treating or housing those with mental disease and those with renal failure. If those with mental disease are not treated or confined, they will roam the streets and prod our conscience. In contrast, those with failing kidney function will die and leave us in peace. The treatment of those with hemodialysis is not so radical an economic venture in the treatment of disease as some have supposed.

A further ethical question to be considered is whether the considerable number of skilled individuals involved in hemodialysis should be utilized in this way, taking into account, for example, the shortage of nurses. Wards in some hospitals are closed because of this shortage. De Wardener estimates that if the present nurse-to-patient ratios in Britain hold ten years hence, some four thousand nurses will be engaged in this activity. Automation as well as the employment of less skilled personnel may help with the staffing problems. But legal problems can arise when care of patients is delegated to "unqualified" staff. The numbers of doctors involved is less important than the number of nurses; but, even so, too few nephrologists are willing to take on the time-consuming demands involved in maintaining a hemodialysis program.

Schreiner has raised the question as to whether the physician might possibly be better occupied with trying to discover how the streptococcus produces glomerular nephritis than with treating the consequences of this infection. This question is really not relevant: Many physicians are quite competent to supervise a dialysis program, but few are competent by native research ability to get at the cause of the kidney failure. Schreiner says it is the old problem of research versus patient care. A more basic problem is the availability of the necessary kinds of talent.

THE AVAILABILITY OF TISSUES AND ORGANS FOR TRANSPLANTATION

In the field of transplantation there are two great barriers to progress: the immunological rejection phenomenon and the great shortages of donor material. At the present time, the rejection phenomenon is beyond our control in any very satisfactory sense, but it is within our power to take a giant step forward in relieving the shortages of donor material. This will require the prior concurrence of those involved, the agreement of society, and, finally, approval in law. The crucial point is agreement that brain death is death indeed, even though the heart continues to beat. Justice Holmes said: "To live is to function; that is all there is to living." This statement applies to organs as well as to the individual.

An *ad hoc* committee of the Harvard Medical School was asked to re-examine the definition of death.[20] Death was, the Committee concluded, much too various in its several aspects to attempt a definition, since death can occur at several levels: cellular (human cells can be maintained alive indefinitely in tissue culture), physiologic or neurologic death, intellectual, spiritual, or social death. In another approach, there is subcellular and cellular life, life of organs, life of the individual, and his life as a member of society. The group chose to define irreversible coma as a new criterion of death. (The ensuing discussion follows very closely that of the Harvard Committee.)

Scarce Resources and Medical Advancement

Such a definition is needed mainly for two reasons: First, improvements in resuscitative and supportive measures have led to increased efforts to save those who are desperately injured. Sometimes these efforts have only partial success so that the result is an individual whose heart continues to beat, but whose brain is irreversibly damaged. The resulting burden is great on the patient who suffers a fate of permanent loss of intellect should he survive, on the family, on the hospital, and on those in need of hospital beds already occupied by these comatose patients. Second, obsolete criteria for the definition of death can lead to controversy in obtaining organs for transplantation.

Irreversible coma has many causes, but *we are concerned here only with those comatose individuals who have no discernible central nervous system activity.* If the characteristics can be defined satisfactorily in terms translatable into action, which we believe is possible, then several problems will either disappear or become more readily soluble.

More than medical problems are present. There are moral, ethical, religious, and legal issues. Adequate definition here will prepare the way for better insight into all of these matters as well as for better law than is currently applicable.

CHARACTERISTICS OF IRREVERSIBLE COMA

As mentioned, an organ, brain or other, that no longer functions and has no possibility of functioning again is for all practical purposes dead. The Committee's first problem was to determine the characteristics of a *permanently* non-functioning brain.

The neurological impairment to which the terms "brain death syndrome" and "irreversible coma" have become attached indicates diffuse disease. Function is abolished at cerebral, brain stem and often spinal levels. This should be evident in all cases from clinical examination alone. Cerebral, cortical and thalamic involvement are indicated by a complete absence of receptivity of all forms of sensory stimulation and a lack of response to outside stimuli and to inner need. The term "coma" is used to designate this state of unreceptivity and unresponsivity. But there is always coincident paralysis of brain stem and basal ganglionic mechanisms as manifested by an abolition of all postural reflexes, including induced decerebrate postures, a complete paralysis of respiration, widely dilated, fixed pupils, paralysis of ocular movements, swallowing, phonation, face and tongue muscles. Involvement of spinal cord, which is less constant, is reflected usually in loss of tendon reflex and all flexor withdrawal or nocifensive reflexes. Of the brain stem-spinal mechanisms which are conserved for a time the vasomotor reflexes are the most persistent, and they are responsible in part for the paradoxical state of retained cardio-vascular function, which is to some extent independent of nervous control, in the face of widespread disorder of cerebrum, brain stem and spinal cord.

Neurological assessment gains in reliability if the aforementioned neurological signs persist over a period of time with the additional safeguards that there is no accompanying hypothermia or evidence of drug intoxication. If either of the latter two conditions exists, interpretation of the neurological state should await the return of body temperature to normal level and elimination of the intoxicating agent. Under any other circumstances repeated examinations over a period of 24 hours or longer should be required in order to obtain evidence of the irreversibility of the condition.[21]

In practical terms, this means that patients who are irreversibly comatose will be unreceptive and unresponsive to applied stimuli and inner needs; they are totally unaware, comatose. There are no spontaneous muscular movements or spontaneous respiration; artificial respiration supports the continuing heartbeat. There are no elicitable reflexes, except rarely stretch or tendon reflexes; the pupils are fixed, dilated, and unresponsive to light. The flat or isoelectric electro-encephalogram is of confirmatory value. All of these findings extend over at least twenty-four hours.

OTHER PROCEDURES

The patient's condition can be determined only by a physician. When the patient is hopelessly damaged as defined above, the family and all medical colleagues who have participated in major decisions concerning the patient and all nurses involved should be so informed. Death is to be declared and *then* the respirator turned off. The decision to do this and the responsibility for it are to be taken by the physician-in-charge, in consultation with one or more physicians who have been directly involved in the case. It is unsound and undesirable to force the family to make the decision.

DISCUSSION

Irreversible coma can have various causes: cardiac arrest, asphyxia with respiratory arrest, massive brain damage, intracranial lesions, neoplastic or vascular. It can be produced by other encephalopathic states, such as the metabolic derangements associated, for example, with uremia. Respiratory failure and impaired circulation underlie all of these conditions. They result in hypoxia and ischemia of the brain.

From ancient times until the recent past, it was clear that the brain would die in a few minutes after respiration and heart stopped; thus, the obvious criterion of no heart beat as synonymous with death was sufficiently accurate. In those times, the heart was considered to be the central organ of the body; it is not surprising that its failure marked the onset of death. This demarcation is no longer valid when modern resuscitative and supportive measures are used. These improved activities can now restore "life" as judged by the ancient standards of persistent respiration and continuing heart beat. This can be the case even when there is not the remotest possibility of an individual recovering consciousness following massive brain damage. In other situations, "life" can be maintained only by means of artificial respiration and electrical stimulation of the heartbeat, or in temporarily bypassing the heart, or, in conjunction with these things, reducing with cold the body's oxygen requirement.

In an address on "The Prolongation of Life," Pope Pius XII raised many questions.[22] Some conclusions stand out: In a deeply unconscious individual vital functions may be maintained over a prolonged period only by extraordinary means. Verification of the moment of death can be determined, if at all, only by a physician. Some have suggested that the moment of death is the moment when irreparable and overwhelming brain damage occurs. Pius XII acknowledged that it is not "within the competence of the Church" to determine this. It is incumbent on the physician to take all reasonable, ordinary means of restoring the spontaneous vital functions and consciousness, and to employ such extraordinary means as are available to him to this end. It is not obligatory, however, to continue to use extraordinary means indefinitely in hopeless cases. "But normally one is held to use only ordinary means—according to circumstances of persons, places, times, and cultures—that is to say, means that do not involve any grave burden for oneself or another."[23] It is the view of the Church that there comes a time when resuscitative efforts should stop and death be unopposed.

Thus, if these new criteria of brain death are accepted, the tissues and organs now consigned to the grave can be utilized to restore those who, although critically ill, can still be saved. To do nothing in this situation is far more radical than to accept the tissues and organs of the hopelessly comatose.

III. *Ethical Problems Arising in Transplantation of Tissues and Organs*

SOME GENERAL COMMENTS

Whenever the transplantation of tissues or organs is concerned, the material needed is in short supply now and will continue to be so into the foreseeable future. Yet, as was evident in the preceding section, we have available a powerful means of overcoming the grave shortages. It is evident that the transplantation of tissues or organs is not purely a medical problem. Perplexing questions abound; some are medical or partly medical, and some are not. The Ciba Foundation symposium was primarily interested in transplantation, but it considered subjects pertinent that are as diverse as how and when can a potential donor be considered to be free of undue influence? How long should "life" be maintained in a patient with irrevocable brain damage? When does death occur in an unconscious patient maintained only on artificial aids to the circulation and the respiration? Are there ever circumstances when death may be mercifully advanced? Can a parent rightly refuse necessary treatment of his child? How can minors, the ignorant, prisoners, be protected in the transplant situation? When may pregnancy be terminated? Is it legal to mutilate a donor for the sake of another person? What protection from society do medical men need in the development of new life-saving techniques? What is the community's financial responsibility in developing and maintaining life-supporting measures? Clearly, problems arising in transplantation are wide ranging.

Nearly all cases of transplantation where homografts are concerned involve experimentation for the benefit of the ailing subject, and thus the ethical problems encountered are usually relatively straightforward. The donor, with reasonable explanatory effort on the part of the physician, cannot help knowing that he is participating in a therapeutic experiment. There are instances of transplantation, however, where the above situations are not present, where transplantation has been carried out in an experiment not for the benefit of the subject. The author has discussed elsewhere a study in which skin homografts were carried out in children who had been subjected to thymectomy in order to see if thymectomy provided a better "take"; it did not.[24]

J. E. Murray believes that the lung is a likely organ to be transplanted and that, of the non-paired organs, the liver is the most promising. Remarkable progress has already been made in liver transplantation. Transplantation of the endocrine organs is being studied.[25] But it is impossible to discuss usefully the ethical problems arising in the rejection phenomenon until it is better understood—beyond acknowledging that its existence must act as a cautionary deterrent in the field. On the other hand, it is difficult to get around the possibility that some organs may be less subject to deleterious action by this phenomenon than others. It seems reasonable to proceed therefore, especially when the only alternative is death.

An especially difficult problem with single organ transplants, such as the heart or liver, is that this is a once-and-only procedure, whereas with the kidney as many as three transplants in a single patient have been carried out. Then, too, in the case of renal disease the fact must be weighed that the man with no kidney function can often be kept alive and functioning for years with intermittent hemodialysis. There are, clearly, basic differences in the problems surrounding the several organs.

If there were no legal or logistical problems, there would be available each year, it is estimated, over 10,600 cadaver kidneys in the United States, for approximately 7,600 kidney recipients, and 6,000 livers for 4,000 potential liver recipients.[26] These data are based on "neurological" deaths when the tissues to be transplanted would be satisfactory.

Some generalizations can be supplied as useful guides in the transplantation field.[27] These have been emphasized for years by responsible investigators in the area. It may be helpful to summarize them: Before transplantation is undertaken there must be a reasonable chance of clinical success. An acceptable therapeutic goal must be present. Adrenal or pancreatic transplants violate this "rule" since acceptable replacement secretions can be obtained. The risks and uncertainties must be presented to the families of the donor and the recipient as well as to the two principals. The protocol for each transplantation must be devised so as to gain and preserve the maximum information. There must be probing evaluation of the results by independent observers. Careful, accurate, conservative information is to be disseminated through legitimate channels, both medical and lay, in order that cruel hopes will not needlessly be raised. The field of transplantation carries great hope for the future; this should not be discredited by unscientific practices or proclamations.

BLOOD TRANSFUSION

In 1668, an eighty-page pamphlet on blood transfusion was published at Bologna. It is fair to call this the first text book on this subject.[28] Thus for three centuries the possibility of the transfusion of blood had been in men's minds, although its widespread practice really dates from about the time of World War II. Between 1668 and World War II, the scene was fraught with animal as well as human experimentation, some of it wild. Blood transfusion has interest and relevance to the present consideration: It represents the greatest and most successful transplantation of tissue. The considerable seventeenth-century interest in blood transfusion was followed by little interest in the eighteenth century, a sequence one often finds in the history of science: Men turn away from insoluble problems, only to return to them when some event or discovery gives renewed hope that they can be solved. In the nineteenth century, several books on the subject published in Europe stimulated an ever expanding interest that has continued to the present.

From the earliest times, blood has been considered to have an almost mystic importance, doubtless because of the plain fact that much loss of blood promptly leads to loss of life. It was believed that the weak could be made strong by drinking the blood of the latter, so the blood of bulls or of gladiators became a popular beverage. Keynes describes the attempt, near the end of the fifteenth century, to rejuvenate the aged Pope Innocent VIII by giving him a drink prepared from the blood of three young boys who thus died in vain.

The history of blood transfusion follows a common pattern of science. First there was the *concept* of introducing various materials into the circulation of an animal, then this was *extended* to blood. *Animal experiments* were carried out. Finally, these were *applied to man.*

Very often before the eruption of a great new advance in science, a *climate* appears wherein many men have similar ideas, and it becomes impossible to be sure who had the new concept first. It is certain, however, that Dr. Wren (later Sir Christopher) must get the credit for first experiments, in 1657, of intravenous injection of foreign substances into animals' veins. Then toward the end of February 1666, Richard Lower first demonstrated to a distinguished company at Oxford that a bled-out dog could be revived at once by the blood from a donor dog. The bled-out recipient "promptly jumped down from the table, and, apparently oblivious of its hurts, soon began to fondle its master, and to roll in the grass to clean itself of blood." This was the first public demonstration of a successful dog-to-dog transfusion. Lower's priority was challenged by one Jean Denys of France, who managed to get *his* claim translated into English and even published in the *Transactions* of the Royal Society for June 22, 1667, without the knowledge of the Secretary, Henry Oldenburg, who unfortunately at the moment was confined in the Tower. He got out just in time to have Denys's letter suppressed, although some copies still exist.[29]

In experiments in 1667, Denys succeeded for the first time in transfusing animal blood into men, first into a sick boy who was made miraculously well by a lamb's blood and then in an experiment in a *well* man, without ill effects. Similar experiments were carried out in England, until inevitably, disaster struck in 1668 in France: A patient died and the widow sued Denys. Denys lost, with the injunction that no further transfusions were to be made unless approved by a member of the Faculty of Medicine at Paris. Opposition there led to discontinuance of the procedure.

Samuel Pepys recorded in his *Diary* on November 14, 1666, comments on an animal-to-animal transfusion and, nimble-witted man that he was, suggested it would be interesting to inject the blood of a Quaker into an Archbishop. On November 21 of the next year, Pepys wrote of a "poor and debauched man, that the College have hired for 20s. to have some of the blood of sheep let into his body." There were no apparent ill effects, although considerable uncertainty as to the outcome had been expressed before the fact. This "poor and debauched" man may have been the first *paid* experimental subject, at least in England. (There is some evidence that the French had preceded the English in this.)

In 1794, Erasmus Darwin proposed the *hiring* of a donor so that frequent transfusions could be made into a sick man. The potential recipient "now found himself near the house of death"; he felt it useless to proceed with the experiment, and it was not carried out. The use of a subject paid to participate in an experiment three hundred years ago and Darwin's suggestion that a donor be hired indicate that some of our modern practices have ancient origins.

The world had to wait until December 22, 1818, for Blundell's account of the first successful man-to-man transfusion. In 1907, Jansky identified four blood groups, and transfusion was well on its way to acceptance as a standardized technique.

O. H. Robertson made use of stored blood in World War I, a practice widely followed in World War II first by the British and then by the United States forces after a tragic error made in Washington was overcome.[30] The American Forces entered North Africa essentially without adequate blood transfusing equipment. Here was human experimentation of a negative sort, but on a massive scale. This incredible mistake came as a result of believing that the newly developed blood plasma, wet or dried, would suffice. It soon became apparent that the infusion of plasma would indeed restore the blood pressure to a level where bleeding would be resumed in those already nearly exsanguinated and much of the remaining essential hemoglobin washed out.[31] (This is not the place to attribute blame. Edward D. Churchill, Consulting Surgeon for the Mediterranean Theatre, is writing the history of this titanic error.) The first blood bank for civilians was established as part of a military effort in Barcelona in 1936. The following year Fantus in Chicago founded the first completely civilian blood bank. Blood substitutes ranging from milk to modified fluid gelatine have been disappointing. Fractionating blood into its components has made it possible to satisfy a patient's needs more accurately than formerly.

G. E. W. Wolstenholme has taken a look at those who give and those who receive blood. He estimates that some seven million transfusion units are presently administered in the United States each year.[32] The donors are usually eighteen to sixty-five years of age, from whom 500 ml. are drawn without ill effect. The use of cadaver blood was suggested by G. Rubin in 1914,[33] and had considerable vogue in Russia during the 1930's. Such a practice is limited by infection developing after death and by the difficulties in obtaining an adequate history to rule out infectious hepatitis, malaria, and syphilis in its early stage. Sometimes blood is taken over a period of weeks, stored for re-infusion into the donor at the time of operation.

Even when infection-free and compatible blood is available, it is not always welcomed. Wolstenholme tells of a press report during World War II of a fanatical Nazi soldier captured at Tobruk who killed himself as soon as he realized he was being given British blood. Some British held a similar aversion. In North Africa, a British general ordered the destruction of one hundred blood transfusion units derived from German prisoners of war rather than have any of it used to save the lives of British wounded. One learns with relief that as soon as the general's back was turned the order was ignored. Arkansas has introduced legislation to control or to prevent the administration of "racially different" blood.[34]

Aside from these bizarre cases, the Jehovah's Witnesses provide a greater and more serious difficulty, one that bristles with ethical problems. One eminent chief of service at a Harvard hospital decided, on the advice of counsel and with Trustee support, to overrule the wishes of an adult "Witness." She was transfused. If one can ignore—overcome—such blood prejudice, can one also force a kidney transplant? What are the limits of coercive therapy? What is to be the end of this complex decision? The rather large group of Jehovah's Witnesses would prefer to lose their life than go against what they believe to be God's instruction (Leviticus XVII, 13, 14): "You shall eat the blood of no manner of flesh for the life of all flesh is the blood thereof." It is customary to accede to such prejudice, but not always. A great ethical problem arises in the case of the children of Jehovah's Witnesses or in the case of a Witness too ill to make a rational decision. If the emergency is not great, legal advice can be sought; if the situation is desperate, some physicians have desisted, some have not. The law is not yet helpful in this area.

It is unquestionably true that blood transfusion is too often too lightly undertaken. One distinguished authority in the field has argued vehemently in the past that blood transfusion should not be carried out during surgery under general anesthesia lest a previously undetected incompatibility or a frank error in matching go unnoticed. To accept as decisive this remote possibility against the undoubted life-saving power of blood transfusion during surgery is sadly unrealistic. When contemplating over-use, one must always remember the possibilities and hazards of sensitization. Wolstenholme estimates the over-all mortality rate for transfusion to be "not higher than three in 10,000."[35]

In extra pay for those who engage in hazardous pursuits, society has accepted the view that risk is reimbursable. One wonders if the question of whether the sale of major organs with the risk this entails will eventually find the same acceptance as the sale of blood for transfusion. When the immunological problem is solved, this question could become a pressing one. Legislation now pending in Italy would make illegal any payment for an organ.

CORNEAL TRANSPLANTATION

In reviewing the history of corneal transplantation, Rycroft has concluded that credit must go to Pellier de Quengsy for attempting in 1789 to stitch a glass disc into the cornea after removing a scarred patch of that tissue; he does not record the outcome.[36] A few years later (1796) Erasmus Darwin, in London, wondered if a "small piece of cornea" could not be trephined out. Such ideas led to the first graft of corneal tissue on a human cornea by Reisinger in 1817. He got the idea from watching Astley Cooper place a skin graft on the stump of an amputated limb at Guy's Hospital. The first successful human corneal graft was achieved by Zirm in 1905. The donor in this case was a small boy who had to have his eye removed because of an intraocular foreign body. Later the Russian Filatov demonstrated that donor material from cadavers could be used, after storage at low temperatures.

Unlike other material where grafting has been attempted, corneal grafts involve avascular tissue, and this undoubtedly accounts for the early and continued success. Since the material can be obtained from cadavers or surgical sources and stored, most of the harassing ethical problems surrounding other tissues or organs are not present here. Prior to World War II, donor material was difficult to find and came mainly from eyes containing tumors. After World War II, when the demand for donor material greatly increased, surgeons turned to cadaver material. Once again the Anatomy Act of 1832 hindered this approach in Britain, and one had to depend on the occasional permission of relatives of the deceased. This situation was improved by the 1952 Corneal Grafting Act, which was later incorporated in the Human Tissue Act of 1961.

The Queen Victoria Hospital's Eye Bank at East Grinstead received in 1965, about fifteen years after its founding, over four hundred eyes. International donor services are now provided. These widespread activities have been made possible by public education through lectures, the press, radio, and television. Such success can doubtless be extended to more complicated transplantation problems by similar educational efforts.

The law concerning what can and cannot be removed from a body and under what circumstances varies with the country or state involved. Much of it is unclear or ambiguous.

KIDNEY TRANSPLANTATION

The general, although not unanimous, view is that an individual with two healthy kidneys can ethically give one, providing the gift is truly voluntary and is given with the full knowledge of the risks, including the information that his sacrifice may turn out to be useless. Still, family pressures are often so great that it is difficult to impossible to determine if the donor is truly a volunteer. Attempts to ensure voluntariness have sometimes led to standardized psychological examination where the examiner attempts to determine if the potential donor is "stable, well-balanced and rationally motivated." Such an examination can also uncover possible pressure from the family. The donor is told that if he does not want to give a kidney, no one will know, for the physician will state that the donor is unsuitable. In these circumstances, about three out of five are found to be genuine volunteers. A major purpose is to prevent external pressure on the prospective donor. There is the recurrent question as to whether one is justified on ethical grounds in refusing to transplant a kidney from a relative who would feel that he had in the refusal failed to save the life of a loved one. One can ask whether it is really ever possible to exercise truly free choice in a situation where the inherent pressures are so strong as they are in family situations. Family pressures can lead to choice of a donor on the basis of his presumed expendability. Family pressure is, however, "consonant with the dignity and responsibility of free life."[37] There are also subtle and strong internal pressures within each possible donor. These pressures are rooted in common religious and social attitudes concerning the propriety of self-sacrifice. It is difficult to see how anyone or any panel of experts could be absolutely certain that free and uninhibited consent exists when the prospective donor is aware that he is making a life or death decision, and that the decision is under scrutiny. The potential anguish of such a situation could be most acute for the identical twin who is a unique donor. But in view of the excellent results after other intrafamilial transplantations, the situation is not limited to twin cases.[38] Excepting identical twins or other close relative donors, the whole issue is clouded by the brief prognosis, in most cases one or two years, at present.[39] It has been estimated that, excluding fraternal twins, there are probably no more than fifteen patients in the world who have survived kidney transplantation for more than three years.[40] It is, thus, not now possible to know the value of the procedure in terms of a five- or ten-year prognosis. Even if the benefit proves to be limited to a few years, this gain is significant for the individual who fills a useful place in society. Starzl asks searching questions as to who is equipped to determine the "usefulness" or "value" of a given individual: "A system of selection based upon such materialistic criteria is founded on the dangerous assumption that a few people are qualified and have the right to adjudicate the value of someone else's years."[41]

Under some circumstances, it is not ethical, or perhaps even legal, for a patient to accept an organ. For example, if the patient knows that the donor's spouse strongly disapproves of the donation, it may be unethical for him to accept. If he knows that a prisoner or a lunatic is giving the organ, it might be not only unethical, but illegal to accept it. A "person under restraint cannot be presumed to consent."[42]

M. F. A. Woodruff finds it curious that so much emotional concern is voiced over a kidney donation, yet during the Battle of Britain no one saw any moral problem in allowing a man to become a fighter pilot.[43] Most would rather give a kidney than become such a pilot. Bentley objects to such an analogy, for moral theologians make a distinction between direct and indirect effects. For the fighter pilot, the possible maiming is never the means of achieving what he wants to do. The maiming, if it occurs, is an indirect effect, foreseen as possible; but in transplantation, the maiming—the loss of a kidney—is the direct means to the end desired. Thus, a moral difference is present.

One can speculate on the consequences of a breach in the present immunological barrier: The transplantation of skin could be life-saving in the severely burned. In another area, with the present population of the United States at 200 million, one can estimate ten thousand kidney transplants each year.[44]

A difficult early period in any specific experimental work is likely to be the time when success is rare. Lord Platt believes the ethical position of removing a kidney from a healthy person when the chance of it surviving as a transplant for a long time is 5 per cent is different from what it would be if the success rate were 90 per cent.[45] "Rarity of success" is a real and complicating factor not usually discussed. In such a situation, whether to continue or to call it quits is a troubling decision. If an acceptable success rate is to be achieved, experimentation must continue. This problem is not limited to organ transplantation; it is common in the development of most complex diagnostic and therapeutic procedures.

Lord Platt takes the view that in certain rare and dangerous developmental procedures, not yet ready for general use, but nevertheless *for the patient's welfare:* "There is a slight danger here, in that one is selecting patients for such procedures partly because they may benefit other people in the future and not wholly because of possible benefit to the present patient."[46] As long as the purpose of the procedure is truly diagnostic or therapeutic for the given individual, there can be little ground for complaint, if at the same time it adds to knowledge or benefit to others. It seems likely that the only questionable situation would grow out of deception of the subject or one's self when there was no true expectation of helping the patient.

Lord Platt is of the opinion that too little thought is given to whether the proposed experiment is really a *sound* experiment.[47] The writer has emphasized for years that the improperly designed experiment, one that cannot give useful data, is an unethical experiment, regardless of whether it is "harmless" or not. There is the requirement in all human experimentation that the ends sought not be trivial.

The next few years may show that kidney transplantation has a better chance of success than has resection of the esophagus for cancer: 15 per cent five-year cures for the lower third; 5 per cent for the middle third; no five-year cures for the upper third.[48] Esophageal surgery would not ordinarily be called experimental, yet kidney transplantation is usually so designated. One may not fairly equate experimental procedures with procedures that have a low success rate. It must be borne in mind that for some diseases— as, for example, cancer of the esophagus—there is no real alternative to surgery, whereas there is an alternative to kidney transplantation: intermittent hemodialysis.

Murray has made the point that an operation on the donor is not a medical procedure at all; it is not making a sick person well, but a well person sick.[49] Any maiming of a patient should be for his benefit. The principle of totality covers this: A part of the body may be sacrificed for the good of the whole. The donor loses a kidney, but has spiritual gain in his sacrifice.

Questions involve both donor and recipient: whether a kidney transplant, for example, will do any good and, if so, to whom. If the transplant lives, the recipient is obviously benefited. Whether the transplant lives or dies, the donor can be benefited psychologically and spiritually. This was affirmed by the Supreme Judicial Court of Massachusetts in the case of the first identical twin transplant.

G. B. Giertz has proposed that a considerable number of persons might agree when healthy, when fully conscious, that a kidney might be taken if certain conditions ensue later in life,[50] or a second solution might stem from a re-evaluation of widely accepted moral principles with alteration of legislation.

HEART TRANSPLANTATION

Transplantation of the heart represents a desperate effort to save a desperate situation. It is a therapeutic effort that will be widely practiced, once the rejection phenomenon is overcome. Just as attention to various unethical procedures has focused our thought on the necessity to straighten out our practices, so also in an opposite sense Barnard's first heart transplant focused attention on a great need. The resultant excitement and the educational effect will in all probability lead to the acquisition of funds and the stimulation of investigators so that the transplant problems—not only of hearts but of other organs as well—will be solved sooner than would otherwise have been the case. While granting a pre-eminent place for the individual's rights, it would be wrong to overlook the fact that society has rights too, especially relevant to the possibilities of successful transplantation.

A considerable debate is at present under way concerning whether or not further heart transplants should be attempted until the rejection phenomenon in general is better understood and better controlled. Another imponderable in the heart transplant situation is that it is impossible to judge with accuracy the prognosis in survival time of the prospective recipient without transplantation. Certainly a heart transplant would not be contemplated if widespread and crippling atherosclerosis were present.

While a great deal has been learned about transplantation in general from work with the kidneys, transplantation of the heart presents certain crucial differences. In the case of the kidney, the donor can survive following the loss of a kidney; the donor of a heart cannot survive. If the transplantation of a kidney is not successful, the subject can be placed on hemodialysis, and two or three attempts can be made at transplantation. No such possibility exists with cardiac transplantation; it is a once and only possibility. The restrictions on this scarce resource are thus more severe with the heart than with paired organs.

A further restriction pointed out by the Board on Medicine of the National Academy of Sciences is that a greater number of surgeons have the knowledge and skill to perform the actual transplantation of the heart "than have available the full capability to conduct the total study in terms of all relevant scientific observations."[51] The Board would restrict cardiac transplantation to those institutions in which there are present not only surgical expertise, but also a thorough understanding of the biological processes that lead to rejection and its control. In this hazardous field it is especially important that careful planning be established prior to the event, that systematic observations be recorded, and that all findings, good and bad, be communicated to the few others engaged in such activity. Rigid safeguards must be established to cover the choices of donor and recipient.

LEGAL PROBLEMS IN THE FIELD OF TRANSPLANTATION

A considerable dilemma is encountered in this area. The rights of donors, alive or cadaver, insofar as the latter can be said to have "rights," as well as the rights of recipients have not been spelled out in law; at the same time experience indicates that it is often undesirable to bring legal decision into a situation that is in a state of rapid change, as this one is.

The use of live donors who have been properly informed, who understand the risks involved and the uncertainty of success, who have agreed in writing, has not led to serious legal problems.

For those who, like G. P. J. Alexandre, believe that the removal of organs is proper in patients after the brain is dead, but whose heart still beats, the philosophy is simpler than for others who do not agree.[52] There is a difference, of course, when one of paired organs is removed and the removal of single organs, like the liver or the heart. Such a situation falls into the category of "statistical morality," for all major surgical procedures have their own mortality rates. When enough operations are carried out, even the removal of one of a pair will lead to death.

Cadaver donors are a special problem. In the first place, true emergency planning is involved so that the kidneys or other organs can be removed and perfused in an hour or less. In such a case, good hope for success is justified. Since the cadaver transplant must be effected in minutes, not hours, what legal procedure can be prepared ahead of time? Eventually, as Giertz has suggested, it may be possible to get enough individuals to agree, when healthy, to organ removal if brain death later occurs.[53]. This procedure could, if extensive enough, make a real impact on the situation. Or legislation might be arrived at whereby tissues might be taken legally after death without further ado, unless the individual

97

or his family explicitly objected or his religion was opposed to such a practice. The situation might also be handled by legal authorization for a previously designated person to give consent to tissue or organ removal after death. Under present legal restrictions, a living person has limited powers to dispose of his body or its parts after death, although some states permit such disposal by will, as in California and recently in Massachusetts.

When Woodruff set about organizing a skin bank in Scotland, he discovered that, under the Anatomy Act of 1832, it was illegal to proceed. The Act had been passed as a consequence of the activities of the Edinburgh murderers, Burke and Hare. The need for a skin bank was appreciated and the situation set to right by the passage in 1961 of the Human Tissue Act. The unethical act (murder) led to restrictive legislation (the Anatomy Act of 1832), a sequence one can often observe when less final ethical violations occur than murder. One can take some comfort from the fact that when need for revision was demonstrated, correction of the law followed.

Another example of the restraining power of the courts was demonstrated in the 1932 case of the rich man who bought a testicle from a young Neapolitan. A surgeon transplanted it with the result that article 5 of the Italian common code of civil rights was promulgated in 1940. This forbade the donation of organs or other parts of the body that could produce a *permanent* deficiency in the donor. Blood transfusion or skin grafts were thus not made illegal.[54] A more enlightened bill is currently before the Italian Parliament for final approval. In the United States, the law has not kept pace with science, but, as suggested above, this may be a good thing until many situations and problems are better clarified than is presently the case.[55]

IV. General Comment

It was a considerable disappointment to the writer, after the examination of more than a dozen areas where scarce resources were involved, to find statements of only the most rudimentary principles of procedure. (One must face the fact that this, too, is a kind of principle.)

The guiding factors encountered (rather than principles in most cases) can be summarized: *Avarice* is exemplified in the secrecy surrounding the Chamberlen forceps. Although lemon and orange juice were in short supply, their effectiveness in treating the scurvy was a matter of record; yet decades passed before the general *ignorance* was overcome. *Self-interest* or dedication to high principle is not clear in the case of anesthesia.

This is not to say that in early times only avarice, ignorance, or self-interest determined the allocation of scarce resources; but it seems evident that these factors were determinants then more often than is now the case.

Continuing with our arbitrary list of examples, the next one, chronologically, is the thyroid hormone. With this, a new and much higher realm of procedure was entered; it could be called a prototype for present action: Myxoedema was recognized as an incurable disease of the thyroid; animals, presumably, had normal thyroids. Seventy-seven years ago the difficulties lying in wait for the transplanter were not known; "transplant" of a sheep's thyroid was carried out. The curative properties of the procedure were evident in a matter of hours, far too soon for grafting to explain the success. It was assumed and later proved true that the infusion of the thyroid "juice" accounted for the good effect. The active element was found to be thyroxine, which was synthesized. The early scarcity of the material and the tedious procedure gave way to the ready availability of the crucial substance as desired for anyone in need. This is a beautiful example of the selfless and effective work of many men, typified also in the triumphs of insulin, penicillin, and the adrenocorticotrophic hormone and cortisone.

There are at the present time plentiful reasons for despairing of mankind, but not in the standards evident in the progress of medicine. In the Western world, at least, the pre-eminence of the welfare of the individual is recognized as an indispensable component in the welfare of society. (It is inconceivable that a healthy society could be based upon exploitation of individuals, a sick use of individuals.) There is a considerable and growing recognition that science is not necessarily the highest value, that it must be placed in a hierarchy of values.

Some may consider these statements rather too grand. Yet what other conclusion can one come to with such visible evidence for them? Consider some major current concerns of today. May children be used in experimental procedures not for their direct benefit? (The answer seems to be "yes" in certain well-defined children's areas, "no" in others.) Relevant to our present interests is the fact that concern for "yes" or "no" *is* present.

It is now recognized that intermittent hemodialysis, as costly and inadequately available as it is at present, can be given to all who need it, at no greater cost than once was required by tuberculosis, even at less cost than mental disease now exacts. These latter unfortunates can add little to the world; hemodialysis can and does add years of productivity to those with otherwise fatal kidney disease.

Moreover, those who were once a grave and growing burden, the hopelessly comatose, can now be the means of extending life for desperately ill, but still salvageable individuals through a new understanding that the brain can die while other parts of the body remain sound and useful. It is also recognized that to *fail* to utilize this material is far more radical than not to use it.

The current requirements of an ethical approach to the transplantation of tissues and organs are a credit to our present standards of morality. All of these concerns, when contrasted with earlier years, offer heartening evidence of the growth of conscience, the advance in philosophical awareness, the gain in spiritual values, the sound growth of medicine.[56]

REFERENCES

1. F. H. Garrison (*An Introduction to the History of Medicine* [Philadelphia, 1914], p. 208) says 1670; A. Castiglione (*A History of Medicine* [New York, 1941], p. 554) says 1647.

2. The usually accurate Garrison says two hundred years. Castiglione says more likely fifty years. *Ibid.*

3. F. H. Garrison, *An Introduction to the History of Medicine* (fourth ed.; Philadelphia, 1929), p. 363.

4. W. Dock, "How the Investigative Scot Foiled the Continental Conqueror," *The Pharos* (April, 1967), pp. 56-58.

5. F. R. Packard, *History of Medicine in the United States,* Vol. 2 (New York, 1931), p. 1096.

6. G. R. Murray, "Note on the Treatment of Myxoedema by Hypodermic Injections of an Extract of the Thyroid Gland of the Sheep," *British Medical Journal,* Vol. 2 (1891), p. 796.

7. A. N. Richards, "Penicillin" (Statement by the Chairman of the Committee on Medical Research), *Journal of the American Medical Association,* Vol. 122 (1943), p. 235.

8. A. Fleming (ed.), *Penicillin, Its Practical Application* (Philadelphia, 1946).

9. G. W. Thorn, Personal Communication by Letter (July 9, 1968).

10. H. K. Beecher, *Research and the Individual* (Boston, 1969).

11. W. J. Curran, "A Problem of Consent: Kidney Transplantation in Minors," *New York University Law Review,* Vol. 34 (1959), p. 891.

12. Geoffrey Edsall, Personal Communication (1968).

13. H. E. de Wardener, "Some Ethical and Economic Problems Associated with Intermittent Hemodialysis," *Ethics in Medical Progress: CIBA Foundation Symposium* (Boston, 1966), pp. 104-125.

14. J. P. Pendras and R. V. Erickson, "Hemodialysis: A Successful Therapy for Chronic Uremia," *Annals of Internal Medicine,* Vol. 64 (1966), pp. 293-311.

15. De Wardener, "Some Ethical and Economic Problems Associated with Intermittent Hemodialysis."

16. G. E. Schreiner, in *Ethics in Medical Progress: CIBA Foundation Symposium,* pp. 100, 118.

17. The Medical Advisory Committee is made up of eighteen physicians. The Admissions Advisory Committee is made up of seven individuals from all walks of life: two physicians, a lawyer, a housewife, a businessman, a labor leader, and a minister. Thus the community participates.

18. De Wardener, "Some Ethical and Economic Problems Associated with Intermittent Hemodialysis." Subsequent allusions to de Wardener in the text are to this article.

19. J. P. Pendras, "Experience with Patient Selection," unpublished data (1967).

20. The Committee members were as follows: Raymond D. Adams, M.D., A. Clifford Barger, M.D., William J. Curran, L.L.M., S.M. Hyg., Derek Denny-Brown, M.D., Dana L. Farnsworth, M.D., Jordi Folch-Pi, M.D., Everett I. Mendelsohn, Ph.D., John P. Merrill, M.D., Joseph Murray, M.D., Ralph Potter, Th.D., Robert Schwab, M.D., William Sweet, M.D., with the author serving as chairman.

21. Report of the *Ad Hoc* Committee at Harvard Medical School to Examine the Definition of Brain Death, "A Definition of Irreversible Coma," *Journal of the American Medical Association,* Vol. 205 (August 5, 1968), pp. 337-40.

22. Pius XII, "The Prolongation of Life," *The Pope Speaks,* Vol. 4, No. 4 (Spring, 1958), pp. 393-98.

23. *Ibid.*

24. H. K. Beecher, "Ethics and Clinical Research," *New England Journal of Medicine,* Vol. 274 (1966), pp. 1354-60.

25. J. E. Murray, "Organ Transplantation: The Practical Possibilities," *Ethics in Medical Progress: CIBA Foundation Symposium,* pp. 54–77.

26. N. P. Couch, "Supply and Demand in Kidney and Liver Transplantation: A Statistical Study," *Transplantation*, Vol. 4 (1966).

27. E. D. Robin, "Rapid Scientific Advances Bring New Ethical Questions," *Journal of the American Medical Association*, Vol. 189 (August 24, 1964), pp. 624-25.

28. Sir G. Keynes, *Blood Transfusion* (London, 1949).

29. *Ibid.*

30. O. H. Robertson, "Transfusion with Preserved Red Blood Cells," *British Medical Journal*, Vol. 1 (1918), pp. 691-95.

31. See H. K. Beecher, "Preparation of Battle Casualties for Surgery," *Annals of Surgery*, Vol. 121 (1945), pp. 769-92; E. D. Churchill, Personal Communication by Letter (June 28, 1968).

32. G. E. W. Wolstenholme, "An Old-established Procedure: The Development of Blood Transfusion," *Ethics in Medical Progress: CIBA Foundation Symposium*, pp. 24-42.

33. G. Rubin, "Placental Blood for Transfusion," *New York Medical Journal*, Vol. 100 (1914), p. 421.

34. Arkansas Statutes 1947 Annotated, 1960 Replacement, Vol. 7A, Chapter 16, "Blood Transfusions":

"82-1601. Blood labeled as to race.—All human blood used or proposed to be used in the State of Arkansas for transfusions of blood, except such units of blood which will have been transported across the State line into Arkansas, shall be labeled with word 'Caucasian,' 'Negroid,' 'Mongoloid,' or some suitable designation so as to clearly indicate the race of the donor of such blood. No human blood not labeled in accordance with the provisions of this act [82-1601—2-1605] shall be used for transfusions in the State of Arkansas. [Acts 1959, No. 482, 2, p. 1923.]

"82-1602. Notice when blood of different race to be used in transfusion.— Any person about to receive a blood transfusion or a parent of said person, or the next of kin of said person shall be informed of the race of the donor of the blood proposed to be used if blood from a person of a different racial classification is to be used." [Acts 1959, No. 482, 2, p. 1923.] Certain emergency provisions are also spelled out.

35. Wolstenholme, "An Old-established Procedure: The Development of Blood Transfusion."

36. P. V. Rycroft, "A Recently Established Procedure: Corneal Transplantation," *ibid.*, pp. 43-53.

37. D. Daube, "Transplantation: Acceptability of Procedures and the Required Legal Sanctions," *Ethics in Medical Progress: CIBA Foundation Symposium*, pp. 188-201.

38. T. E. Starzl, "In Discussion: 'Organ Transplantation: The Practical Possibilities,' by J. E. Murray," *ibid.*, p. 98.

39. W. E. Goodwin, "In Discussion: 'Transplantation: The Clinical Problem,' M. G. A. Woodruff," *ibid.*, p. 17.

40. Starzl, "In Discussion," *ibid.*

41. *Ibid.*

42. Daube, "Transplantation: Acceptability of Procedures and the Required Legal Sanction," *ibid.*

43. M. F. A. Woodruff, "Transplantation: The Clinical Problem," *ibid.*, pp. 6-23.

44. Murray, "Organ Transplantation: The Practical Possibilities," *ibid.*

45. Lord Platt, "Ethical Problems in Medical Procedures," *ibid.*, pp. 149-70.

46. *Ibid.*

47. *Ibid.*

48. E. W. Wilkins, Personal Communication, 1967.

49. Murray, "Organ Transplantation: The Practical Possibilities," *Ethics in Medical Progress: CIBA Foundation Symposium.*

50. G. B. Giertz, "Ethical Problems in Medical Procedures in Sweden," *ibid.*, pp. 139-48.

51. Statement Prepared by the Board on Medicine of the National Academy of Sciences, "Cardiac Transplantation in Man," *Journal of the American Medical Association,* Vol. 204, No. 9 (1968), pp. 147-48.

52. G. P. J. Alexandre, "In Discussion: 'Organ Transplantation: The Practical Possibilities,' by J. E. Murray," *Ethics in Medical Progress: CIBA Foundation Symposium,* pp. 68-71. Compare also in this connection Report of an *Ad Hoc* Committee at Harvard Medical School to Examine the Definition of Brain Death.

53. Giertz, "Ethical Problems in Medical Procedures in Sweden," *ibid.*

54. R. Cortesini, "Outlines of a Legislation on Transplantation," *ibid.*, pp. 171-87; "In Discussion, 'Transplantation: The Clinical Problem,'" *ibid.*, p. 16.

55. C. E. Wasmuth and B. H. Stewart, "Medical and Legal Aspects of Human Organ Transplantation," *Cleveland-Marshall Law Review,* Vol. 14 (1965), pp. 442-71; also, C. E. Wasmuth, "Law for the Physician: Legal Aspects of Renal Transplantation," *Anesthesia Annals,* Vol. 46 (January-February, 1967), pp. 25-27.

56. In preparing this article, the author also had occasion to use the following sources not directly cited: Charles H. Best, Personal Communication by Letter (June 28, 1968); E. D. Churchill, "Wound Shock and Blood Transfusion" (in preparation); Editorial, "Ethics in Research," *Hospital Medicine,* Vol. 2 (April, 1968), p. 759; C. S. Keefer, Chairman, F. G. Blake,

E. K. Marshall, Jr., J. S. Lockwood, and W. B. Wood, Jr., "Penicillin in the Treatment of Infections. A Report of 500 Cases"; Statement by the Committee on Chemotherapeutic and Other Agents, Division of Medical Sciences, National Research Council, *Journal of the American Medical Association*, Vol. 122, No. 18 (1943), pp. 1217-24; S. Krugman, J. P. Giles, and J. Hammond, "Infectious Hepatitis," *Journal of the American Medical Association*, Vol. 200, No. 5 (May, 1967), p. 365-73; P. Lieberman, *Medico-legal Monograph*, Law Department, American Medical Association (1966); F. Mariceau, "Des Maladies des Femmes Grosses et Accouchées" (Paris, 1668; also English edition: "The Diseases of Women with Child and in Child-bed," trans. Hugh Chamberlen [London, 1672], see translator's note concerning the Chamberlen secret); J. R. Mote, Personal Communication by Letter (June 26, 1968); *Report of the Medical Research Council for 1962-63 (Cmnd. 2382)*, "Responsibility in Investigations on Human Subjects," pp. 21-25; D. H. Russell, "Law, Medicine and Minors—Part I," *New England Journal of Medicine*, Vol. 278, No. 1 (1968), pp. 35-36; D. H. Russell, "Law, Medicine and Minors—Part II," *New England Journal of Medicine*, Vol. 278, No. 5 (1968), pp. 265-66; D. H. Russell, "Law, Medicine and Minors—Part III," *New England Journal of Medicine*, Vol. 278, No. 14 (1968), pp. 779-80; P. White, Personal Communication (1968); R. M. Zollinger, Jr., M. D. Lindem, Jr., R. M. Filler, J. M. Corson, and R. E. Wilson, "Effect of Thymectomy on Skin-homograft Survival in Children," *New England Journal of Medicine*, Vol. 270 (April 2, 1964), pp. 707-710.

PAUL A. FREUND

Legal Frameworks for Human Experimentation

A CONSIDERATION of possible legal frameworks for human experimentation ought to rest on an appreciation of certain characteristics of the legal order. In 1954, Columbia University took as the motto for its bicentennial celebration, "The Right to Knowledge and the Free Use Thereof." Noble as the sentiment is, a lawyer might be inclined to invoke Justice Holmes' regular challenge to his law clerks: "State any proposition, and I'll deny it!" The law values the free use of knowledge, but it values also a right of privacy and of literary property; it makes accommodations through distinctions between public and private figures, published and unpublished work, research and plagiarism. The law is dialectic in a deeper sense than its adversary process. It mediates most significantly between right and right.

The law is highly solicitous of physical integrity—a sentiment whose lineage can be traced historically to both religious and royal concerns. Even self-willed injury, if destructive enough, is made illegal, like mayhem and attempted suicide; to that extent, an individual is a trustee of his own person. Even trivial injury caused by another, like an offensive touching, if deliberate and not consented to is also unlawful. In the great range of unintended injuries, legal liability ordinarily depends on a calculus of risks and benefits of the injury-causing activity and the relative capacity of the classes of parties involved to bear and distribute the costs. The spectrum of this calculus may run from absolute prohibition of fireworks, to liability for want of ordinary care in driving a car, to absolute liability for marketing packaged food that causes illness—a compensatory liability, irrespective of blamelessness, like workmen's compensation for employees' injuries, which is regarded as properly an inherent cost of carrying on the enterprise. The last example, that of a warranty of fitness for the intended use, carries us into the borderland of tort and contract: There is liability for unintended physical harm, but it can be viewed as resting on the breach of an implied term of the undertaking. This is seen most vividly, perhaps, in liability where harm results not from any impact, but from a failure to take affirmative action, as in the case of a passive lifeguard or nursemaid in a situation of peril. Because of a relationship of trust and dependency, fiduciary duties of single-minded loyalty arise. The relevance to the doctor-patient relationship of all these categories of unintended harm is plain enough.

The dialectic in the law's solicitude for physical integrity is supplied by the concomitant ideal of free individual choice and self-assertion, within socially approved bounds. The concepts of assumption of risk, waiver, consent, or voluntary participation, whether in playing football or tying oneself to a mountaineering guide, reflect this countervailing social and legal value. This is, in turn, qualified by the reservation that consent to procedures that are negligent will not be binding, and that a fiduciary relationship imposes special obligations of disclosure and good judgment in accepting consent or participation. This would be particularly true where the fiduciary is a member of a class that enjoys a legally granted monopoly, putting the subjects in something of the position of a captive audience.

In addition to its dialectic quality, law has the capacity to adapt to a changing order of values. To recognize this capacity, one has only to think of the traditional rule of *caveat emptor* and of its current transformation through implied warranties by the seller. The relation between social values and the law in bringing about change is surely a reciprocal one. If the medical profession simply waits for clear directions from the law in a period of shifting moral judgments, medicine and law will be playing an Alphonse-Gaston game. We quote Arthur Hugh Clough's lines as a straightforward ethical precept:

> Thou shalt not kill, yet need not strive
> Officiously to keep alive.

It is a measure of ethical change in the face of a new scientific environment—not, to be sure, an ethical change at the deepest level, but at the point of middle-level rules—that Clough's verses were in their day sharply ironic, part of his "New Decalogue," a kind of Black Ten Commandments.

One further characteristic of law central to our inquiry is its arsenal of resources, or patterns, for ordering affairs. To speak simply of legal prohibitions would be misleading, for a legal order can function primarily to facilitate (as in the law of contracts or wills) rather than to limit (as in the law of crimes). Of course, it is a matter of emphasis: To facilitate requires rules of order, and to impose controls will serve to facilitate; but the difference in priorities is significant for the choice, or the admixture, of legal patterns of order.

Two such patterns seem particularly relevant to medical experimentation with human beings. One is the model of the voluntary association or community. The other is the imposition of extrinsic standards and sanctions for their breach. The two models may be found together—as in a constitutional order—in structural provisions like separation and distribution of powers, and in extrinsic controls like a Bill of Rights, enforceable through the courts. A convenient framework for considering the role of law in human experimentation is afforded by these two models of order.

The creation of a particular model is likely to be conditioned by organization structures that are at hand, in the same or other fields, and by the polemic or at least optative purpose of the model-builder. Whether I describe a pitcher as half full or half empty may depend on whether I am combating the illusion that it is completely empty or completely full. The model of the voluntary association or community for medicine would probably not have occurred to an observer before the modern teaching hospital came into being, any more than the model would have served for higher education while it was conceived of as Mark Hopkins on a log. To the extent that the model is an apt one, it reflects the problems arising from the organization of medical care, the proliferation of drugs and therapies, the interrelation of investigatory and therapeutic roles within the profession, and the powerful lodestone of scientific method.

It is now easy enough to deride the canon, found in some court opinions a generation or more ago, that a physician experiments at his peril. Rightly understood, the maxim is sound enough: that where there is a satisfactory and accepted form of treatment, a physician who departs from it to pursue an idiosyncratic therapy is responsible if it does not succeed. Today, it is said, we recognize that most medical treatment is experimental. That statement, too, needs interpretation. If it means that the standard of what is satisfactory and approved has expanded with the development of new and more powerful drugs, that more options are open to the physician, and that he should be prepared to shift from one to another in light of the patient's reactions, there can be no quarrel with the statement about experimentation. But if it means that the physician is an experimentalist in a more precise sense, as one engaged in a collaborative enterprise with his patients to advance the frontiers of knowledge, as a university professor may be engaged with his graduate students, genuine legal and ethical problems are exposed.

The problems of the community model revolve around the possible confusion of roles and are not peculiar to medicine. If, for example, a corporation's directors conceive its function to be not the maximization of profits for investors, but a combination of profit-making and public service (as through charitable contributions or the employment of redundant personnel), investors may feel that the directors are unfaithful to their fiduciary duty and hence untrustworthy. Some rationalization can, of course, be made in terms of long-run benefits to investors through better community relations. This justification diminishes when the tenure of stockholdings is short-term. An analogy to the hospital would have to stress the short-run relationship of most patients to the enterprise. Here again distinctions can be drawn between the patient who may suffer a recurrence of his ailment and thus possibly benefit in the long run and the one whose ailment is non-recurring. Should one who is unlucky enough to suffer an attack of measles be regarded (apart from obvious availability for the study) as a pre-eminently appropriate participant in experimentation that will not benefit him, but may benefit future sufferers? Perhaps there is a fellow-feeling that would warrant this identification. On the other hand, there may be a feeling that while an individual is seeking to be relieved of a disease, he should be peculiarly immune from any moral pressure to contribute to the greater mastery of the disease— that he should be entitled to the single-minded fidelity of the physician to his recovery and viewed as an end, not a means. If it be answered that the fundamental good is the quality of medical care, and that this is enhanced for all through the whole complex of research, experimentation, and patient care in one community, the question to be answered is whether encouragement of participation by the patient is indispensable to this fruitful combination of functions, or whether other subjects may be procured for experimentation that is not for the direct benefit of the participant. The question is meant to be real and by no means rhetorical.

If the analogy to other communities of participants is to be pursued, certain structural characteristics ought to be examined. The voluntary community is signified at a minimum by the open window and the open door. Its procedures should be open to scrutiny, and participation should be freely terminable. Whether a patient is free, as a stockholder or a club member is, to terminate his participation will depend realistically on the freedom, in an informed sense, of his physician to withdraw the patient from the experiment. Moreover, the voluntary community is marked by a measure of reciprocity of duties and powers. The duty to cooperate persists until legitimately ended, and there should be corresponding authority, by voice or vote, to have a share in the governance of the community. What that share ought to be in the case of students or of stockholders poses thorny enough issues; in the case of patients, the problem is complicated because they are in a status of dependency. Nevertheless, two observations can be made. First, whatever the role of the physician in approving both an experimental procedure and his patient's participation, a final veto should rest with the patient so far as his part is concerned. Secondly, the concept of participation in decision-making may point up certain weaknesses in the concept of the constituency of patient-subjects. If it were the fact that patients on the wards were more freely used, or involved, in experimentation than those on the private floors, some explanation would be called for as part of the open-window policy. It may be that with the advent of Medicare any such differences will tend to disappear. If so, the tendency would seem to be a wholesome one, just as a broadly based compulsory military service affords a fairer foundation for a test of popular approval of a war than does a narrowly selective system.

The model of the community or the association calls for structural safeguards that will serve to promote the highest quality of medical care, preserve the integrity of the patient as an end, and at the same time facilitate useful experimental endeavors. Ideally such structural provisions are self-motivating, like the rule of the nursery that the boy may cut the piece of cake in two and the girl may have the choice of pieces, or the rule that the dividend rate of a gas company may rise as its charges to consumers are reduced. Analogues are not easy to find in the field of experimentation, but they ought to be sought after. An approximation might be the practice of rejecting scientific papers for publication when they disclose unethical elements in the procedures employed; overreaching would be to a degree self-defeating. This suggestion may be thought to place too great a power of censorship in the editors, particularly if the editors retained discretion to publish papers deemed to be of outstanding importance, regardless of ethical shortcomings. A useful alternative, avoiding the censorship issue, would be to require each published paper to contain a statement of the method of securing the subjects' participation and the form of professional approval secured for the procedures.

The point just mentioned—professional approval—assumes another kind of structural safeguard, through checks and balances. A profession accustomed to consultations and to review by tissue committees will understand the value of corroborative procedures for experimentation. These center on the hospital staff committee, whose approval is required prior to the conduct of an experiment on human subjects. How this committee should be constituted is itself, at this stage of experience with the device, a proper subject of experiment. At the least, the committee should include persons from other medical specialties than that of the experimenters. Whether it should include lay members, in particular a lawyer, can hardly be answered *a priori*. There would be an advantage in early participation by one who might press for clearer analysis of the ethical issues—the soundness of the design, the hazards, the potential benefits to the subjects, direct or remote, and the extent of disclosure to them in obtaining consent. The naïveté of his questions might occasionally furnish a useful component in the discussion. On the other hand, a lawyer whose judgment was so conservative that to keep away from the risk of trouble was his touchstone of wise judgment could prove to be too leaden-footed for the assignment. Studies of staff committees in operation are badly needed at the present time. Apart from such committees, a review committee on a higher administrative level is a useful tribunal, providing a check on the procedures of the staff committee as well as a source of guidelines for the institution. Questions raised by this administrative group, with remand of protocols for clarification or modification as seems necessary, will serve as a feedback and as a kind of common law of the subject. At this level, the case for non-medical representation is clearer. There should, of course, be liaison between the two echelons, and it would be useful if individual members of the administrative committee sat occasionally with the staff committee to get a closer feel for the actualities of the process than is possible through written abstracts alone.

110

Guidelines, to which reference has just been made, should be both substantive and procedural in their coverage. They stand midway between general homiletic maxims and detailed codes of ethical behavior. Of the making of guidelines there is seemingly no end. Although many analytical improvements and refinements have been produced since the *Nuremberg Code* (as, for example, in identifying the spectrum from direct therapy to therapy with longer-range experimental ends to experimentation with non-patient volunteers), even the most thoughtful sets of guidelines are subject to certain ambiguities. For example, the statement of the British Medical Association, issued in 1963, contains the following critical provision:

No new technique or investigation shall be undertaken on a patient unless it is strictly necessary for the treatment of the patient or, alternatively, that following a full explanation the doctor has obtained the patient's free and valid consent to his actions, preferably in writing.

The passage seems to state that full explanation and free consent are not required for a new technique employed on a patient if, and only if, the technique is "strictly necessary for the treatment of the patient." Does this really mean that the new technique must itself be essential for the patient, thereby precluding a new technique where other modes of treatment are not wholly adequate or safe and the new technique offers promise of better results without unduly greater hazard? Or would the latter be categorized as "strictly necessary"? Perhaps the statement quoted means only that some form of treatment is strictly necessary for the welfare of the patient and the new technique is to be judged solely from that standpoint, without regard to other possible values of its employment experimentally. In that case, the statement would not offer a guideline for the circumstances in which the new technique would be appropriately used for the patient's well-being. In short, the statement seems to be either excessively severe or insufficiently informative.

The discussion thus far has been shaped by the concept of an association or community. Some awkward fits have been noticed, as well as some suggestive lines of analysis in terms of participation and structural devices for both facilitation and safeguards. Attention has been focused within the community on the patient-subject, whose status raises the most complex issues of possible conflict of roles. Much of what has been said is also relevant to the position of the volunteer subject, whose status is less complex, but who may have special vulnerability because he is not buffered by a caretaking physician. Possibly such a role could be created by assigning to the non-patient volunteers a medical adviser whose responsibility would be the well-being of the subjects both in respect to initial consent and ongoing participation. This office would somewhat resemble that of a consumer's counsel (but, it is to be hoped, be more effective) or a civil-rights division in an attorney general's office.

The complementary legal framework, in addition to structural measures within a community, is furnished by extrinsic controls. This is the model of the Bill of Rights, as distinguished from separation and distribution of powers.

The legal requisites for legitimate, liability-free experimentation can be described in threefold form: the exercise of due care in administering the procedures; soundness of the experimental design, in that it must not be incapable on its face of producing significant results and its known hazards must not be disproportionate to the ends sought; and informed, voluntary consent, unless the subject's participation is enlisted for his direct benefit and explanation would be detrimental to his well-being, in which case it will be prudent to secure the informed consent of a member of the family.

The sanction employed by the law is typically the action for monetary damages, charging violation of one or more of the standards just described. In states where hospitals, as charitable corporations, enjoy immunity from tort liability, the staff members themselves may have even greater reason to apprehend the risk of personal liability on their part.

The overhanging threat of litigation from the investigator's standpoint and, from the subject's, the uncertainties of the outcome of a trial of the issue of blameworthiness create an atmosphere satisfactory to neither class. Attention should be given to plans for the compensation of subjects for harm resulting to them irrespective of the blamelessness of the investigator. This could be done on a voluntary basis through hospital or other institutional funding, or it could be imposed by statute. Contested claims under such a plan could be heard and determined by special tribunals established for the purpose; whatever the tribunal, the issue of causal nexus between experiment and injury is likely in many cases to be a vexing one.

More fundamentally, a rule of compensatory liability without fault raises a question of the adequacy of incentives to follow the high standards of performance that, in principle, obtain. If liability for fault is eliminated, will carelessness and overreaching flourish in a few places and perhaps bring the general development of experimentation into disrepute, as was threatened by the highly publicized New York cancer-cell episode? The question is an instance of a pervasive confrontation between two social philosophies —the one putting primacy on responsibility, blameworthiness, rewards, and penalties for behavior, the other stressing security of the victims against the impersonal dooms of modern life. The conflict marked the early days of unemployment compensation, when debate centered on employer or plant funds versus pooled funds— the former providing an incentive to a firm to regularize employment, the latter providing greater assurance of compensation to the unemployed. Of course, liability without fault and insurance to cover it need not produce a general slackening of care and prudence. Reputation counts for something; and in the case of fire and theft insurance, the underwriters have exerted valuable efforts to raise the standards of care. In medicine, it would be necessary to assure that the underwriters' representatives were not indeed too restrictive and cautious in their standards of approval. The claims of progressive medicine, no less than of fiscal conservatism, would have to be given a voice.

A combination of the two forms of liability, with and without fault, is possible, as the current Keeton-O'Connell plan for automobile accident compensation demonstrates. Under that plan, compensation would be due, without inquiry into fault, for expenses and loss of wages, up to $10,000; recovery for pain and suffering would require a lawsuit involving proof of the defendant's fault. In the field of experimentation, a similar combination might be tried, perhaps with the variation that the recovery based on fault would require proof not simply of fault but of gross fault, in order to discourage speculative claims while retaining some extrinsic deterrent against recklessness. The existence of the basic compensation plan might serve, furthermore, to improve the general attitude of judge and jury toward the experimentation itself.

Throughout this discussion of legal frameworks the criterion of consent has emerged in one guise or another. It may sound for investigators a jarring note, as if a *prima facie* assault were proposed, which was made lawful by the victim's consent. The concept of participation may have greater semantic appeal, suggesting as it does a common enterprise in which the various parties share.

Nevertheless the concept of agreement in one form or another seems inescapable, as an earnest of the law's concern for voluntarism in private hazardous undertakings that, in fact, serve public purposes.

The concept of consent has been much derided as unrealistic and artificial, and of course it embraces a range of responses that differ in their degree of autonomy and understanding. The psychological constraints or compulsions that operate on a seriously ill patient are different from those that affect a person attracted to an experiment through an advertisement. Nevertheless a requirement of "voluntary, informed consent" does have values beyond the symbolic one of respect for individual autonomy and personality. It is far from the be-all and end-all of legal and ethical safeguards, but it is a valuable ultimate check, reminding one of Keynes' rationale for the gold standard: that it is a safeguard in case the managers of the currency should all go mad at once.

Not the least of the functions of consent is its reflexive effect on the management of the experiment itself. To analyze an experiment in terms of risks and benefits to particular groups by way of presentation for consent is a salutary procedure for self-scrutiny by the investigator—like the preparation of a registration statement by a corporation issuing securities.

An example in the field of medical experimentation can be taken from the tests of magnesium as a remedy for a serious form of nutritional deficiency in infants, which is fatal in perhaps 20 per cent of the cases and for which no effective treatment had been found. Magnesium appeared to give good results, but had not been subjected to a controlled experiment on human infants. Assume that such an experiment is, in fact, considered. What is the role of consent? Four possibilities suggest themselves. First, no consent might be required, in the view that a physician could conscientiously employ or decline to employ the drug in the interest of sound patient care. Secondly, consent might be thought irrelevant for an opposite reason, that good practice would call for use of the drug even without a controlled trial, in view of the seriousness of the illness, the drug's promise, the lack of an alternative, and no indication of deleterious side effects. The drug might thus be accepted, like aspirin or digitalis, on a basis lacking in scientific rigor. Assuming the experiment is to be tried, two further alternatives are open. The patients' parents, after an explanation, might be asked to consent to the use of the drug or to its non-use. It seems likely that it would be more difficult to secure the latter consent than the former. Finally, the parents might be asked to consent to the inclusion of their children in a randomly designed experiment.

One additional element of consent might enter into the calculus —namely, termination of consent. How should a physician measure his responsibility to continue the experiment for the sake of scientific rigor against preliminary indications during the experiment that the drug is effective and safe? There is an inescapable element of choice, judgment, or will in every inductive experiment; there is no "logical" stopping point so long as the hypothesis tested has not (yet) been disproved. Consequently scientific rigor is at best an imprecise canon, to be weighed along with economy of time, effort, and other pragmatic judgments concerning appropriate termination. The making of this kind of analysis does not, to be sure, depend on a requirement of consent, but that requirement will make more vivid to the investigator the options that he must weigh in order to be candid with himself and his patient.

TALCOTT PARSONS

Research with Human Subjects and the "Professional Complex"

THE ETHICAL problems involved in research that makes use of human subjects are by no means new, but they have become intensified in recent years through a number of circumstances. In the medical field, which has stood at the center of the discussions leading to this book of essays, the rapid technical advances have raised many ethical issues. Not only new but more daring and, presumptively at least until fully tested, riskier procedures are increasingly being employed. Organ transplants are, of course, the most commonly discussed example today.

Another reason for the increasing concern with these problems is the rapid growth of research in the behavioral and social sciences. Almost in the nature of the case, such research makes use of human subjects over a wide range. For example, the concern with child development and various aspects of education involves very sensitive areas. Survey research and various forms of participant observation have been expanding rapidly, and these matters will undoubtedly call for careful scrutiny in the future.

This paper will not be concerned specifically with the medical problem, but will stress the continuity of the impingement of medical research on human subjects with that of research in other areas. There is a sense in which our tendency to underplay such ethical problems arises from the early predominance in research of the physical sciences, where injury to the chemical substances in the test tube does not raise ethical issues, though the cost of the substances may be relevant, as may also be the possibility of an explosion that would injure persons or property.

Medical research, on the other hand, has a direct and obvious impact on persons. Also, the ethical problems involved in medical research are closely related to those raised in the therapeutic care of patients. Indeed, a large proportion of research subjects is drawn from patient populations. The ethical problems of therapy are very old indeed, and tradition provides a frame of reference from which to consider new aspects of medical research involving human subjects. There is also an important continuity with other professional fields. The legal profession, for example, has a long tradition dealing with the relations between lawyers and their clients.

Research and practice are two principal functions of what I shall call the "professional complex" in modern society: The first is concerned primarily with the creation of new knowledge and the second with the utilization of knowledge in the service of practical human interests. Since, however, this complex is grounded in important ways in various forms of competence, there is a third salient function—namely, that of teaching, or the transmission of knowledge to those classes of persons with an interest in its acquisition.

It is significant that a large proportion of medical research clusters around medical schools. Though, of course, oriented to research and to practice (for example, through their teaching hospitals), medical schools are primarily concerned with the training of future physicians. At the same time, the central locus of "pure" research in the modern intellectual disciplines is in the "academic" world, notably the faculties of arts and sciences where research is typically combined with teaching, but where there is much less emphasis on practice than in the professional school or those organizations specifically oriented to practice.

I suggest that the ethical problems of research with human subjects possess important continuities not only with the relations of professional personnel to patients and clients in the realm of practice, but also with the relations of teachers to the "subjects" on whom they perform certain kinds of "operations"—namely, their students. Just as patients often serve as research subjects, so do students, particularly in the behavioral sciences.

This paper will attempt to deal with the ethical problems of human experimentation in research in the context of the professional complex as a whole. The discussion will focus on the interdependencies of the three principal professional functions of practice, research, and teaching. In modern systems, the interrelations among the institutional provisions for these functions are complex. They overlap to a great extent, however, since the same organizations and the same personnel are frequently involved in at least two, if not three, of the functions. In all three cases, a "professional" element must establish an appropriate pattern of relationship to a "lay"

117

element—whether the latter consists of patients, clients, students, or research subjects, and the former of practitioners, professors, or investigators.

By some kind of informal consensus, two focal points of this relationship have crystallized: the problem of "voluntary informed consent" and that of "protection of privacy." I suggest that these problems are continuous between the three principal functional contexts of the professional complex, and that none is altogether new. In my analysis, I shall interpret the two "standards" in terms of their bearing on the functioning of the professional complex as a whole.

I shall treat the question of ethics here as essentially one of *social* responsibility—that is, responsibility to promote or at least do no harm to the values and welfare of the societal system and the various classes of its members. The investigative activities in question are part of this system, and I conceive this social reference in sufficiently broad terms to include protection of rights more or less fully institutionalized. (Violation of the rights of individual or collective units is not usually the result of the implementation of a value or interest of the society.) Allowances must be made, of course, because legitimate values and interests are often difficult to interpret, and conflicts of values and interests are exceedingly pervasive in all complex and rapidly changing societies.

For the sociologist, the desirability of "enforcing" high levels of responsibility immediately raises the question of the "mechanisms" of "social control" by which relative conformity with normative expectations is or can be achieved. A brief outline of a classification of such mechanisms may serve as a useful introduction to a more detailed analysis of the mechanisms of particular interest here.

Mechanisms for Favoring Accountability

In one sense, the most elementary mechanism is the "discipline" of the market. This device maximizes the chances that participating units will act responsibly by following the dictates of their own self-interest, as measured in terms of monetary gain or loss. Generally speaking, this balance cannot hold unless markets are normatively regulated at least at two levels. The first is the framework of legal institutions and moral sanctions in such matters as property, contracts, and honesty; the other is the more specific level of regulation, which often attaches particular monetary consequences to certain classes of acts. (Guido Calabresi has analyzed such regulation in accident control through traffic laws and insurance systems.)

Legal sanctions and mechanisms, defining rights and obligations as well as enforcing them, back up systems of market control. These mechanisms operate in many fields other than the market, but in the present context they appear first at this point. An interest of a person—or a collectivity—can be protected if he has both the right and the realistic opportunity to seek "remedy" in the courts and thereby hold accountable those who have injured or might injure his interests. Both these modes of control have serious limitations for many classes of cases, but they are, nevertheless, of great importance in establishing a broad framework within which expectations of accountability are established. Thus, the importance of the adjudicatory system is by no means confined to the cases in which formal court decisions are made, since anticipation of such decisions serves as an exceedingly important guide to action.

A second set of mechanisms concerns the more direct use of collectively sanctioned authority (in principle, that of any collectivity, but especially public authority).[1] The first level of this process involves the operation of administrative or executive agencies that implement policies or other decisions binding on the members of a collectivity. Here, of course, responsible administrators or executives have authority, according to established rules, to "enforce" the agency's policies either on non-members (for example, taxpayers in the case of the Bureau of Internal Revenue) or on its own members.

The question is bound to arise as to who holds the administrators accountable. The most important mechanism for such a check is the authority of elective office, whereby executive implementers are responsible to elected officials who, in turn, are responsible to an electorate. This set of institutions is particularly conspicuous in the field of private organizations within the limits of the latters' jurisdiction.

Just as the first pair of mechanisms leaves important gaps in necessary or desirable controls because it is difficult to insure that the self-interest of acting units will effectively coordinate with the objectives of such control, so the second pair just mentioned leaves gaps in the "enforceability" of controls through the exercise of authority. One of these of special interest to us concerns the "competence" of untrained persons, whatever their position of authority, to evaluate either the individual or the collective interest in a mode of action, in the sense that only medically trained people can competently judge the therapeutic effects or dangers of certain procedures.

Within the gaps left open by all the control mechanisms so far discussed, but still in the category of institutionalized mechanisms rather than movements of revolt against the institutionalized order, we may speak of still a third pair. Both of its members operate through *persuasion,* mobilizing "opinion" in favor of or in opposition to courses of action, but without invoking either inducements for self-interested compliance or coercive or compulsory sanctions.

For the first, the mass media constitute the most tangible as well as largest scale example. They "broadcast" to indefinitely general publics, most of whose members do not claim any special expertise in judging the content of the communication. This mechanism undoubtedly exerts important pressure in bringing to bear sanctions of approval and disapproval with respect to many kinds of action. Thus it has been claimed that the immediacy of experience of televised actions involving violence has introduced a new factor into the evaluation of the role of violence in modern society.

The second of the currently relevant pair narrows the "public" within which persuasion is attempted. There are many bases of qualification, such as commitment to a specific religious or ideological position, but that of special interest here is some order of technical competence importantly, if loosely, validated by status in a professional group. Such a group is defined by qualifications for membership that combine functions in and on behalf of the society with levels of technical competence to perform them which require grounding in some phase of the general intellectual tradition.

Competence is conceived to be an essential condition of effective performance of this combination of functions. In addition, however, there must be integrity of institutionalized responsibility of a fiduciary sort. To some extent, this integrity insures that such competence will be used in the interest not only of the societal "clients" to whom these functions are important, but also of the wider collective systems. This combination of criteria implies, of course, that technical functions are to some degree specialized. Most of the interests on which their performance impinges lack, to a greater or lesser degree, the competence not only to perform these functions, but to evaluate the way in which they are being performed. Thus, the ultimate responsibility for standards both of competence and of integrity must rest with the professional complex itself.

To use the medical case for reference, the principle of *caveat emptor* for the purchaser of health services will scarcely be adequate as a basis for accountability. Nor will legal liability be sufficient, if this must be enforced by judges and attorneys who are not technically competent at professional levels in anything but the law, and if the initiative is left to litigants who conceive themselves to be injured and are willing and financially able to assume the burden of litigation. Nor can accountability reside with administrators who are not themselves professionally competent in the subject matter in question, nor with grievance procedures, nor, finally, with the "decent opinion of mankind" as expressed through the mass communication system. Professional groups must, to some essential degree, be self-regulating, taking responsibility for the technical standards of their profession and for their integrity in serving societal functions.

In concluding this sketch of mechanisms for implementing accountability, two points must still be made. First, the six mechanisms just outlined should be regarded as ideal types. In reality, several—if not all—are involved in most concrete situations. My central purposes here are, namely, to focus on the indispensability of fiduciary professional responsibility in insuring accountability in the ethical contexts that involve professional function in important degrees and, secondly, to give a rough frame of reference for characterizing the alternative, complementary, and supplementary mechanisms for the concrete cases where professional responsibility alone will not suffice.[2]

All such mechanisms—being attempts to "control," to enforce compliance with norms—imply some common background of legitimation, which will be differently structured in the different cases. Where a division of labor is involved, as is true of our interest— this will always have to include the legitimation of the functions of the groups and types of activity in question, of the ways in which the standards of performance of those functions are upheld, and of the protection or enhancement of the rights and interests of those outside the groups of performers of the functions on whom the actions of such groups impinge. The paramount question in this context, of course, is that of the basis of legitimation of the *function* itself.

The Professional Complex

In modern societies generally, and rather especially in the United States, the research function has, as we have suggested, come to be institutionalized as part of what we have called the professional complex. This is a complex of occupational groups that perform certain rather specialized functions for others ("laymen") in the society on the basis of high-level and specialized competence, with the attendant fiduciary responsibility. Since the competence of their members, along with components of special skill and "know-how," is grounded in mastery of some part of the society's generalized (intellectual) cultural tradition, the acquisition of professional status is almost uniformly contingent on undergoing training of a relatively formally approved type. In our society, such training has come increasingly to be acquired in the university, whatever special provisions for *practicum* experience there may also be (for example, in hospitals).

These specialized functions range widely—from dealing with the spiritual welfare of persons by the clergy (the original contrast with "laymen"), through the ordering by law of the relations of people to one another and to public authority, the management of conditions of health and illness, and the control of the physical environment through technology. On another and crosscutting basis, professional functions (besides participation in the government of professional organizations) may be classified in three categories: *practice* (for example, the provision of services to predominantly lay groups who are ill or threatened with illness); *teaching* of the knowledge and skills important to the practice of one's own profession; and *contributing* to the advancement of knowledge, or research. Since professionals are trained in the general cultural tradition, specialized teaching of future professionals is closely articulated with the more general function of teaching, especially what is often called "general education."

In American society, the center of the professional complex has come to be the university—"flanked" by other components of the system of higher education. The university is the focal center of the research function, especially in its most prestigious sector. Graduate schools of arts and sciences are the main training organ for the academic profession itself, including that sector primarily concerned with the teaching of undergraduates. University professional schools are now the primary locus of the training of members of the "applied" professions, including not only practitioners in the narrower senses, but future teachers in such schools and many future research workers.

One of the main bases of this clustering of professional functions around the university lies in the crisscross relation between the pure intellectual disciplines and the fields of their application in practice. So far as one can speak of a "science of medicine," it is not a discipline, but a mobilization of the relevant parts of a whole group of sciences (in the discipline sense) in terms of their bearing on problems of health and illness. The teachers of and researchers in the "basic sciences" in medical schools, and indeed increasingly in teaching hospitals, are not in the practitioner sense "medical men." They are scientists whose expertise is similar to that of their brethren in arts and sciences departments. Concentration in the university facilitates the cultivation and exploitation of such linkages.

The university is not simply a congeries of discrete individuals, departments, and schools, but an interwoven nexus of relationships. The great majority of its members at professional—faculty—levels perform in varying combinations all three of the principal substantive functions of the professional complex. That most of them are teachers almost goes without saying, since teaching is historically the primary "academic" function. Nevertheless, an increasing proportion are at the same time engaged in research. At university levels, such people are now the overwhelming majority. Furthermore, not only are many of the members of professional faculties engaged in the practice of their professions, but members of faculties of arts and sciences are generally engaged in performing a variety of services for laymen, such as "consulting," writing, or lecturing for lay audiences.

Since there is such concentration of multiple functions among university faculties, it would seem likely that there should be some important common themes in the social organization of the settings in which these functions are carried out. These common themes should include both the relational systems in which such members are related to one another in their work and the discharge of their common responsibilities as well as their relations to the classes of laymen with whom they are—in their specialties, in professional terms—brought into contact.

It is fairly well known that the structure of faculties and their constituent departments is of a relatively distinctive sociological type, which some of us have called *collegial*. This is a subtype of the associational pattern of structure and stands in strongest contrast to the hierarchy of authority characteristic of administrative bureaucracies. It is distinguished from other associational types, above all, because its membership is typically determined by occupational role, the performance of which is a "full-time job." On the other hand, the members constitute, in ideal type, a "company of equals." Power tends to be widely distributed within such a group, and each member has relatively protected spheres of autonomy—a major aspect of what we call "academic freedom." Corporate action is typically taken by the "democratic" procedure of one member, one vote. Such decision is, moreover, generally preceded by discussion conducted according to "rules of order." In both cases, there is sharp contrast with "executive" decision-making.

The collegial pattern of organization of professional groups is, in turn, linked with another common structural theme permeating the complex. This involves the professional individual in membership in a common solidary collectivity. This is most obvious in the case of the teaching function. The student is "admitted" to the college or school. To continue to function as a student, he must retain his membership "in good standing" until graduation. Similarly, however, patients are "admitted" to hospitals in what is, in some sense, a membership status. The case of the private patients of "individual" physicians is not so different as it seems on the surface; physician and patient join together for a common therapeutic task.[3] Hence we suggest that the research subject is also "selected," perhaps because he has characteristics of technical interest that are presupposed; but he also participates in a solidary relationship with the investigators.

Thus if this feature of inclusion of the "client" in a relation of common collective solidarity with the professional person or agency applies to the roles of practitioner and of teacher, it should also apply to that of researcher whose "client" is the human research subject. This possibility has probably been obscured by at least three factors. First, we have tended to treat research in the physical sciences as the prototype, but there the objects of investigation are not human beings with whom the investigator has to establish *any* kind of social relationship. Second, on the whole, the research function has received less attention from social scientists than have the other two primary professional functions. Third, there are deep-seated tendencies in our cultural tradition to define the relation in other ways. To many students, including for long the present writer, it seemed only "natural" to conceive the practitioner-client relationship as a special case of the market relationship, especially where it is performed on an individual fee-for-service basis. The professional offers his services on a market, and they are purchased by the client. This account of the process highlights certain aspects of a complex relationship while underplaying others. In particular, perhaps, it makes elucidation of the role of the research subject difficult. The typical client, including the medical patient, expects relatively immediate "value received" from the services of his physician, whereas there is usually no comparable *quid pro quo* in the case of the research subject. Thus, it is more difficult to see how the latter is in any sense assuming obligations by serving as a subject.

Again, a certain suspicion about the adequacy of this point of view might be aroused by various features of the market for professional services. But one factor in particular stands out. Though some professional services are given on a contingent fee basis (notably in law), the rule applying both to medicine and to teaching is, rather, that fees are due regardless of the success of the endeavors. Even though the patient dies, his medical bills must be paid; even though the student "flunks out," his tuition is not reimbursed. Failure in the common endeavor does not absolve either party from making a fair contribution on the basis of *capacity to contribute* and not value personally received. In this respect, the relationship is more like marriage with the definition of obligations in terms of "for better, for worse," and not of specific benefits received from the relationship, which is the guiding principle of the commercial market relationship.

As we have suggested, the market perspective tends to dissociate the client role from that of the research subject and, indeed, to treat that of the student as a case altogether separate from either of the two. A striking empirical fact, however, is the extent to which there has actually been a coincidence of two or more of these roles on the "lay" side, as there has been on the professional function side. In medical research, where subjects are humans rather than animals, they are *also* patients in a very large proportion of cases. I suggest that more than considerations of pragmatic convenience underlie this state of affairs. If patients are conceived as "cooperating" with their physicians or therapeutic "teams" in a common enterprise within a framework of solidarity, and if, furthermore, the therapeutic agency is engaged in the distinct but closely related function of research, then it would seem positively appropriate that there be a presumption of willingness to cooperate in the research enterprise as well. The basic principle is that fellow members of solidary groups are disposed, and in some sense obligated, to help

125

one another whenever they can, subject to their basic rights and the possibility of conflict with other obligations, usually in other solidary contexts.

The problem of "what each gets out of it" involves certain complexities. Uncertainty is a fundamental feature of the medical situation generally. Careful diagnostic investigation in particular cases aims to reduce this uncertainty to a minimum, but it remains considerable in a large proportion of cases, especially the more "serious" ones. In addition, of course, many therapeutic procedures impose other burdens on the patient, such as suffering and disability, in the hope that these burdens will eventually prove to be the cost of favorable outcomes. Uncertainty, then, is a particularly prominent feature of research. If it were fully known in advance what the consequences of research procedures would be, there would be no point in instituting them—except, in the medical case, for therapeutic reasons. Hence the primary problem of justifying use as research subjects concerns the positive benefits to be gained, rather than the costs and burdens.[4]

Before entering into this, however, a word should be said about the coincidence of student and research roles. Certainly this coincidence is relatively common in the case of medical students, but it has also been much practiced in psychology and the social sciences, where many researchers have drawn their subjects from their own college classes. There is, of course, an important sense in which both patients and students constitute "captive audiences," a circumstance that introduces certain constraints on the more absolute versions of the standard of "informed voluntary consent." I shall postpone more general discussion of such constraints, but perhaps the direction the discussion will take is evident from the above argument.

Solidarity and the Problem of Trust

We have suggested that social control in the professional complex cannot rest mainly on the common sanctions of economic inducement as this operates in market systems, nor on authority and power in the ordinary administrative sense. The discussion of solidarity was meant to suggest that the most important mechanisms of social control in this area are to be found in the operation of solidary groups relatively independent of the above classes of sanctions. Commitment to values on the basis of a sense of moral obligation is an indispensable basis of control, but—though a central one—this is *one* factor in the disposition of members of solidary groups to *trust* one another. A somewhat further analysis of the nature and bases of such trust, as it operates in the professional complex, should bring us closer to a useful interpretation of the principal current discussions of ethics in this field.

Relative to its relevant "laity," the professional relation is by its nature asymmetrical and thereby drastically different from the democratic associational relationship among "peers." In one essential aspect, the primary axis of this asymmetry lies in the superior competence of the professional, without which there would be no legitimizing sense for a layman to enter into any one of the three basic types of relationship we have discussed. The process of learning "with" peers (in ignorance) is different from that of learning "from" a teacher who has superior competence in the subject matter. Seeking the services of a competent physician or lawyer is different from peers "agreeing" about what should be done in a distressing situation. And "cooperating" in the research plan of a trained investigator is different from a group of (non-expert) peers in the subject discussing what would be interesting to "find out."

In all three of these basic respects, there exists a "competence gap" between professional and lay persons. The variations in the specific nature of this gap are endless in different relations, but this is pervasive. *If* the necessary lay cooperation with the professional is to be assured, it cannot rest on the layman's full understanding of "what the professional is doing" in a sense presupposed by the slogan *caveat emptor* in the market field. There must be bases of trusted validation of competence other than the typical layman's personal competence to evaluate it. But this issue also raises the fundamental question of integrity—namely, not only whether the pretension of competence is justified, but whether, if it exists, it will be used to exploit or benefit the participating lay elements or, as I much prefer to put it, be used in a higher-order *common* interest.

Such a competence gap must be bridged by something like what we call trust. We suggest the following principal factors on which the generation of such trust depends: First, it must be believed on both sides of the gap and, of course, by a sufficient proportion of the participants that the enterprise in question is in the service of *common* values. This is generally the case with respect to the valuation not only of good health but also of education. Second, this sharing of common values must, within the requisite ranges, be translatable into common *goals,* such as the curing of a particular form of ailment in an individual patient or in a class of patients. In the achievement of such common goals, patients are more likely to be asked positively to cooperate than passively to "submit" to the ministrations of their physicians.[5]

A third condition is the successful fitting of the expectations engaged on both sides of the relationship into the balance of the plural set of solidary involvements in which all actors, individual and collective, are involved. Just as it is scarcely possible for a concrete individual to be "only" a sick person and thus a patient—except in extreme conditions and temporarily—so it is not possible to be only a student or only a research subject, to say nothing of the corresponding conditions on the other side. This, as we shall argue below, is the focus of the "privacy" issue. A fourth condition is that the acceptance of a relation of trust should not be grossly incompatible with known facts and conditions of feasibility. A physician who had been known to be guilty of various kinds of malpractice would certainly forfeit a good deal of trust, as would a teacher who had grossly misinformed his students about the subject in question. Thus, there must be some adequate "symbolization" of both competence and integrity.

In the favorable case, these four factors mutually reinforce one another. Sharing values makes agreement on common goals easier, and "confidence" in competence and integrity makes commitment to mutual involvement in such goals easier. Integrity includes respect for the interests of the layman outside the technical concerns of the professional context. All these considerations focus mutual trust in the conception or "feeling" of the solidarity of collective groups.[6] However dependent this "feeling" may be on "input" factors, once established, it acquires a certain autonomy of its own. People defined as sharing one's values or concrete goals and in whose competence and integrity one has "confidence" come to be thought of as "trustworthy individuals" or "types." Because of these aspects of belonging together, such people can be relied on, within limits of course, not only to respect one another's interests, but more critically to give certain benefits of the doubt to the importance of a common interest that transcends the interests of the individual unit members. Thus, we mean by the solidarity of a collectivity the "pull" of a common interest that can motivate actions which, while not necessarily in conflict with unit interests, at least are not fully "dictated" by them.

Beyond this, we suggest that solidary groups exert "pressure"— through leadership, ideology, norms, and the like—on their units to play the expected role in the process of interaction. They exert such pressure by means of sanctions that come to focus in appeals to loyalty to the values, goals, and collective solidarity of the group in question. Such a sanction system depends, of course, on participants in some sense defining themselves as belonging to the group: hence the importance of the concept of membership and the voluntary principle.

The "interests" that are served in the professional functioning of the three categories may be classified under three rubrics. The first has been the main point of reference of much general discussion—namely, each participant receives in a short run a *quo* for the *quid* that he contributes. The usual model here is that of the market. The patient pays for the value of the services he receives from his physician. We are, however, all aware that there are important sources of "satisfaction" other than monetary gain or the relief of a particular distressing condition.

This exchange of relatively immediate benefits, however, merges into broader contexts primarily in two ways. The first is the extension of the set of collective interests that are involved on both sides. Thus a patient's recovery benefits not only himself, but his family and the organization that employs him. A physician's record of therapeutic success not only brings him income from practice and personal satisfaction, but it redounds to the benefit of the reputation of his profession and the subunits of it that he is associated with. Certainly in the teacher role, what the individual student has specifically learned is not the only aspect of the successful performance of the function. The class, the department, the college, or the school all have genuine interests in successful teaching. Indeed, morale in a class is enhanced when some of its members learn effectively. In outstanding cases, people treasure the experience of having been a member of an unusually effective teaching-learning system. Indeed, the ramifications of this "Chinese box" of increasingly extensive collective inclusions go far to provide an essential base of operations for performance of the various kinds of professional functions.

One major indication that such institutionalization is important is the persistent ambivalence that exists in public attitudes toward all the main professional groups. The medical profession, in general, enjoys a high level of public confidence. Nevertheless, a persistent minority regards the whole system as a pious fraud that exists only to line the pockets of its practitioners at the expense of helpless and gullible people. To take another example, the wave of radical student protest in our universities expresses profound distrust of that part of "the system." This protest is partly significant precisely because of the high esteem in which higher education is *generally* held.

The second direction of the extension of the "interest base" of professional function is temporal. Generally speaking all but the more trivial benefits of professional function take time to materialize. Many therapeutic regimes are of long duration, and the course of learning is proverbially not only hard but long. "Instant education" is deservedly felt to be unlikely to be worth much. Research, however, is at the extreme of a range in this respect. Indeed, the values of the scientific world make it clear that research oriented to relatively immediate and specific practical goals is likely to be less "fundamental" and less productive of practical benefits in the long run than is more "basic" research concerned with general and often largely theoretical problems of science.

The "logic" of investment in the economic sense is the most familiar example of the general principles involved in the use of resources without reference to short-run utility and in the interest of larger benefits in the long run. Education is, of course, such a process of "investment" of present resources in the interest of a future. Research is simply a further step along the same path. Instead of imparting what he now knows to students, the investigator himself assumes the "student" role and attempts to learn things which nobody yet knows, but which, when known, could subsequently be taught to others. The dissociation between the research function and the two other primary professional functions obscures these continuities.

If we accept the general proposition that the research subject, like the client or the student, is in a fundamental sense included in the professional system, then the question posed above—"what does the research subject get out of it?"—can immediately be answered in principle. According to his status in the system, he gets the same *kinds* of rewards that all other participants get and, in particular, that the investigators get. The highest order of reward is the prestige and satisfaction of having made a "contribution to the advancement of knowledge."

We refer to this reward as the highest, but by no means the

only one. Thus, investigators are generally also paid in money, essentially because they are performing more or less full-time jobs and must make their living that way. Research subjects are sometimes paid, sometimes not. In the other sectors of the professional system, clients are generally not paid, but themselves pay. Some students or their parents pay tuition, but it is not too farfetched to say that many, especially the more advanced students, are paid through various kinds of fellowships and stipends. Nevertheless, the pay, where it exists, is not conceived primarily as matching the economic value of the contribution, as a commercial price is. It is thought of as an "honorarium," itself a contribution to getting the primary contribution made.

"Bracketed," in a sense, between this highest motive of the sense of contribution to knowledge and the "lowest" of financial remuneration is a whole series of other motives that are relevant. In the medical field, the research interest in the advancement of knowledge is, of course, closely linked to the valuation of health and hence to the interest in the conquest of preventable and curable disease and of premature death, though eventual death is surely recognized to be inevitable and even in some sense desirable.[7] Another important cluster of motives concerns the fact that the sick person is, in the nature of his position in society, relatively isolated and deprived of the opportunity for normal functioning. Thus, if the sick person has the opportunity through an active contribution to be more than the passive "object" of treatment or investigation, he may gain a sense of meaningfulness that would not otherwise be available to him.

Interaction with respect to professional function is not nearly so one-sided as it is often held to be. Clients are not, in general, simply passive recipients of service; they are contributors to the common output of the cooperative system. Indeed, students are rather loudly insisting that they be considered active participants in the learning process, not just "receptacles" into whom information is poured by their teachers. Research subjects must be thought of in the same way, as has been particularly vividly brought out by Renée Fox. In all three categories, there are, of course, cases where the role of the nonprofessional is overwhelmingly passive, but it is legitimate to regard such cases as relatively marginal rather than definitive instances of the main structural relationship. Thus, the role of active participant seems to us clearly to presuppose a positive bond of solidarity across the professional-lay line.[8]

Voluntary Informed Consent and the Protection of Privacy

The two formulae included in the title of this section have come, by a kind of informal consensus, to be the main foci of the discussion of the ethical problems of human experimentation. I should now like to attempt to show how the considerations advanced above throw light on the problems involved in these two formulae, singling out the elements of legitimacy in them as well as showing some of the limits on their too-sweeping use.

We have suggested that the professional complex belongs basically in the associational sector of the structure of modern societies. In this connection, we have stressed that inclusion in some sort of membership status is important for the "lay" contingent in the system. Certainly, then, the voluntary principle is much involved with this complex, as is indicated by the key term "voluntary association." But voluntariness involves two-way consent. Certain associational structures impose no qualifications for inclusion, but such qualifications are of central importance in the professional complex. Thus we have emphasized, on the professional side, validation of competence through training and certification. On the lay side, for example, one cannot ordinarily be a patient without being defined as ill or potentially so; nor can one be a lawyer's client without having a "legal problem." Otherwise, the professional may simply refuse to spend time and effort over that person.[9] To enter various courses of study, a student often has to meet qualifications independent of his mere desire to pursue those courses, as well as to be "motivated" to learn in them. Finally, a research subject must be evaluated as to whether he is a suitable source for the information that would contribute to the success of the investigation.

The reciprocal of professional consent to inclusion, often phrased as "admission" to a program, is "lay" consent to participate. Clearly, by no means all potential students consent at various levels—for example, to accept an offer of admission to a college, to undertake a program of study, or to "take" a particular course. So far as the client relationship is concerned, the most salient case is the strong medical emphasis on the importance of the patient's right to choose his physician. The voluntary aspect of participation in the capacity of research subject should be placed in essentially the same framework.

In this framework, however, there is both the stress on the desirability of voluntary consent and the problem of defining certain limitations on it. The framework of admissions to institutions of higher education and those to hospitals and clinics implies that the collective entity the layman is "joining" can, in part, define the new member's range of choice and thereby limit it in certain respects. A first-year medical student simply cannot impose his conception of a good medical education, including a perfectly free choice among the teachers currently functioning at his school. He must somehow fit into a program. The same is true of the patient in a clinic or hospital. If he entrusts his interests to the collective entity, he must "adapt"—within limits, of course—to the exigencies of the organization, though he can refuse to accept service or even leave against medical advice. The clinic or college is in command of scarce resources that cannot be made indiscriminately available simply on "demand." Thus, to take one familiar case, a particularly popular teacher cannot pay equal attention to all students who might like to receive his attention.

Research subjects, like the other two classes of laymen, are both selected and select, and the voluntary principle has its applications on *both* sides of the relationship. Not infrequently there is an element of conflict between the two sets of interests. Thus students who desire admission are sometimes rejected, and clients who desire the services of particular practitioners cannot obtain them. Although it is not yet common, it is relevant that potential subjects are often denied opportunity to participate in important research because of selective procedures. Similarly the right of students, clients, and subjects to refuse opportunities of participation often imposes frustrations on the professional element who would like to secure their participation.

Conflicts at the threshold of participation and involving a membership status are complicated because constraints of other elements in the relational nexus restrict the voluntary principle. Thus, we have suggested that neither patients nor students are wholly free to refuse reasonable requests to serve as research subjects. They tend to retain a "formal" right to refuse, but seldom exercise that right in normal circumstances.[10] Scarcity factors also play a part, as in shortages of hospital beds or places in the "better" colleges.

The standard of voluntary consent should rightly be regarded as a decision on *both* sides of the relationship to "admit" to and to accept a membership status, but certain circumstances impose legitimate exceptions. The standard usually makes explicit only part of the relational complex discussed—namely, the voluntariness

133

on the part of the research subject. On the professional side, there is selectivity, and certain presumptions may be created by multi-functional role relations or the distinction between formal rights and informally legitimate expectations. In any case, the maximization of voluntariness may be said to apply at the point of decision as to whether or not to participate.

It can be fairly said that our society strongly values rationality of action, and that we wish to create conditions of action where people know, so far as possible, what they are doing when they make commitments. I can see no general objection to the obligation to inform subjects, as well as members of the other two relevant categories of laymen, as fully as possible in advance about "what they are letting themselves in for" in deciding to participate. To modify too naïve and literalistic interpretations of "being informed," however, three sets of considerations need to be kept in mind: uncertainty, cost, and relative competence.

We generally use the term "risk" where uncertainty is calculable to some fair degree of approximation. Where risks in this sense are rather clearly known, certainly prospective participants should be informed of them, though this obligation can easily be overformalized. Admissions officers do not usually give applicants precise statistical estimates of the probabilities of their successfully completing a course of study, nor do physicians overformalize the risk of treatment. There is a cost factor involved here in which the expenditure of time and effort by the professional should certainly figure prominently, but there may be a similar expenditure on the other side.

There is, however, more to uncertainty than risk in the above sense. Student performance can only be predicted within considerable margins of error; the same is true of decisions of courts as well as of the course of various forms of illness and research. The essential point is that *nobody* in the system can be *fully* informed about what participants "may be in for," except in the more trivial kinds of situation—which is one of the primary reasons why mutual trust is so important in such relational systems. Thus, there is the danger that the criterion of being informed may introduce undesirable constraints on the performance of the professional function if it is too strictly construed.

The importance of the cost factor should also not be underestimated. When Gerald Platt and I sent out questionnaires to members of the American academic profession, we certainly did not in any sense "fully" inform our prospective academic respondents in detail, question by question, about our reasons for asking them what we did. Even to approximate such a standard, we would have had to prepare a long and complex document that they would have had to read carefully before deciding whether or not to accede to our request. Such a measure would probably at least have doubled, in both time and trouble, the burden imposed on the respondent and would have reduced greatly the rate of return. Hence, the cost factor applies on both sides of the relationship and is far from trivial.

In this and many other cases, the factor of cost merges into that of competence. In a short time and at relatively low cost, it is often impossible for the professional to inform the layman fully, if by that is meant giving him as good an understanding of what is involved as he, the professional, has. Being informed, like the voluntary component, cannot be absolutized without imposing severe impediments on all three of the primary professional functions. *What* it is important for the student, the client, or the research subject to know must be selectively defined in terms of the function he performs in the system and the ways in which the activities of the others impinge on his role and functions. Only in limiting cases does sufficient knowledge constitute in any absolute sense *full* information about everything involved.

To return to the standard of voluntariness: Once a decision to participate in an associational collectivity has been made, the participant becomes entitled to the rights of membership in the collectivity, but he also becomes subject to the corresponding obligations. Perhaps the most important single protection of his rights is his freedom to resign his membership status at any time or to use the threat of doing so as a source of leverage for protection of his rights—individually or in concert with others. This is indeed the actual case of the bank depositor; withdrawal of all deposits comes close to being a form of "resignation."

On the other side of the coin, however, no complex collective system can operate unless there is a relative concentration of authority and power by virtue of which many decisions binding on the collectivity as a whole are taken without the full consent of *all* participant members. However many problems there may be today about the authority systems impinging on students, there would seem to be little serious defense of the view that *no* authority system whatever needs to be involved in the teacher-student rela-

135

tionship, a position that would be tantamount to eliminating all "requirements" from courses of study. The same clearly holds true for the professional-client relationship—whether the use of authority be rather nakedly stated in such a phrase as "doctor's orders" or more subtly as "legal advice." Surely if we are correct about the parallelism of the three professional subsystems, the role of research subject, once assumed, cannot be totally immune from authority and power.

Thus, there must be constraints on the voluntariness of cooperation from moment to moment as the process unfolds, except in the important sense of freedom to "resign." The research program, like the program of study and the therapeutic regimen, has "requirements" that someone is authorized to enforce.[11] Put a little differently, the status of membership in a collectivity is not compatible with an act-by-act reservation of rights. The member cannot refuse to comply with the requests of legitimate leadership and authority within the collective system of reference—except, again, in the sense of his right to withdraw. Such authority, of course, should be exercised sparingly and with an understanding of sensitivities, but it cannot be dispensed with altogether.

Thus, the voluntary principle in associative relationships is of truly fundamental importance. At the same time, however, it cannot operate effectively if it is not balanced in the *same* collective system by a system of obligations that are enforced by authority. Compliance with this authority—in the *ad hoc*, act-by-act sense— cannot be wholly voluntary.[12] In professional collective systems, the need for this involuntary aspect stems primarily from two sources. The first is the role of special technical competence in such systems and the presence of a competence gap. The second, however, is the simple exigency that effective action in complex collective systems necessitates differentiation on an axis of leadership and followership, or relative concentration of authority and power. Associational *collectivities* on the whole, relative to other types, minimize this concentration, but do not eliminate it.

In this "dialectic" situation, by stressing one side to the total exclusion of the other, the operation of the factors on the other side may be impeded even though they are essential to the functioning of the system. There should, in my opinion, be *no* total burden of proof on either side—either that *any* limitation on voluntary informed consent, as judged by the strictest criteria, is presumptively illegitimate, or that *any* limitation on the exercise of professional prerogative or authority in the interests of the autonomy and free-doms of the "lay" element is presumptively illegitimate.

There is a similar "dialectic" in the professional complex be-tween the rights of privacy and the obligations to sacrifice privacy —most obviously, but by no means exclusively, through the dis-closure of information.[13] It is, of course, well known that a doctrine of privileged communication is deeply embedded in the tradition of the practicing professions. It is one of the principal features of the Hippocratic Oath and is also central to the legal profession. The privileged communication between attorney and client, however, is connected with an institution of obligatory disclosure as one of the fundamentals of procedure in systems of adjudication. Admissible evi-dence is restricted to what has been *publicly* stated under oath and subject to cross-examination. Witnesses, usually including litigants themselves, are obliged to answer counsel's questions in public.[14]

This relation surely obtains in medicine, where "case records" available publicly *within* the professional system constitute an es-sential part of the professional decision-making system. The rela-tionship also applies within the teaching system, but is a little more difficult to see there. But on the disclosure side, a teacher is surely not entitled to withhold from students "personal" opinions touching on the subject matter of his teaching; he is obligated to answer to the best of his ability any legitimate questions put to him by his students, often exposing thereby his "shameful" ignorance, bias, or prejudice. On the other hand, the privacy of his "personal" life is protected. A sociologist teaching a course in marriage and the family may legitimately refuse to answer students' questions about his *own* marriage situation on the ground that they are "too per-sonal." The teacher also enjoys an area of privacy in his profes-sional capacity. An obvious example concerns the preparation of materials for use in teaching. He may retire to his study "free from interruptions," as we often say, consult such books and other sources as *he* deems appropriate, organize his thoughts in the man-ner he considers best, and then "present" the subject in the way he thinks most satisfactory. Student "participation" could not reach the point where the teacher could not prepare a lecture without securing student consent to every decision on what was to be presented, what sources were to be used, or how the material was to be pre-sented. This clearly would be "invasion of privacy." Students, of course, enjoy similar prerogatives of privacy when they are writing a term paper or preparing for an examination.

Both teacher and student, however, eventually come to the "moment of truth" when they *must* perform "in public." The teacher must actually present the subject to his class, if only in the concealed sense of "setting the tone" for an ostensibly free discussion, and the student must submit the paper or write the examination.

It would, indeed, be strange were the research function totally outside this general pattern. There has been so much talk about the rights to privacy of research subjects that a word needs to be said about the rights of investigators. Clearly the research process itself is in some respects privileged in that the laboratory or the office in which research operations are being carried out is certainly not open to any wanderer who might be "curious."

There is, however, a particularly telling example on the professional side of this process. The researcher is exposed to a stringent test of *public* evaluation, the most important aspect of which follows the publication of the results of his work. Especially in the more rigorous of the sciences, this evaluation usually takes place in journals that have a special fiduciary relation to the professional group in question. Publication, in this sense, may be regarded as a particularly prominent case of "obligatory disclosure" of professionally relevant information. Like the witness in court, the author will be evaluated almost ruthlessly, in terms of what he "reveals" in the article he publishes. Interestingly enough, however, not only are the earlier phases of the investigative process relatively free from "invasions of privacy," but in general the privacy of the decision to publish is elaborately protected by professional institutions. The core of this protective process is the "referee" system whereby manuscripts submitted to technical journals are "entrusted" to the editor and then anonymously evaluated by referees of the editor's choice. The editor or sometimes a board takes sole responsibility for the decision.

This process very frequently does not result in an either-or decision—to publish or not—but in a decision as to the "form" in which material should be published. Thus articles usually undergo extensive revision in the editorial process, in which anonymous referees play a considerable part. We suggest that the "privileged" process of preparation for publication—including, of course, reaching negative decisions—is analogous to the preparation of a legal case, in which the "ordeal" of presentation in open court is not undertaken without an important process of preparation in private.

These examples occur on the professional side of the relationship. In accord, however, with our general principle that the patterns should be basically reciprocal, we can say in general that research subjects, as selected members of the professional community, undertake obligations to "disclose" information that would not be disclosed in the ordinary course of daily life. Of course, the rule of anonymity frequently protects their privacy by limiting the "personal" repercussions of this disclosure, but the more important point is that the rights of privacy are dynamically linked to an obligation to disclose things which, apart from the professional nexus, would not be disclosed.

For the clinical practice of medicine, in addition to confidential information, access to the body presents an especially important aspect of the problem of privacy. It is merely necessary to recall that not much more than a century ago in most of the Western world the notion of a male obstetrician dealing with cases of pregnancy and childbirth was at least frowned upon, if not widely forbidden. The concept of privacy also extends to information about people's medical conditions, so far as they are not fully evident. Hence, the doctrine of privileged communication applies even where these conditions are in no sense shameful.

A particularly interesting point, however, concerns the extension of the concept of privacy, and in a related form of consent, to the situation of death. Renée Fox, in her illuminating analysis of the autopsy situation, has emphasized the ways in which the corpse is treated as a sacred object.[15] Permission to dissect it is a special privilege, one which for long was totally forbidden in official religious doctrine, forcing medical teachers and students to raid cemeteries to procure cadavers for the study of anatomy.

A new phase of this problem has, however, developed recently with the technical possibilities of organ transplants in cases where removal from the "donor" would be fatal. There is consensus that consent, in this case consent of the next of kin, must be given. But the problem of the medical definition of death has arisen in a new form because of the relation of timing to the condition of the organ to be transplanted. There seems to have been a strong movement to the conception put forward, especially by Dr. Beecher, that "brain death is death indeed," which justifies earlier intervention than the older conceptions emphasizing heart action and respiration would have permitted. This possibility of earlier intervention presents a particularly important ethical problem in the American setting where the desirability of the conquest of disease is so strongly emphasized.

Thus, like voluntary consent, the protection of privacy is not an absolute, but is linked with a complementary obligation of otherwise "unusual" disclosure. "Privileged communication" commonly applies to relatively early stages in the genesis of results that in turn must, for various reasons, be placed in what is in some sense a legitimate public domain.

The common factor between the voluntary consent context and that of protection of privacy thus appears to be concerned with the outcome of the temporal genesis of values. The granting of consent, in this sense, may be taken to mean a "commitment" to participate in a specially important kind of professionally collective enterprise. On the "lay" side, protection of privacy defines certain limits to the claims that participation in the enterprise may impose on individuals. But the reciprocal is that such participants also have their privileges of privacy in being free to "work on" their contributions without unnecessary interference.

Voluntary consent is in its most important aspect a grant of freedom to the professional complex to advance those interests that are most central to that complex. The privacy issue, on the other hand, concerns the definition of the limits of the legitimacy of such commitments to the professional enterprise—but, be it noted, defining the privileges not only of the lay, but also of the professional elements involved.

Summary and Conclusion

Ethics is, in one primary aspect, a system of control of human behavior in the interest of maintaining and implementing values. For this reason, we began the substantive analysis of this paper with a sketchy classification of the principal types of mechanisms of social control on which ethical considerations may impinge. The emphasis was on social control because this paper has been primarily concerned with the social level of the problem.

Although our classification of six types is a description of components—all of which may, in principle, operate in every situation of social control—their combinations vary greatly in different kinds of social context. To the sociologist, the present problem belongs in the distinctive sector of modern social organization that we have called the "professional complex." The emphases in the field of social control distinguishing this sector differ especially from commercial markets and bureaucratic-administrative organizations, which depend much more directly on economic inducements or on authority and power, rather than on persuasion.

We therefore turned next to an outline of the professional complex with an attempt to locate the research function and some of the forms it takes within this complex as a whole. From one perspective, this complex is the main point of articulation between the primarily cognitive aspect of the cultural tradition and the concrete organization of modern societies. Its structural core lies in systems of higher education understood in a broad sense. This core has become much more highly differentiated in recent times, both internally and from other sectors of the society. Not only has it incorporated the extended range of the modern intellectual disciplines, but it has differentiated the functions of teaching—both of "educated citizens" and of professional practitioners—establishing an important relation to practice in the application of knowledge itself and, most important for us, developing an extended and highly differentiated research function.

All of these functions necessitate structured relations between members of professional groups and "laymen," the difference being defined in terms of the special competence of the former gained through training and experience. Corresponding to the classification of professional functions is a categorization, again in ideal type, of the lay personnel involved—clients (including the patients of medical practice), students, and research subjects. We have noted, however, that the categories often overlap, and that, for example, patients often serve as research subjects.[16]

Our general suggestion with respect to these three categories of laymen is that they must, by and large, be brought into some kind of membership status with the professional personnel, in common solidary collective structures. Although this membership status is highly tenuous in some cases, it dominates the social structure of the relational systems involved. Thus, the sociological nature of these relational systems becomes of vital importance.

We have further suggested that the predominant structural type of internal professional relationships is a special form of the collegial. This associational category stands in sharp contrast with both the market type and that of administrative bureaucracy, especially in its egalitarian emphases. Though clients, students, and research subjects are not "colleagues" of the professionals they deal with, the relationship still belongs emphatically in the associational category. This is true despite the element of inequality deriving from differences of competence. This factor does, however, draw a crucially important line between such relational systems and those in which the members are strictly peers—as colleagues, members of many voluntary associations, and indeed citizens generally are.

It is in this setting that we raise the question of the importance of mutual trust, its conditions, and its relations to associational solidarity. That such trust is problematical is indicated by the general ambivalence toward professional function present in the undercurrent of hostility to medicine and in student distrust of the educational "establishment." Trust in the presently relevant sense is the attitudinal ground—in affectively motivated loyalty—for acceptance of solidary relationships. These confer not only the enjoyment of the rights of participating membership, but also the corresponding obligations. We suggested, as one major implication of this point of view, that the rewards enjoyed by research subjects are, qualitatively, essentially the same as those of investigators. The most important, though by no means the only, reward is the satisfaction of having helped in making a "contribution to the advancement of knowledge," with the corresponding recognition of this contribution.

We have suggested that the achievements of the professional complex are essentially collective achievements, including the contributions of both professional and lay elements. For the latter, however, given both the presumptively voluntary basis of participation (especially marked since the typical layman does not have a career stake in the function) and the competence gap, there is a particularly important problem of the legitimation of the process as a whole and of the professional element's role in it. One primary focus of this legitimation problem we have called the context of the integrity of the professional element and, assuming its leadership, of the collective organization as a whole, including lay contribution. It is in this context that we consider the ethical problem to focus and the problems of voluntary informed consent and of protection of privacy to center as two primary foci of the ethical problem.

It is particularly important to be clear that this ethical problem does not focus on the most general levels of acting in terms of the values of "common honesty" or elementary "good will." The standards worked out must take full account of two further factors. The first is the technical nature and complexity of the issues at stake. Thus, there is no common-sense solution to the question of *when* a person has died, for the ethical purposes of a decision to remove his heart. The second is the *social* problem of the balancing —by the same units that bear ethical responsibilities—among plural, partly conflicting, and potentially competing ethical obligations.

This moral complexity, which goes beyond common sense, can be handled only insofar as it is grounded in an ethic of the professional complex. This ethic goes beyond the levels of differentiation of the more general ethic of the society. What is often referred to as "professional ethics" is part of what is needed. It is insufficient, however, because it does not take adequate account of the role of the laity in all three of the respects discussed in this paper. There is considerable consideration of the ethical obligations of professionals, especially toward clients but also toward students, yet there is relatively little discussion of the reciprocal obligations of the lay components—not only toward the professionals, but toward the effective performance of the functions of the relevant part of the professional complex as a whole.

The problem is, perhaps, particularly acute with respect to the research function for two reasons. The first is its relative newness, at least on anything like the recent scale. The second is the relative absence or secondary significance of tangible, immediate rewards for participation in the role of subject. In any case, the two contexts of consent and of privacy clearly relate to the associational pattern, since the participation for which consent is sought and given implies a membership status. Further, the requirement of being informed is of a piece with the role of information in the research function. What the investigator requires of his subject is always, in some sense, information, though the techniques of acquiring it may go far beyond simply asking the subject questions or passively observing his behavior; much of the relevant information the subject himself may not know, as in the case of states of his internal organs.

The dynamic connection between consent and privacy may be brought out at one level by pointing out that consent to participate actually constitutes consent to relinquish certain areas of privacy that might otherwise have been enjoyed and protected. Indeed, this is patently true in many kinds of research with human subjects such as eliciting intimate details of personal history.[17] Hence, the canon of protection of privacy is thereby importantly relativized.

It is not *all* privacy that has to be protected, but those areas that are not included in the relinquishment to which explicit or implied consent has been given. One example of such protection is the anonymity device, by which confidential information is kept within a small, responsible professional group and diffusion takes place only in forms that eliminate identifiability of individuals. Another device is the exercise of care not to invade areas of privacy not germane to the program of research.

We have insistently argued that both the consent and the privacy criteria not only apply to ethical standards for the protection of research subjects, but also define important rights of *both* professional and lay participants in *all three* of the primary professional functions. Thus, we noted "admission" as the counterpart of consent and also the professional's right to privacy in certain phases of his work as a counterpart of the subject's right of privacy.

Similarly, however, neither the right to consent nor the right to the protection of privacy can be considered to be absolute on either side of the professional-lay relationship. Each is one side of a more or less "dialectic" structure that includes elements of its opposite in the *same* structure. Consent applies with maximum salience to the decision whether or not to accept a proposal to participate in any one of the three lay capacities. Even here, however, there may be presumptive obligations, as in the case of patients in a research-oriented medical institution. Once participation has been consented to, however, there is considerably greater constraint to accept collectively legitimized decisions—including those made by legitimate leadership—without having consented to them in advance in detail. This is a consequence partly of special exigencies of the professional complex and partly of the nature of effective social organization more generally. Thus, there is an especially important linkage between the protection of privacy and the institutionalization of obligatory disclosure.

In the internal "dialectic" of the consent and the privacy problems as well as in the relation of the two complexes to each other, a temporal order suggests functions that are not readily understandable on common-sense bases. The right to consent is presumptively maximal at the stage of the decision whether or not to participate, which in general means to accept a membership status. After this stage, however, in all three contexts of lay participation, the relative absoluteness of the right to consent becomes modified by the exigencies of effective collective action (subject to the continuing residual right to "resign"). These exigencies include performances of superior competence by professionals, legitimized by standards of integrity as well as of competence and also, where needed, by assertion of authority. This, of course, is one of the most important contexts in which the factor of trust operates. One way of putting it is to say that trust is a necessary basis for the operation of effective leadership, which in turn is an essential ingredient of the success of complex collective enterprises.

Similarly, however, certain protections of privacy seem to constitute prior conditions of the mobilization of information and of other resources through processes that eventually entail various forms of obligatory disclosure. Thus we cited the preparation of legal cases for trial and of academic materials both for teaching purposes and for evaluation of research results.

Further, there is the interesting sense in which the consent complex is "bracketed" within that of privacy. The essential meaning of "invasion of privacy" seems to be "intervention" in the lives of persons and, we add, of collectivities. Consent is a kind of legitimating mechanism that attempts to distinguish the interventions which are legitimate from those which are not. Hence we have spoken of the voluntary relinquishment of privacies under institutionalized conditions that often involve privileged communication, anonymity, and so forth.

Neither privacy nor intervention can reasonably be confined to an informational context. The relevance of information as the core desideratum, however, is deeply grounded in the societal functions of the professional complex, because this complex is the primary "interface" between the cognitively primary component of the cultural tradition and the main structure of modern societies. The professional complex is the primary location of the three primary modes of ordering the relations inherent in this interface—namely, *utilizing* available rational knowledge or information in the interest of a multiplicity of functional needs of the society and its subunits; *transmitting* available knowledge from those who already have mastered it to various classes of people who may need it; and *extending* and *improving* the state of knowledge beyond that given at any specified time.

Thus, the three main professional functions lie on an important continuum that certainly relates to the temporal dimension. The first function—practice—is defined mainly by the utilization of available knowledge and its embodiment in technologies for the

145

solution of *relatively* current and immediate problems. The sick person has a "condition" that calls for remedial action, and he turns to a physician or health agency for help. The time-span may be considerable, but it is far from indefinite. The second function— teaching—is a process of generating resources for the future performance of applied functions. This function may be called the generation of competence, though presumably competence does not exhaust the desired outcome of teaching. The assumption, however, is that the teacher imparts what is known. Hence, the typical contribution is distinguishable from the research function— which is to improve the cognitive base underlying both practice and teaching.

Thus, the continuum runs from utilization of given resources to relatively proximate increase of resources for such utilization to the genesis of still more "ultimate" resources. This continuum is associated with increasing time-spans necessary for the fulfillment of the conditions of societal "payoff." Students, while in a course of training, cannot be fully competent practitioners, and their training requires rather extended periods of time. Programs of research involve, in general, still longer periods of time before significantly usable results can be attained. Often, research processes must take the "detour" of concern with problems of "pure" science without reference to immediately practical results. Moreover, there remains in the research function the inherent factor of uncertainty.

The increasing importance of time along this continuum, however, is connected with that of autonomy. The professional practitioner can only be subjected to detailed accountability through the intervention of lay agencies. At every step, such intervention is made at the expense of sacrificing the benefits of special professional competence. In teaching, this relative immunity from immediate accountability must be extended to the student as well as to the teacher. For many purposes, a half-trained student is less useful than one without any training. Only after the period of "gestation" has been completed is direct accountability appropriate. This situation clearly is even more true of the research function, which requires a longer "moratorium" from payoff accountability and is generally more esoteric than most of the practice and teaching functions. Clearly lay participants in research are also in a relatively difficult position: It is difficult for them to be nearly fully "informed"; tangible and immediate rewards are relatively secondary; and the incidence of uncertainty factors is high.

It seems to follow from these considerations that what we refer to as academic freedom is part of a larger complex of institutionalized autonomy that may be called professional freedom—the institutionalized focusing of the more immediate responsibilities for the upholding of standards of competence and integrity on the individual professional and on various practices and agencies within the professional complex, rather than on the lay groups on whose interests the consequences of these functions impinge.[18]

This freedom complex is characteristic of institutions whose functions are associated with growth and development of societies for the future, with the genesis of new resources rather than the utilization of present resources. In the creation of credit and the stimulation of economic growth, banking operations belong to the same general family of social phenomena and have many of the same basic properties as a system—including the institutionalization of special freedoms based on trust as well as similar vulnerabilities (financial panic, for example).

These considerations, taken together, illustrate why the common-sense level of ethical orientation is not only "inadequate," but potentially dangerous in the conditions of a pluralistic modern society. On the lay side of the relationship, in our particular subject matter, insistence on the more absolute versions of the right to voluntary informed consent and the protection of privacy has the high probability of putting pressure on lay participants to exercise their residual "rights to resign" or to refuse to participate except on terms of the most stringent guarantees that their putative interests will not be injured.

This is a familiar pattern. The rigid insistence on "rights" is essentially a declaration of distrust in the professional complex. Its effect will ordinarily be a "deflationary" or "fundamentalist" restriction of developmental potential.

The inclusion of the "lay" element in the positive functioning of the professional complex is the primary mechanism by which this tendency to withdraw or implement the right to resign is counteracted, and the basis of trust preserved and strengthened. The positive participation of the research subject and its ethical regulation hence are of special salient significance, because research has become the most important single spearhead of the trend of progressive advance of modern societies.

The problems of this study, thus, concern the exceedingly important interface between one main sector of the professional complex and the laity on which it impinges in one direction—that of performance of professional function. It is not surprising that the ethical problems have become acute with respect to the "highest" level of these functions—that of research. It has been our endeavor to go beyond analyzing this interface as such and to place it in the context of the social organization and functioning of the professional complex as a whole. We have particularly emphasized the continuities of structure between the lay and the professional sides of the relation with respect to both the consent problem and that of privacy. We have also stressed the broad nature of the pattern of social organization into which both sides fit, and which extends, with the appropriate modifications, to all three of the principal professional functions.

In this context, one can see the sense in which the standards of voluntary informed consent and of the protection of privacy may prove to be double-edged swords. The perspective from which the present discussion arose concerned the protection of the lay element against abuses and exploitation emanating from the professional side. Such protection, if carried too far in terms too rigidly defined, however, can easily encroach on the rights of consent and privacy that are essential to the professional's performance of *his* functions and those of the complex as a whole. The operation of the professional complex depends on certain balances, both among its internal components (most emphatically including the lay elements) and in its relation to the nonprofessional social environment. It is my conviction that only by seeing the professional complex as a system can one cope with pressures that are threatening to distort either the internal or the external balances. Society has a profound stake not only in the successful operation of the professional complex, but also in the rights of the laity to minimization of injuries from this operation. Balancing of these interests within a workable and appropriate societal framework is a paramount societal interest.

REFERENCES

1. I am thinking of "legal" accountability, as just sketched, as involving an indirect rather than direct use of public authority. Put in sociologically functional terms, the system of courts and the processes of adjudication perform more integrative than executive functions in the operation of a society.

Research and the "Professional Complex"

2. An interesting development in recent years combines the factor of fiduciary responsibility on the part of members of the profession with that of certain important lay elements. This is the system of review boards which in hospitals and various other institutions that engage in research with human subjects pass on the ethical admissibility of research projects undertaken within their organization. Often, in somewhat the manner of boards of trustees, lay citizens of important standing are enlisted along with the professional contingent. It is significant that among these laymen two groups figure prominently, namely lawyers and clergymen, who in general have a rather high reputation for readiness to assume such responsibility.

3. For the argument in favor of this point of view, see Talcott Parsons, "Some Theoretical Considerations Bearing on the Field of Medical Sociology," in *Social Structure and Personality* (Glencoe, 1964).

4. Dr. Renée Fox has made particularly illuminating contributions to the sociological understanding of the combination of the roles of patient and research subject. See her book *Experiment Perilous*, which reports a study of a metabolic research ward, where the patients had been subjected to especially drastic and risky procedures. (See especially pp. 85-109 and 243.) She has generalized this analysis, with much additional material, in the article "Some Social and Cultural Factors in American Society Conducive to Medical Research on Human Subjects," *Symposium on the Study of Drugs and Man*, Part IV. In a personal communication Dr. Fox has suggested the following paradigm of types of subjects as a function of lessening degrees of uncertainty: 1) research on animal subjects, where uncertainty and risk are at a maximum; 2) research on moribund, terminally ill subjects, who have "little to lose"; 3) research on patients somewhat less desperately ill, in degrees to those with more or less "normal" expectations of health and longevity.

5. In a striking oral statement, the head of a pediatric service in a major hospital once said in my presence that in his opinion fully one half of the therapeutic failures on that service were attributable not to the lack of available knowledge and therapeutic measures adequate for success in the case, but to failure of the staff to secure the *cooperation* of "patients"— that is, children and members of their families—which was necessary for the successful implementation of a therapeutic program. Such noncooperation is grounded in deficiency of trust in the present sense. It can, of course, reach into unconscious psychodynamic levels.

6. See Fox, *Experiment Perilous* and "Some Social and Cultural Factors in American Society Conducive to Medical Research on Human Subjects," for the way in which Dr. Fox has analyzed these relationships in a concrete case of medical research.

7. Compare Talcott Parsons and Victor M. Lidz, "Death in American Society," *Essays in Self-Destruction*, ed. Edwin Shneidman (New York, 1967).

8. Often, even where it is not clearly intended, reflection and analysis can bring out the appeal to values and solidarity. If a personal example may

149

be permitted, Dr. Gerald Platt and I have been engaged in a rather large-scale study of members of the American academic profession. Our basic data are derived from a long questionnaire which was mailed to over 4,500 individuals. Sixty-six per cent, slightly over 3,000, of them responded at the expense of about 2½ hours of time and effort each. No honorarium was offered, but the covering letter appealed explicitly not only to the valuation of research, but to long-run professional interests. Also prestige symbols such as the location of the investigators at Harvard University and the blessing of the American Association of University Professors on the project were explicitly used. Our basic appeal could be phrased "Fellow academic men. . . ."

9. This is very different from a relation of friendship in which such specific qualifications are not essential criteria of a claim to "help" or, more generally, participation.

10. There is a particularly important parallel here in the relation of bank depositors to the lending operations of banks. The "contract of deposit" leaves the depositor full rights to withdraw his total deposit on demand at any time. But the function of the bank as a creator of credit in the interest of economic efficiency depends on the probability that the large proportion of depositors will "trust" the bank and leave considerable balances in it. Indeed, if most of them exercise their legal rights, the "good" bank which is doing its job is necessarily insolvent. We are suggesting that both students and clients, and of course research subjects, are in the role analogous to depositors, and that they in a similar sense are under a kind of obligation to trust the professional elements with whom they associate. This obligation is a kind of "citizenship" of the collective system in question, not a "formal" obligation.

11. The right to resign is, of course, restricted in a few cases—such as legal commitment of patients to mental hospitals—but these cases are not of central significance to this analysis.

12. In the sense that *every* participant's desire to have it done "my way" has no claim equal to that of legitimate leadership in determining collective decisions.

13. In the medical case, access to the body is an exceedingly important "privilege" of the physician that "invades" otherwise operative privacies.

14. I am especially indebted to Lon L. Fuller for insight into this set of connections. See his book *The Morality of Law*.

15. Dr. Renée C. Fox, "The Autopsy: Its Place in the Attitude-Learning of Second-Year Medical Students," unpublished paper.

16. It should, of course, be noted that there are other important categories of laymen with whom members of the professional complex must establish relations. These are not categories in relation to whom the professional functions are performed, but those who in different ways undertake responsibility for the support of the professional function—shading into tol-

erating its performance in the face of actual or potential disturbances by it or opposition to it. These include persons and collective agencies involved in financial and political support outside professional organizations as such, trustees and other members of professional organizations with fiduciary functions on their behalf, administrative personnel whose functions are facilitative of the professional, and, not least, many kinds of subprofessional supportive personnel such as secretaries, technicians, orderlies, and simple caretakers of physical facilities.

17. A good case here would be the Kinsey studies.

18. Some such qualification as "more immediate responsibilities" is of course essential because the kinds of autonomy and support which are essential to the functioning of the professional complex cannot be taken for granted by its members as a matter of right without *any* corresponding responsibilities or accountability. The latter cannot, however, be immediate and detailed without stultifying effects. It can be seen here again how important the factor of trust is in bridging the gap.

MARGARET MEAD

Research with Human Beings: A Model Derived from Anthropological Field Practice

"ANTHROPOLOGICAL RESEARCH does not have subjects. We work with informants in an atmosphere of trust and mutual respect." This was the opening sentence of my attempt to draft a response to the request of the National Institutes of Health for a statement of procedures in research on human subjects. This position stands in extreme contrast to the assertion that fully informed consent for the experimental analysis of a complicated piece of medical research would require four years of medical school.[1] It stresses not only the importance of the relationship between a research worker and those among whom he seeks new knowledge, but also the possibility of substituting voluntary participation for "informed consent" as a precondition of ethical research work. I shall approach the problem from this extreme contrast, as the most useful contribution that anthropology can make to the development of a model in this field.

The model presented by Talcott Parsons[2] stresses the possibility of regarding human subjects as participants in a collective enterprise and presents as an ideal what has long been anthropological field practice.

It is necessary to spell out the forms used in field work in the study of the culture, the language, or the physique of isolated primitive peoples on which anthropological research styles have been developed and which are still used as reference points when anthropological research is undertaken in complex societies.[3] In this situation, the people to be studied have lived within an extremely isolated human environment, have no written language, and only the most superficial knowledge of either the paraphernalia or the concepts of civilization. They live in self-contained communities, and their assent and active help are necessary if the field worker is to live among them. He must live among them, within sight and sound of their twenty-four-hour activities throughout a normal annual cycle (which may include periods of nomadism), if he is to give the required account of their lives. For permission to live among them and for such cooperation as he needs to obtain a house, food, and transport, he must convince them that his intentions are friendly, and that the difficulties he may cause are in some way compensated for by benefits. These benefits may be material—the bringing of money into the community, the promise and supplying of routine medical help, or the importation of goods that can otherwise only be obtained by long expensive expeditions. But although all of these inducements are useful supplements, in the end the anthropologist is dependent upon enlisting intellectual curiosity that complements his own research interests, enjoyment of the research enterprise, and—today with modern methods of recording—an interest in tape, film, and photography. Ideally, and this practice is easy to follow among recently contacted peoples, the anthropologist does not pay for information, nor does he pay anyone to dictate a text or take a test or stand correctly while being measured, or repeat a chant three times so that it can be perfectly recorded. He pays for time and for work; if he wants a man to spend an allotted number of hours as guide, interpreter, companion, or domestic worker, this payment is phrased as compensation for the time that would otherwise be spent in hunting, fishing, or gardening. Among the interested and available members of the community in which he has succeeded in settling, he selects those with sufficient intellectual interest and talent to be principal *informants*—that is, systematic collaborators into the nature of the language and culture. With the help of such informants, he gradually builds a conceptual model of the language and culture. As he does so, the informants increase their own capacity to understand the grammar of the language that they speak and the culture within which they live and act. The field worker is continuingly dependent upon testing out his abstractions by concrete applications, either provisionally—as in such questions as: "Would it be possible to say. . .?" or "Could a mother's brother . . .?"—or by proposing explanations of observed behavior and having these explanations criticized by his informants.

A relevant aspect of this process is the high level of intellectual performance that can be evoked from an uneducated but able mind when the subject matter is personal and relevant. An abstract idea of linguistic form takes considerable teaching, but a New Guinea Arapesh linguistic informant could learn rapidly to deal with the idea of formal gender in his own language, which has thirteen noun classes, and to recognize anomalies and exceptions within the language. Similarly, today first-generation Manus schoolboys with an equivalent of a sixth-grade education and very halting English are able to read my discussion of Manus kinship—with its full complement of their own terminology[4]—where they would have difficulty with much simpler concepts without the backing provided by experience. In physiological or psychological investigations, much of the same thing might well prove to be true were it fairly tested; the ability to give introspective reports on one's own state might be found to be greatly in advance of the ability to deal with descriptive materials that lack personal relevance.

The cooperative enterprise in which anthropologist and informants engage is the framework within which information is collected about other individuals and observations are made of the behavior of those members of the village who are less closely involved in the work. The informant's judgment is relied upon when it is a question of continuing the making of a film after the head of a sacred puppet has fallen off or of recording during a quarrel or mourning. Within the context of the practical imperative that one must be able to continue working in the community and so do nothing that will interfere with that work, a healthy caution is dictated. It is not worthwhile to violate the sensitivities of the people with whom one is working. A second and principal imperative is the enjoined respect for the people among whom we work, as members of the human race comparable in abilities and dignity with our own, carrying a culture that is the object of our greatest scientific solicitude. There is also the obligation not to damage the chances of other anthropologists to work in the same area, under the same authorities, or with other members of the same tribe. Even failing the full operation of this value system, the constraints provided by the situation itself are useful and should be considered in any research model that draws upon the anthropological field situation.

The field situation within which almost all anthropologists have worked has also prevented the practice of deceit and falsification that tempts the social scientist working within his own language and culture. Usually of a different race and always with a different standard of living, the anthropologist cannot conceal his research identity and carry on his work. He may have to temper some of his research efforts to local fears and prejudices if a people object to certain kinds of note-taking for fear of taxation,[5] for example, but in general he is constrained to tell the truth.

He must give an account of himself that is creditable and acceptable to the people among whom he works and is congruent with the activities that they will see him carry out. Although some subsidiary explanations can sometimes be used, and others are sometimes supplied by local imagination, the only explanation that is completely reliable and not likely to be contradicted by governmental authority, gossip, the accounts given by a colleague who is working with a nearby tribe, or his own behavior is the truth—that he has come to find out how the people live, what is the language they speak, what they believe. Pure scientific inquiry, for its own sake, thus becomes the easiest way to explain what the anthropologist is doing. Wanting to know, when what one wants to know is valued by those from whom one must learn it, is an appeal that few human beings can resist—whether it is a desire to know how their kind of house is built, how they trap game, how they pray to their ancestors, or how many of their children have got their second teeth.[6]

The problem of communicating to a primitive people what will be done with the information that they have helped develop is of a different order. They may have no conception of printing or of what the publication of details about their social forms and individual behavior may mean. Consent in such cases would be even more ridiculous than it has been shown to be in the case of complicated experiments in our own society. Furthermore, it is not only their own current reputations that are at a risk they cannot estimate, but today, as primitive peoples are rapidly entering the modern world, it is the dignity and sensitivity of their descendants that must be considered. The situation is somewhat comparable to consent given by parents for the use of films made of their children in a modern country, without any real ability to predict how the children will feel about such continuing exposure to the public eye. Here, in the case of primitive peoples, of children, or of any individuals who are not in a position to evaluate the effects of publication, a heavy responsibility falls upon the research worker (see Appendix IV).

This responsibility for the effects of publication of any given piece of anthropological work takes several forms. There is first of all the responsibility to individuals who, if identified, must not thereby be exposed to legal sanctions, to ridicule, or to danger.

Second, there is the responsibility to the group as a whole. Where customs are portrayed that contrast with the ethical standards of those who govern them or with the missionized or educated members of their own society, these must be represented in such a way that full justice is done to the cultural framework within which a given practice, however apparently abhorrent, occurs. A classic example is the way in which the aged among the Eskimo asked to be walled up and left to die. Their voluntary sacrifice—which was all that they could do, under such primitive conditions, for the well-being of their children and grandchildren—can either be portrayed as the dignified and voluntary act they conceived it to be or it can be transformed into killing grandmothers by using the terminology of peoples who have both a superior technology and a different ethic about suicide.[7]

Different levels of protection of the identity of individuals, villages, and tribes are called for by different degrees of discrepancy in the observance of traditional or imposed custom. It may be permissible to say that polygamy is still practiced, provided no census is published, by a tribe within which it is forbidden by law, but in that case it might be necessary to conceal the village in which one had worked. In some cases, tremendous sacrifices of important exact knowledge that would come from fuller identification of individuals, or groups, have to be made. The alternative that is possible in cases where individuals may not be exposed to legal sanctions but may feel that their privacy is invaded is full discussion of the details which are to be published with those concerned. Instances of such anthropologically responsible discussions are Ted Schwartz's publication of the details of the Paliau movement in the Admiralties, which he discussed at length with its leader Paliau (see Appendix IV),[8] Oscar Lewis' publication of the autobiography of the Mexican family reported in *Children of Sanchez,*[9] and Rhoda Metraux's case histories of educated Chinese who had volunteered to be part of the medical cultural study on Human Ecology and Health, at New York Hospital, Cornell Medical Center (see Appendix II).

But the Oscar Lewis case raises a further issue, the obligation of the research worker to his own discipline and to the general public image of scientific work.[10] Where feelings run high, and where the research may expose conditions that are unacceptable to others, the consent of the individuals actually involved, although quite genuine, may not be enough. Public exposure of situations that they wish to conceal or deny—either the behavior of their ancestors, their less educated neighbors, the poor, the exploited, and the criminal in their own society—may raise grave questions. But if such exposure has been accompanied by a scrupulous seeking of informed cooperation by those studied, and a full and responsible recognition of the social issues involved, the situation, although difficult, remains ethical. The research worker may feel that the exposure of some evil transcends his obligation to the image of his science that will be formed by angry resentment of his disclosures.

Finally, there is the responsibility of the anthropologist for the way in which his findings are interpreted and articulated into the ongoing understanding of human behavior in the human sciences of his day. Acute problems are raised, for example, by the question of active research in some field that is being politically distorted, such as constitutional type and race. During the Nazi period and for many years afterwards, studies of human constitutional type were branded as Nazi, and today, where there are such determined segregationist efforts to establish racial inferiority to explain the low achievement levels of Negro Americans the same type of argument is used against studies that explore differences among different racial groups. Recent discussions suggest that failure to continue to do research in a field may actually do serious damage by reducing the impact of previous research that was well established and actually has not been challenged in any way.[11] In other words, it is suggested that knowledge must continue to live through new research; without the new research, it will die. This is the more significant because it is in those fields where the results have the highest degree of social relevance—such as race, the effects of socio-economic deprivation, population control—that research efforts are sometimes inhibited or the results withheld because of imagined ill effects.

I have discussed this anthropological model from the standpoint of the position of the research population; the ethical position of the investigator; the effect on the nature of the research; the impact on the discipline in terms of the effect on the work of other and subsequent investigators; and the effect on the relationship between science and society. We may now examine how this model, here based upon anthropological field work practice and proposed as a desirable form by Talcott Parsons, fits into our contemporary American attitudes toward experimentation with human subjects.

I will draw specifically upon the series of papers for earlier parts of this project, upon reports of the November 3-4, 1967, conference and the working groups that led up to it, upon researches conducted by Dr. Rhoda Metraux and myself on the image of the scientist in American culture,[12] and upon an exploration of the problem of professional ethics that has concerned me for many years.[13] American cultural attitudes are, of course, closely related to British attitudes and very much influenced by historical connections with Europe, by response to Nazi wartime experimentation, and to some extent by reported Eastern European activities. It is interesting that the discussions prepared for the earlier conference (November 3-4, 1967) used the word "experiment" with the popular ambiguity that surrounds it—as a trial, a test, something not based upon true and tried methods (as in the discussion of the effects upon a large group of people of a new form of housing or sewerage disposal), and as something deliberately done *to* human beings in order to obtain or validate new knowledge. The term covers such various activities as the introduction of a new form of government, when George Washington spoke of the United States as an experiment, through the use of a previously untried decontaminant in water, a new method of teaching reading, the deliberate withholding of a drug from half of a special group of subjects or injection of subjects with substances whose action is unknown, the creation of psychological states by hypnosis, falsification of the social environment. The key attitude toward all of these activities, from the largest and the least planned to the most precise laboratory situation, is the word *guinea pig*. The relationship between the experimenter and those upon whom he operates is thus compared to a power relationship in which human beings are reduced to the status of *experimental animals,* animals kept caged in laboratories for scientific purposes. Even answering a questionnaire for a mass survey may be spoken of as being made into a guinea pig. The mad scientist and the evil scientist are typically portrayed with a set of caged animals in the background and with a prostrate human being on whose head or body the scientist is operating.[14]

The laboratory animal is seen as bred for purposes of experiment, deprived of freedom, tortured, and killed, thus exemplifying the terrifying limits to which scientific experiment can go. Human beings placed in the position of laboratory animals are reduced to the condition of powerlessness, stripped of their individual rights and dignities.

Seen in this way, experimentation on human beings is placed in a wholly negative light; the knowledge the experimenter seeks is a cold impersonal knowledge identified with destructiveness, particularly the destructiveness of the bomb.

This view of the scientist-experimenter contrasts sharply with the view of science as the benefactor of Mankind, and, interestingly enough, the importance of experiments to mankind is most frequently invoked in defense of experiments on human beings. So in discussions the emphasis is on weighing the costs and benefits to the individual and to mankind, with the insistence that we can only arrive at certain kinds of wholly beneficent and life-saving knowledge by taking risks with individuals in the experiments that establish that knowledge.[15] And in the discussions of medical research, the continuum that is recognized is that between the physician and his patient for whose well-being he may even take the risk of using an untried method and of being censured by his peers, through the clinical experimenter who is governed by considerations of concern for a group of patients for whom, however, he has less individual concern than would their own personal physicians, through the experimenter who is primarily aiming at future benefits for large, unspecified populations of beneficiaries, to those research workers who, although they may hold medical degrees and work in a hospital setting, are nevertheless only interested in some piece of knowledge that has no known applicability to the Welfare of Mankind.

Through this series of repeated characterizations runs the theme that the new and untried is always dangerous, but that its use can be condoned if the risk is shared by the practitioner who employs it. So we move from danger to the patient and the practitioner, in acts undertaken out of dedication and concern, to danger to the subjects as the acts become increasingly divorced from specific concern for human welfare. In the most extreme cases, the impersonal experimental scientist is seen as a bad father and husband, as a dangerous neighbor who might "blow up the whole apartment house."

Throughout runs the ambivalence toward one who has special knowledge and skill that give him powers over life and death, powers which in primitive societies frequently resulted in healing and death-dealing powers being joined in the same practitioner. This ambivalence recurs in modern societies in the demand that a physician should exercise his power to end suffering in terminal cancer or prevent a deformed infant from living, and reaches political dimensions in Stalin's fear of doctors, in the doctor's plot, and in the experimenting physicians in Nazi concentration camps.[16]

To the fears and hopes that are associated with the extraordinary powers of the physician over pain and death are added, by extension, the fears and hopes toward other sorts of power and other sorts of loss of individual rights. So we find the belief that the psychiatrist "can see right through you," that the social scientist "can tell just what you are thinking or what you are going to do," the fear that fluoridation in the city water system will lead to mass poisoning, and that the government will be able to brainwash an entire population. All of these fears, by the possible victims, are of course matched by hopes—differently phrased—that increased knowledge will make it possible for the psychiatrist to give a more perfect diagnosis, for the social scientist to prevent a riot or an economic depression, for the city planner to combine the water system and the sewerage system into one whole, and for the political scientist to design a world system of order that will prevent nuclear war and provide for peaceful relationships among nations. Just as at the very most primitive level, fear of the shaman's powers was matched by the claims he made, so our contemporary attitudes toward experiments of all kinds are focused on the question of power: How to attain it, how to limit it, how to hedge it about with sanctions so that it is beneficial, not detrimental, to mankind.

The inclusion of questions of human rights and civil liberties within the context of allowable experimentation is, of course, completely congruent. Discussion rages over the areas of the autonomy of the experimental subject, the need for full consent, and the ideal subject who is fully informed because his education matches that of the experimenter, and the inadmissibility of experiments on children, the mentally defective, the institutionalized, prisoners, and so forth. The more powerless the subject is, *per se*, the more the question of ethics—and power—is raised.

Congruently, the question of the ethics of experimentation reaches its height in those cases where the research worker has the highest standing and works with the greatest academic and social sanctions. The researcher in a university teaching hospital is faced with demands that would never be made of the general practitioner; the trained nurse is hedged about with requirements that would never be made on the unlicensed local old granny; the pharmacist is forbidden to take an eye winker out of the eye of a passerby, but no odium attaches to the chief accountant who has a reputation for "being awfully good at taking things out of people's eyes." As status and public attestations of that status increase, greater accountability is demanded. It is assumed that trust will follow status, and therefore that more precautions must be taken to see that the trust is not abused.

For this reason, it seems to me that it is difficult to combine discussions of rules governing experimentation on human beings by those who have been officially pronounced to be responsible scientists with discussions about how many people Society is willing to let be killed because no measures are taken to prevent window-washing without harnesses or dangerous grade crossings. In the models presented by Guido Calabresi of collective and protective measures, the issues were statistical ones in which the public acted when the risk to any one of them seemed great enough.[17] The willingness to take measures or spend large sums to prevent diseases that may strike anyone anywhere (of which poliomyelitis is a prime example) and the unwillingness to take comparable measures where the incidence of disease or accident is concentrated in one class or one part of the population are striking. But the issue of rules governing experimentation seems much more a question of the sanctions that control the specialist in a society becoming ever more specialized, in which the power derived from scientific knowledge is becoming ever greater. It is not a question of how dangerous it is to drive on American highways on weekends or how much pollution the population of a town is exposed to, but rather of how much power a specialist should have and how trust in his essential benevolence can be preserved. The assurance that no experimentation will reduce human beings to the status of experimental animals but instead will be dignified and modulated by the concern of the physician for his patient and the dedication of the researcher to the well-being of his particular science and subjects and to the welfare of mankind is an assurance that the researcher, awesome in his great knowledge, can be trusted. Any uncovering of unethical methods—inoculation of patients without their consent, exposure of a group to unnecessary hazards—in the course of experimentation is detrimental to this trust and arouses fear that may assume paranoid proportions. In complementary fashion, controls over the procedures arouse anger in many research workers, who are distressed by any suggestion that the trust they place in their own professional ethics and that of their colleagues needs such external controls.

In the light of these contemporary cultural attitudes—and I must emphasize that I am not making ex cathedra or general statements about research or medicine, but comments on the contemporary American attitudes we all share—I do not believe that considerations of cost benefit or of the extent to which society is willing to pay a price in some human lives in order to save many more human lives are the most useful direction in which to look for solutions to our problem.

Rather, I would say that the issues are how the scientist, sanctioned by society, is to maintain the trust that accompanies that sanction, and how contemporary views about human experimentation affect this trust. Obviously all experiments in which advantage is taken of the helplessness of another human being—whether it be of his status as a child or as a prisoner, whether he is a patient dependent on his physician or a student fearful of not receiving a good grade—are violations of trust. Equally obviously, deceit of any sort or, in the current phrase, increase in the creditability gap lowers trust. Conversely, any way in which research can enhance the status of the subjects and so increase their human dignity endows the investigator with a beneficent and trustworthy role. The suggestion made by Talcott Parsons that subjects be treated as collaborators—the position of those with whom an anthropologist works—then becomes a highly important one, and one which, at the present time, is congruent with the demand that students, patients, and clients have more of a role in any activity in which they are involved, rather than continuing their past role as passive recipients on whose behalf power is delegated to the specialist practitioner.

The model of the research participant, who is also a collaborator of the research worker, is a valuable addition to our criteria for a properly designed experiment. In the first place, any simple use of a stooge is ruled out, as are disguised participants in flying-saucer cults or aberrant religious sects (see Appendix I), or adolescent gangs. On the other hand, where the nature of the experiment requires a certain amount of surrender of autonomy on the part of the subjects, this can be accorded with dignity, as a group agrees to participate knowing that placebos may be used, that there may be apparatus involved which may falsify some aspect of the situation, or that observations of a sort of which they have no awareness may be made. Here assent to the conditions of the experiment becomes identical with the kind of assent that a psychologist would accord a fellow psychologist, or a physiologist a fellow physiologist. What is an indignity without participation is transformed into something of which the subject may be proud. At the same time, the experimenter is necessarily forced into abandoning simple deceit and the invalidation of the experiment by the unconscious giving of cues to the subject. His attention is turned to devising ingenious methods that reduce these sources of error.

In the previous discussions, it was also suggested that more exacting criteria for the use of human subjects in experiments would produce better science, as the experiment itself would be subjected to sharper scrutiny. This would also be so if the purpose of the experiment had to be explained to participants treated as intelligent, responsible, although not necessarily scientifically knowledgeable human beings. Some of the traps into which experimenters fall would be avoided, such as rivalry traps or the uncritical pursuit of fashion.[18]

The participant research subject bears the same relationship to the captive, deluded subject that the conscientious objector volunteering for research on the effects of starvation or hazardous blood diffusion bears to the prisoner or the charity patient experimented upon without his knowledge or consent.

It is also useful to inquire why more stringent rules have to be promulgated when government funds are involved. There is, of course, the cynical and often true explanation that politicians may use inflamed public feeling simply as a political weapon to destroy an opponent or cut down the executive budget, so that distrust of research, accusations of cruelty to animals, or interferences with privacy may simply be used as weapons, as misuse of public funds. But there are other, more reputable reasons why government participation should raise the levels of scrutiny. The investment of public funds in any act implies public support as well as sanction. When the law supports the demands of a professional association for the fulfillment of certain requirements, one public sanction is given. When public funds are appropriated to give professional training to members of that profession or to support their research, additional sanction is given. Thus, greater precautions were demanded for the astronauts in the space program, in which a large amount of public funds and therefore a larger amount of public responsibility were involved, than when it was expected that several test pilots would be lost in testing a new airplane under a system where pilots were licensed but not publicly financed. Similarly, the standards for day nursery care, or for adoption, that accompany federal grants may seem exorbitant and even ridiculous when compared with current unfinanced practice, but the same conditions apply. For that for which society pays, it must also take collective responsibility. It is vitally important that society should be on the side of life and concern for individual lives; the greater the investment of public funds, the higher the demand for ethical supervision. But there would not seem to be any comparable need for rigid rules, as opposed to standards of retrospective accountability.

Such a model of research participation can deal effectively with such questions as informed consent. If any sort of exploitation of the powerless is ruled out, including payment to those in financial need for acting as subjects and persuasion of students in need of recommendation and backing, then a truly cooperative enterprise can be inaugurated in which there is a partnership in the socially sanctioned search for knowledge, both the knowledge the benefits from which are already predictable and the knowledge which has no immediate rewards beyond the extension of man's understanding of the universe and his place within it.

Such a model of voluntary participation in research brings us back, by a circuitous route, to Mr. Calabresi's discussion of collective choices.[19] If we recognize that the scientific enterprise is of the greatest importance to modern society, then it will be possible for those who represent that society to endorse, sanction, and underwrite the conditions, training, and research facilities that give the highest protection to that enterprise. Instead of thinking of research on human subjects as something to be avoided when possible and controlled when it cannot be avoided, we can begin to think of participation in scientific research as a form of education for students and a form of responsible citizenship activity for adults. If all participation is voluntary and treated as a privilege, if participants in the research are given adequate information on the purposes for which the experiment is made and the results which come from their participation, this can have profound repercussions in the whole public understanding of science. The present humanitarian urge to contribute to blood banks and to eye banks might be supplemented by active participation such as that of a group of volunteer faculty members near one great medical school who have not only willed their bodies for post-mortem use to the medical school, but agreed to take part in annual medical examinations that will enhance the scientific usefulness of their contribution. The contrast between such an active participation and the fear of body snatchers of the last century dramatizes the possible wide changes in public attitude that might result.

Research *on* human subjects calls up images of repugnance and terror: The subject is seen as a victim, the experimenter as brutalized, the results compromised by the methods through which they were obtained; and the public view of the scientist is one of suspicion and rejection. Participation in research by human beings who are enthusiastically related to the explorations of new knowledge not only for the benefit of Mankind, but for the sheer enjoyment of being a part of great intellectual adventures calls up exactly the opposite set of images.

The related models that Talcott Parsons and I have presented rely, it has been argued, on a level of participation that cannot be expected within many of the ward situations of our urban hospitals. But I submit that the intense willingness of an individual of any level of education to participate in an enterprise—because he himself is suffering, has suffered, or may suffer, because his child is suffering, has suffered, or may suffer, because he himself is dignified by an order of social participation not readily available to him, or because, being intellectually alert, he is given a part in an intellectually stimulating exercise—is related to the degree of the involvement of the subject. Because he is personally involved through his experience, his fears, his solicitude, his desire for recognition as a socially valuable person, or his satisfaction in using his mind, he is by any one or all of these routes removed from the demeaning status of *guinea pig*. Guinea pigs are not able to invoke their experience or fears or cognitive powers in this way. These are distinctively human and noble aspects of humanity.

We can further adopt the position that the failure to do research, to experiment, and to learn is reprehensible. We can cease to try to limit and curtail experiments on human beings, while we devise more and better experiments *with* human beings who, as participants, are collaborators.

Appendix I: Problems of Falsification

In recent years there have been a great many experiments and investigations reported in which deliberate falsification has been introduced. Instructed stooges have been directed to deny sensory evidence, or to mimic pain that they did not feel, or to obstruct situations planned by their peers. Investigators have posed as possible converts to flying-saucer cults. Under the guise of "participant observation," various forms of "cover" have been developed for social investigators, which have later been revealed to the public in the reports on the experiments. These are, I believe, all deeply unsatisfactory in several ways: (1) the effect of the observation or disclosure or publication of the results of such scientifically—or humanely—motivated activities on the subjects; (2) the effect on the investigators; (3) the effect on the validity of the experiment itself; and (4) the effect upon the whole culture of the presence of methods of observation and experimentation in which human dignity is violated as contrasted with methods in which human beings are fully respected and protected, or in which human beings are asked to knowingly sacrifice their own safety or privacy for the benefit of others or later generations. Failure to distinguish among these effects is responsible for some of the confusion in this field.

Effect on the Subject: To fail to acquaint a subject of observation or experiment with what is happening—as fully as is possible within the limits of the communication system—is to that extent to denigrate him as a full human being and reduce him to the category of dependency in which he is not permitted to judge for himself. The various ethical ruses that are used—such as telling the subject he has been tricked, deluded, spied upon, or lied to immediately after the experiment is over—fail to take into account that when such a subject is debriefed, he can accept such debriefing only by some other ruse, such as in the identification with the lying experimenter or in the decision that social science is a bunch of confidence tricks and now he also knows a few. Alternately, if he cannot make use of satisfying self-protective devices, his dignity will have been abused and affronted. If he decides that being lied to or tricked is the price he must pay for some other benefit—health, education, political preferment, employment, or a graduate education in a social science—he will nevertheless invest these very benefits and those who confer them upon him with some negative effect.*

---

* Allowance must be made here for those who are so sophisticated in the use of tests and instruments of various sorts that they take a professional pleasure in undergoing them. It was striking to observe the differential response of the psychologically- and physiologically-sophisticated to tests like the Cantril-Ames demonstration of optical illusions formerly displayed at Princeton, through which psychologically trained individuals moved with enjoyment, while historians—trained to trust their own eyes and ears and judgment—came out feeling demeaned and abused. A failure to take this particular double-take into account is often responsible for violent disagreements on method. This was true also in discussions of the Kinsey report; some scientists were willing to discuss the rather limited details of their sexual lives with the same scrupulous honesty that they accorded to records of archaeological excavations or weather testing; they became particularly angry if more sophisticated social scientists suggested that some of the respondents to the Kinsey questionnaire had lied.

Research with Human Beings: An Anthropological Model

Effect on the Investigator: But perhaps even more serious than the effect upon the subject or object or unwarned collaborator, which in most cases is brief and transitory, is the effect upon the investigator himself. Ethically, it means that he becomes accustomed to tricking, deceiving, and manipulating other human beings and, to that extent, to denigrating their humanity. Besides the ethical consequences that flow from contempt for other human beings, there are other consequences—such as increased selective insensitivity or delusions of grandeur and omnipotence—that may in time seriously interfere with the very thing which he has been attempting to protect: the integrity of his own scientific work. Encouraging styles of research and intervention that involve lying to other human beings therefore tends to establish a corps of progressively calloused individuals, insulated from self-criticism and increasingly available for clients who can become outspokenly cynical in their manipulating of other human beings, individually and in the mass.*

Both of these undesirable consequences are prevented to some extent by the honest belief that the deception is absolutely necessary to the conduct of an experiment and that the experiment itself must be performed. Arguments of this sort can be advanced for both laboratory and field tests of new drugs: Elimination of other factors of suggestion and belief must be made by the use of placebos, and so forth. When astronauts are being selected, it is vital to know their ability to withstand various kinds of strain, and this can only be found out by tests involving deception of various sorts, such as simulation, secret observation by long-distance TV, concealed indicators, and so forth. The ethical difficulties involved in even these situations are attested to by the number of cases where the experimenter with a new drug, for example, will insist on trying it on himself first.

Many of the situations where concealment is genuinely necessary and the experiment cannot be performed in some other way can be handled by general assent from the subjects, who know that they are agreeing to being deceived for the purposes of the experiment itself. Individuals who have particular diseases, conscientious objectors who wish to make a contribution to human welfare, candidates for dangerous secret activities or especially exacting forms of warfare or exploration, and students of psychology may volunteer to participate in activities where

---

* Here again, we should mention the other effect. Instead of being cynical about his manipulations, the experimenter or interventionist who deceives may also take refuge behind the great good that he is doing to the subject as a patient or to other men who will benefit from his activities—in developing a new drug or writing advertising copy that will induce people to spend their money more wisely. Here the need to justify demeaning other human beings, in particular respects, is compensated for by another kind of delusion of grandeur: that of becoming someone who benefits mankind on a large scale, the omnipotent theorist, the all-knowing teacher, the scientist working for the intelligence agency of a particular government or conspiring with some secret plot to save the world.

they consciously abrogate some of the dignities and freedoms that are associated with the status of a fully healthy, free citizen of a free society. The medical profession demands this of many patients, lawyers demand it of clients—"just put yourself in my hands and trust my judgment" —priests demand it of penitents, and parents demand it of their children. Such a status is not ennobling; it may be necessary; and it can be defined so that consent is given in such a general way that the particularities of placebos, stooges, and fabricated situations are left intact to test the physiological or psychological behavior of the subject. But the crucial question must be whether the deception is absolutely necessary in order to perform an experiment which is itself necessary. By the automatic inclusion of deception in a research or treatment plan, many research workers are simply relieved of any obligation to make new research designs which would not involve any deception at all.

The Effect of Deception on the Experiment Itself: This topic is usually considered only in the way I have discussed it above. Does the experimental design require that the subject be deceived or that the observer be concealed or disguised? This is the first question, which is sometimes qualified by considerations of the benefits to the subject himself or to mankind that may result. Thus, it may be argued that an astronaut who could not stand some sort of strain that could only be produced by dissimulation would lose his life, or that democracy will be able to protect itself better if it knows how innately cowardly or subject to sadistic suggestion the average citizen is.

Important as such considerations and rationalizations are, there is still a further and relevant question: Is any experiment in which one human being lies to another—either as to the chemical composition of a pill, the meaning of a test, the purpose of an inquiry, or his own responses if he is operating as a stooge within an experimental situation— ever a *valid* experiment? There is sufficient evidence from clinical observations to suggest that many, if not all, human beings are able to pick up, often at an unanalyzed level, multisensory cues that other human beings are not aware they are giving. If an experiment or observation situation contains one human being who knows that he is lying, we have no way of preventing some knowledge of this from being communicated to the participants, and therefore no way of controlling this factor, which may take many forms: lowered sense of danger, heightened discomfort, fear, and distrust, a sense of unreality, distrust of the self. To this provision of cues by the experimenters and "participant" observers must be added such matters as contexts. In a recent experiment reported at Yale,[1] subjects were involved in acts of inflicting apparent suffering, at the orders of the experimenters, on subjects who simulated pain. The results were presented as evidence of the lengths to which Americans would go in torturing others under orders—from Yale University! In another experiment on panic, students at a lecture were subjected to the sounds of an air raid—while the lecturer continued to lecture.*

---

* Under some circumstances, there may of course be a reverse effect, in which a medical school or a discipline comes to be regarded as a place where ani-

Research with Human Beings: An Anthropological Model

The danger of distortion by cues unconsciously given by the experimenters and stooges and unconsciously picked up by the subjects is so great that it can be categorically said that if deception is a necessary and intrinsic part of the experimental or observational design, then human investigators must be removed from the experiment and other means found for giving instructions, faking situations, and making observations. In the simplest case, if the purpose of work required from competitive teams is not to beat each other, but to manifest to observers their behavior when given insoluble tasks, the instructions should be written or at least tape-recorded after careful scrutiny; the observers should be operating with *absolutely concealed* long-distance TV. In the Asch experiment,[2] student participants were paid to lie about their perception of the relative length of two lines, so that Asch could study conformity, as first one and then more and more of a group were instructed to report a false perception. The results could have been accomplished better and more validly had the participants been given, in some automatic fashion not involving a human deceiver, distorting spectacles, so that at first one and later all but one would report a "false" perception, yet—as is the case in the real-life situation that Asch was attempting and failing to simulate—honestly reporting what they saw. The same kind of criticism can be made of the cross-cultural experiment[3] in which small boys, in several countries, were instructed to say "I won't" when their playmates wanted to undertake some activity. The fury expressed by the others, regardless of culture, which was supposed to prove the cross-cultural occurrence of the same responses is impossible to separate from a covert recognition of being duped. The creation of fool-proof, free-of-human hands, and free-of-human cue-giving experiments only requires a little patience and experimental imagination—as, for example, an experiment (devised by Alexander Bavelas) in which two partners who think they are working together in matching the levels of colored liquids in glass tubes are actually and quite honestly working at cross purposes because the buttons which control the levels of colored liquid are reversed. If the subjects have entered freely into a general agreement to undergo a variety of tests and are permitted to respond honestly, no stooges are used, and the situation is free of human cue-giving experimenters and observers; the need for debriefing, one of the rather lame methods used by human experimenters who lie, is also removed. The subjects need never be told what the mechanical devices were since their trust in other human beings has not been violated, as it is when human stooges or deceiving experimenters have to be involved in the experimental design. Our technology is sufficiently far advanced to make such mechanical surrogates for human involvement feasible. If the potential invalidity of all experiments where lying occurs is recognized, this will stimulate the use of other kinds of experiments. In the case of observation, it may take more time to gain the confidence of a group, or it may take more train-

---

mals are mercilessly tortured, and human subjects manipulated and brainwashed; in such cases where deep trust has been replaced by deep distrust, the experimental results will also be distorted.

ing to photograph without guile or intrusion; there *may* be cases where the observer must be disguised, as in the investigation of criminal or treasonable activities. These do not fall under the heading of science, but of civil rights.

Appendix II

*Study Program in Human Health and the Ecology of Man—China: Measures Taken for the Protection of Confidentiality in an Interdisciplinary Study of Health and Cultural Adaptation Based on Retrospective Life Histories**

by Rhoda Metraux
The American Museum
of Natural History

Certain problems of protection for human subjects are well exemplified by a study carried out with Chinese informants in the Study Program in Human Health and the Ecology of Man, New York Hospital-Cornell Medical Center, over a four-year period in the mid-1950's. This research, concerned with cultural aspects of health, was based on life-history data obtained through open-ended interviews, medical examinations, and projective tests administered by an interdisciplinary team of physicians, psychiatrists, clinical psychologists, and anthropologists. The one hundred informants, all of them unpaid volunteers who were fully briefed in the purposes of the research, had been reared in mainland China and were, with a few exceptions, living in New York City. They were highly educated business or professional men and women or students, selected through a liaison member of the small interacting community of Chinese exiles, and each of them was highly visible within that community. While the research was in progress, no report was given at a scientific meeting at which at least one member of the community was not present and no publication appeared that was not immediately circulated among Chinese readers. Protection of the subjects was crucial both for the sake of the informants themselves, who had shown considerable fortitude in volunteering, and in order to uphold confidence in the still ongoing research.

From the beginning, research reports necessarily dealt with intimate and often carefully guarded details of individual and family life history as well as data on the estimated intelligence and the medical, psychiatric, and psychological well-being of specific informants. Clearly the light disguises ordinarily used in medical reports were totally inadequate as a protective device. They were also inappropriate, as falsifications would

---

* The research program was carried out under the direction of the late Harold G. Wolff, as part of a series of studies relevant to cultural aspects of health.

inevitably distort findings that were based on the complex mosaic of individual characteristics and life experiences.

Two methods of presentation were devised to meet these difficulties. The first method is based on distantiation. It was used, for example, in an analysis of informants' ways of handling their relations with officers of the Immigration and Naturalization Service—an extremely touchy subject at that time. Using this method, descriptive and illustrative data were presented anecdotally, while the significant, highly individualized details that differentiated adaptive and maladaptive styles of response were codified and presented in tabular form. In this case, discussion is removed two steps from the original data, and further analysis would require taking a step back to the unpublished case-by-case comparisons. Nevertheless, the method permits one to make statements about the findings and to present the details, dissociated from individual life histories, that entered into the actual analysis.

The second method involves participation of the subjects themselves in the formulation of statements about their own life history and, inevitably, in the phrasing of conclusions. Using this method, the writer explained the purpose of the paper and in what way the information given by the subject was relevant to the problem under discussion. A draft version of the paper was given to the subject to read. Then, phrase by phrase, the author and the subject worked out how the data were to be treated in the formal presentation. Although it was a time-consuming process, it also became an invaluable research tool (particularly in a study in which informants were constrained to use a language not their own, in which subtle points of meaning were often mistranslated initially by the subject or the interviewer). Here, the context and phrasing of the informant's original interview statement (usually tape-recorded) provided a check against elaborations and rephrasing in the later discussion. In no case where this method was used was it impossible to find a way of wording a statement for publication.

But some understanding of Chinese culture and special cultural vulnerabilities was a necessary background for deciding which method was the appropriate one for handling various kinds of detail. Thus, for example, it was possible to discuss with a Chinese informant who had a classical, not a modern, education the difficulties he had had in adapting himself to a modern style of living or the break that this change in life style brought about in his relations to his parents, siblings, wife, and children. But it would not have been possible to discuss the hypothesis that estimated low intelligence played a part in a family's rejection of an eldest son and in their indifference to his increasing difficulty in carrying on an ordinary adult life. This was a hypothesis that could be discussed only indirectly with uninvolved informants and could be presented only in a form that protected the subject from the indignity of a public judgment of his incapacity and privately recognized loss of status in his family.

The most difficult cases to present were, on the whole, not those involving information that might dismay or anger Chinese subjects. The difficulties of getting access to certain kinds of information in interviews were enough to alert researchers to potential problems of public presentation. For example, Chinese informants were exceedingly reluctant to discuss illness in infancy; to do so was an implied attack (and it was used in this way) on their parents. Yet when this was clearly understood, informants could recollect and present relevant data, as they recognized that this is not an American viewpoint.

Much more difficult were situations that an American audience thought might be demeaning to a Chinese or that struck Americans as painful or ridiculous. Thus, once rapport was established, a Chinese subject had no difficulty in discussing a polygamous household, or a father's background as a warlord, or the effect of circumcision on later virility, or the effect of long years of celibacy on intellectual effort. The problem here is essentially one of protecting subjects belonging to one cultural tradition in terms of the sense of security and dignity characteristic of a different tradition. There is a kind of double-take involved in this. On the one hand, it is essential to be clear and to make clear to others what is, and what is not, demeaning within an alien tradition. But at a further remove, when working with highly sophisticated subjects, it is necessary to assume that they will find demeaning or shameful whatever is so regarded in the culture of the research worker who does not take into account the sensitivities of an audience of his own society. The problem comes down to this: how to present data about a subject in which he takes pride, but which *he* himself recognizes will be very differently regarded in another class, caste, or cultural setting. It is the most difficult, but today perhaps the most important form of protection that must somehow be given to human subjects.

Appendix III: The Case of John Howard Griffin, Author of *Black Like Me*[1]

During the discussion at the September, 1968, conference the question was raised as to whether John Howard Griffin's darkening his skin by a biochemical method so that he would be taken for a Negro and be able to explore the treatment of Negroes in the Southeast was an inadmissible type of deception. At the conference no details of that case were presented by the participant who raised the question. It is an interesting, perhaps crucial case in many ways.

John Howard Griffin is a novelist, who became blind during the early days of World War II, when he had to abandon a medical career and became actively involved in helping Jewish children escape from the Nazis. He returned, completely blind, to Texas with his family and lived on a small farm for twelve years, where he wrote six successful novels. In 1957, he regained his sight and was horrified, when he could *see*, to realize how close the caste relationships in the South were to the racial attitudes that he had abhorred when practiced by the Nazis. His attention became fixed on the question of color and the responses which white and black people made to color. In order to explore

172

this more thoroughly, he took a treatment that darkened his skin, was highly dangerous, and, in the form in which he took it, did him some irrevocable harm although the skin coloration was reversible. He then traveled through the South, finding out not what it was like to be a Negro, but how the indignities heaped on anyone suspected of being a Negro, and the help freely given by Negroes to others with a black skin, looked to a white man reared as he had been, protected from this knowledge.

As a commentary on this case I would say: (1) he was not a scientist but a writer with an ethical mission searching for material, as writers do search for material; (2) he took tremendous risks both with his personal safety, his sanity, and ultimately, after the book was published, with the life and the safety of his family—far out of proportion to any risk to which he exposed any of the people whom he met; (3) as his goal was to probe a situation—as a white man taken for a black man—his means were completely appropriate to his ends. Individuals whom he deceived in passing were not experimental subjects or part of any experimental situation, nor were they identified in a way through which they could even recognize themselves again.

I believe this case falls quite outside the range of those scientific explorations which I have condemned, in which (1) the deception is unnecessary, (2) is damaging to subject and experimenter, and (3) when revealed is damaging to the trust of the public in scientists as such.

Appendix IV

The Problem of an Unpredictable Future Position of an Individual Identified in a Research Project: 1953-1968 A Melanesian Leader in Papua, New Guinea

In 1953, Theodore Schwartz and I made an extensive study of a political movement in the Admiralty Islands, I as part of a restudy and Dr. Schwartz as a specific study of the movement and its native leader Paliau. At that time, Paliau had become known in many parts of the world, especially in Australia and in Roman Catholic circles, as a leader who had transformed a cargo cult into a successful political movement. He was well known as a sergeant in the police force of the Mandated Territory of New Guinea. During World War II, he found himself behind the Japanese lines and took the responsibility for organizing the food and living arrangements for indentured laborers from other islands who had been left on New Britain when Rabaul fell to the Japanese. After the war, it was impossible to try as traitors Melanesians from the Mandated Territory of New Guinea who had worked under the Japanese administration: members of the Trust Territory that owed no allegiance to Australia. An attempt, however, was made to punish them as war criminals. Paliau maintained that he and others arraigned with

173

him had been instructed by the Australians, when they evacuated Rabaul, to obey the Japanese. He successfully refuted the charges of being a war criminal, but his career in the police force was over. He returned to his own island of Balowan, and with many vicissitudes—a cargo cult, imprisonment for involvement in the cult under the heading of "spreading false rumors," an attack on his life by the insane former husband of a new wife, a trip to Port Moresby for "indoctrination"— he maintained a hold on some five thousand people whom he had succeeded in uniting in his new movement. He was first permitted to become chairman of half of this population, a local Council compound. While we were there in 1953, the local government Council authority was extended to the entire five thousand people, out of an estimated twenty thousand Admiralty Island inhabitants. It seemed unlikely at that time that he would increase his political importance further. Many local government officials were hostile; his original dream of operating in a larger sphere, including the entire Bismarck Archipelago, seemed completely incapable of realization.

In 1954, I wrote *New Lives for Old*,[1] and in 1958, Theodore Schwartz completed the manuscript of *The Paliau Movement in the Admiralty Islands, 1946-1954*.[2] In 1957, I discussed Paliau in one of the Terry Lectures at Yale as a man of unusual ability, comparable in quality to Churchill or Roosevelt, astonishing in a man who came from a small island group of only six hundred preliterate people. The Terry Lectures were published in 1946 under the title of *Continuities in Cultural Evolution*.[3]

In 1964, in the wake of the newly established electoral proceedings in New Guinea, Paliau was elected a member to the new House of Assembly for the Admiralty Islands, in spite of active opposition. In September of that year, on my way back to the Admiralties, I was interviewed in Sydney, Australia, by a reporter for the *Pacific Island Monthly*, who had taken the trouble to look up *Continuities in Cultural Evolution*, a book of a type not usually presented in the popular and highly politicized periodical. As a consequence, *Pacific Island Monthly* published Paliau's picture with a full-page article entitled, "Paliau Compared to Roosevelt." This article might have been a hazard to a man who continued to be the target of much local mission attack. But Dr. Schwartz and I had written our descriptions so that they could be read by anyone interested in the Paliau movement, and because Dr. Schwartz had painstakingly gone over the text with Paliau (who was now operating on a wider, much more politically important stage than when we had done our original writing), he could be proud, rather than hurt, by the discussions that had been published.

In 1967, National Education Television made a film[4] of anthropological work in Manus from 1928 to the present and included Paliau as a prominent figure. The filming ended in the autumn of 1967, and it was clear then that it would take approximately a year to complete the editing. The next election for the General Assembly was coming up in May-June of 1968. Had Paliau lost, it might have been said, then or later, by commentators on the responsibilities of social scientists working

174

Research with Human Beings: An Anthropological Model

among emerging peoples, that the film had lost him the election and his chance to be a significant molder of the future of Papua-New Guinea. However he was re-elected!

This case is presented in illustration of the vicissitudes of social research on living persons whose future roles cannot, in the nature of the case, be predicted.

REFERENCES

1. *Compendium on the Ethics of Human Experimentation.* Conference on the Ethical Aspects of Experimentation on Human Subjects, sponsored by *Dædalus* and the National Institutes of Health, November 3-4, 1967 (mimeographed; Boston, 1967).

2. Talcott Parsons, "Some Sociological Considerations Bearing Upon Research with Human Subjects," this volume.

3. Margaret Mead and Rhoda Metraux (eds.), *The Study of Culture at a Distance* (Chicago, 1953).

4. Margaret Mead, *Kinship in the Admiralty Islands* (New York, 1934), pp. 183-358.

5. Ethel J. Lindgren, "An Example of Culture Contact Without Conflict: Reindeer Tungus and Cossacks of Northwestern Manchuria," *American Anthropologist*, Vol. 40, No. 4 (October-December, 1938), pp. 605-621; Ethel J. Lindgren, "Field Work in Social Psychology in Eastern Asia," *First Congrés International des Sciences Anthropologiques et Ethnologiques,* London, 1934 (London, 1934), pp. 152-53; Michael Polyani, "Scientific Outlook: Its Sickness and Cure," *Science,* Vol. 125, No. 3246 (March, 1957), pp. 480-84.

6. Many social investigators in our own society will dispute this finding because the way in which scientific research has been presented has muddled the issue among ourselves and among ethnic groups within or in contact with larger societies. But I am presenting here the actual situation before these deformations of scientific work have been introduced, when genuine intellectual interest in something valued by those studied is quite sufficient to enlist cooperation.

7. Polyani, "Scientific Outlook: Its Sickness and Cure."

8. Theodore Schwartz, "The Paliau Movement in the Admiralty Islands, 1946-1954," *Anthropological Papers of The American Museum of Natural History,* Vol. 49, Part 2 (1962).

9. Oscar Lewis, *The Children of Sanchez* (New York, 1961).

10. John Paddock, "Oscar Lewis's Mexico; a review of *Five Families* and *The Children of Sanchez;* a review of Pedro Martinez; Private Lives and Anthropological Publications; Appendix: *The Children of Sanchez* in the Headlines," *Mesoamerican Notes,* Vol. 6 (Mexico City, 1965), pp. 3-144.

11. Margaret Mead, Theodosius Dobzhansky, Ethel Tobach, and Robert E. Light (eds.), *Science and the Concept of Race* (New York, 1968).

12. Margaret Mead and Rhoda Metraux, "Image of the Scientist Among High-School Students: A Pilot Study," *Science*, Vol. 126, No. 3270 (August 30, 1957), pp. 382-90.

13. Margaret Mead, "The Ethics of Insight-giving," *Male and Female* (New York, 1949), pp. 431-50; Margaret Mead, "The Social Responsibility of the Anthropologist," *Journal of Higher Education*, Vol. 33, No. 1 (January, 1962), pp. 1-12; Margaret Mead, Eliot D. Chapple, and Gordon G. Brown, "Report of the Committee on Ethics," *Human Organization*, Vol. 8, No. 2 (Spring, 1949), pp. 20-21; Margaret Mead, *The Changing Culture of an Indian Tribe* (New York, 1932).

14. Margaret Mead, "The Dangerous Godless Brain," *Look*, Vol. 22, No. 2 (January 21, 1958), pp. 20-27.

15. *The Biological Effects of Atomic Radiation: Summary Reports for a Study by The National Academy of Sciences* (Washington: National Academy of Sciences-National Research Council, 1966). C. H. Waddington, "The Biological Effects of Bomb Tests," *New Statesman and Nation* (June 8, 1957), pp. 725-28.

16. *AAAS Committee on Science in the Promotion of Human Welfare.* Margaret Mead, Chairman: Privacy and Research Involving Human Subjects, December 28, 1967. Program of the AAAS 134th Annual Meeting in New York City, December 26-31, 1967, p. 51; Herbert S. Dinerstein, "The Soviet Purge: 1953 Version," P-370 (Rand Corporation, 1953), pp. 1-25; Irving Ladimer and Roger W. Newman (eds.), *Clinical Investigation in Medicine: Legal, Ethical and Moral Aspects* (Boston, 1963); Margaret Mead, "From Black and White Magic to Modern Medicine," *Proceedings of the Rudolf Virchow Medical Society*, Vol. 22 (1965), pp. 130-31. This paper has been abstracted from lectures given at Harvard Medical School in 1960 ("The George W. Gay Lectures Upon Medical Ethics") and at the Rudolf Virchow Medical Society in 1963.

17. Guido Calabresi, "Reflections on Medical Experimentation in Humans," this volume.

18. John R. Platt, "Diversity," *Science*, Vol. 154, No. 3753 (December 2, 1966), pp. 1132-39.

19. Calabresi, "Reflections on Medical Experimentation in Humans."

APPENDIX I

1. Stanley Milgram, "Some Conditions of Obedience and Disobedience to Authority," *Human Relations*, Vol. 18, No. 1 (1965), pp. 57-76.

2. S. E. Asch, "Studies in the Principles of Judgments and Attitudes. II. Determination of Judgments by Group and by Ego Standards," *Journal of Social Psychology*, Vol. 12 (November, 1940), pp. 433-65.

3. Stanley Schachter, "Cross-Cultural Experiments on Threat and Rejection," *Human Relations*, Vol. 7, No. 4 (November, 1954), pp. 403-39.

APPENDIX II

Lawrence E. Hinkle, Jr., John W. Gittinger, Leo Goldberger, *et al.*, "Studies in Human Ecology: Factors Governing the Adaptation of Chinese Unable to Return to China," *Experimental Pathology* (New York, 1957), pp. 170-86.

Lawrence E. Hinkle, Jr., Norman Plummer, Rhoda Metraux, *et al.*, "Studies in Human Ecology: Factors Relevant to the Occurrence of Bodily Illness and Disturbances in Mood, Thought and Behavior in Three Homogeneous Population Groups," *American Journal of Psychiatry*, Vol. 114, No. 3 (1957), pp. 212-20.

Rhoda Metraux, "Life Stress and Health in a Changing Culture," *Family Mental Health and the State* (London, 1955), pp. 113-26.

Rhoda Metraux, "Childhood Security and Adult Adaptation: Some Effects of Culture Change on Health Among Chinese." Paper presented at the annual meeting of the American Orthopsychiatric Association, New York, 1956.

William E. Mitchell, "Persistence and Innovation of Cultural Behavior in an Alien Society: A Study in Behavioral Adaptation Based on Perceptions by Twenty-Six College Educated Chinese Living in New York City 1955-56, of United States Immigration Law and Procedures," Master's Thesis, Columbia University, 1957.

APPENDIX III

1. John H. Griffin, *Black Like Me* (Boston, 1961).

APPENDIX IV

1. Margaret Mead, *New Lives for Old: Cultural Transformation, Manus 1928-1953* (New York, 1956; reprinted with a new preface, New York, 1966).

2. Schwartz, "The Paliau Movement in the Admiralty Islands, 1946-1954."

3. Margaret Mead, *Continuities in Cultural Evolution* (New Haven, 1964).

4. Craig Gilbert, producer and director, *Margaret Mead's New Guinea Journal* (National Educational Television, New York, 1968), 16 mm, 90 min., sound, color.

GUIDO CALABRESI

Reflections on Medical Experimentation in Humans

THE PROBLEM of experimentation on humans necessarily looks rather different to one who has concentrated on accident law than it does to the doctor or even to the jurisprude. The torts professor sees the possibility of a choice between the life, well-being, or comfort of a given patient and the lives or well-being of unknown future patients. He is immediately struck that the issue in medical experimentation is the risking of lives to save other lives while in accident law, almost always, the issue is the taking of lives simply because saving them costs too much.

In torts law, we have become accustomed to the fact that many activities are permitted, even though *statistically* we know they will cost lives, since it costs too much to engage in these activities more safely or to abstain from them altogether. We have grade crossings, even though we know that with grade crossings a certain number of people will be killed each year and even though grade crossings could be eliminated relatively easily. We use automobiles—knowing that they cost us fifty thousand lives each year—because to use safer, slower means of transport would be far too costly in terms of pleasures and profits foregone. Worse even than that, we use automobiles with relatively cheap (but relatively dangerous) tires, airports with relatively cheap (but relatively dangerous) control systems, and so on *ad infinitum*. And we do this because we deem the lives taken to be cheaper than the costs of avoiding the accidents in which they are taken.

From the perverse standpoint of accident law, then, the whole fury about medical experimentation would seem to be a tempest in a teapot. Surely it is more justifiable to take some lives in order to save more lives than it is to take lives simply to save money, as we do in the accident field. But this view, I fear, is far too superficial. Even in the accident field, there are many occasions when we do treat life as a pearl beyond price. When a known individual is trapped in a coal mine, we try to rescue him at enormous money cost and even at the risk of many other lives. Yet if we always gave human life the value we give to the life of the man in the coal mine, we would surely abolish grade crossings, make cars and airports much safer, and perhaps even forbid "non-essential" driving completely. What is the meaning of this apparent paradox? And what does it tell us about medical experimentation?

The first possible explanation has to do with statistics. Somehow a man is less a man to us when he is simply a number. We know the man trapped in the coal mine, just as we often know the patient subjected to experimentation. The statistical accident victim we do not know, and so we can ignore him. But that is not in itself an adequate explanation. The statistical victim is just as real as the man in the coal mine. If we want to be fully rational, we must admit to ourselves that he has as much of a family as a known victim, that he and they suffer as much when he is killed, and that only a willful ignoring of reality enables us to treat him as less real than the man trapped in the coal mine.

But perhaps this willful ignoring of statistical victims is less foolish, though no more "rational," than it might seem at first glance. We are committed to "humanism," to the dignity of the individual, and to human life. Much of the fabric of our society depends on our belief in this commitment, as do most of our traditional and "cherished" liberties. Accident law indicates that our commitment to human life is not, in fact, so great as we say it is; that our commitment to life-destroying material progress and comfort is greater. But this fact merely accentuates our need to make a bow in the direction of our commitment to the sanctity of human life (whenever we can do so at a reasonable total cost). It also accentuates our need to reject any societal decisions that too blatantly contradict this commitment. Like "free will," it may be less important that this commitment be total than that we believe it to be there.

Perhaps it is for these reasons that we save the man trapped in the coal mine. After all, the event is dramatic; the cost, though great, is unusual; and the effect in reaffirming our belief in the sanctity of human lives is enormous. The effect of such an act in maintaining the many societal values that depend on the dignity of the individual is worth the cost. Abolishing grade crossings might save more lives and at a substantially smaller cost per life saved, but the total cost to society would be far greater and the dramatic effect far less. I fear that if men got caught in coal mines with the perverse frequency with which cars run into trains at grade crossings, we would be loath to rescue them; it would, in the aggregate, cost too much. Lest this remark seem unduly cynical, we might consider our past unwillingness to keep all but a few victims of renal failure alive by use of artificial kidneys. Until now, artificial kidneys have cost too much, and people perversely have suffered kidney failure too frequently, so even though the victim was as clearly known to those who had to decide whether to save him as is the man in the mine, the answer quite frequently was no.

It should be clear that the foregoing does not mean that individual human life is not valued highly. Nor, certainly, does it suggest that we are indifferent to when and how society should choose to sacrifice lives. Quite the contrary; it indicates that there is a deep conflict between our fundamental need constantly to reaffirm our belief in the sanctity of life and our practical placing of some values (including future lives) above an individual life. That conflict suggests, at the very least, the need for a quite complex structuring to enable us *sometimes* to sacrifice lives, but hardly ever to do it blatantly and as a society, and above all to allow this sacrifice only under quite rigorous controls. (This last desire to control individual takings and yet to keep society from being the blatant taker itself reflects a conflict of desires.) I suggest that the problem with human experimentation lies in the fact that, unlike accidents, it has seemed to be quite unamenable to most of the complex "indirect" controls over takings of lives we have so far developed in our society.

In the field of accidents, much of the control over the taking of human lives is accomplished by what economists call the market. Limbs and lives are given a money value; the activities that take lives or limbs in accidents pay the victims; and people quite coldly decide whether it is cheaper to install a safety device or to pay for the accidents that occur because the safety device is missing. Despite the enormous oversimplification of the foregoing example (the effect of "fault" in determining accident payments, for instance, is ignored), it indicates how "accidents" are controlled in an indirect fashion which, nonetheless, takes into account both the values of lives taken and the cost of saving them.

Reflections on Medical Experimentation in Humans

The beauty of the market device is that no one seems to be making the decisions to take lives and, therefore, no blatant infringement of the commitment to human life as sacred occurs. Moreover, when society *does* enter into the accident field directly, it is usually to impose more stringent prohibitions, regulations, or safety standards than the market would bring about. We do not allow drunken driving—any more than we allow murder—even though the drunk may be perfectly willing to compensate his victim. The consequence is that collective societal action seems always to be directed toward preserving the individual life rather than taking it, and our commitment is further strengthened. (Only a few professors worry that failure to go beyond the market in areas where the individual choice to take lives is less obvious than in drunken driving or murder is also a societal decision, but one which lets lives be taken. Such ratiocinations of professors happily do not destroy the picture of a self-contained system in which almost all collective decisions are life-saving ones.)

Other elements of accident law serve to reduce still further the blatantness of the taking. In many situations, the victim can be said to have, to some extent at least, consented to the risk. Consent is often actually very dubious. Are we, in fact, free to avoid driving cars? Is a tunnel-digger free to engage in a safer occupation? And is there any consent at all when a pedestrian is run down by a car? But these questions are neither here nor there. They would be crucial were free consent the keystone of the system (as it may have to be in medical experiments). Where, however, consent serves merely to lessen further the directness of a taking that is already controlled by a seemingly impersonal system, even semi-free consent suffices to support the belief that our society prizes individual lives above all.

The same is true about the introduction of moral elements like fault into a system of accident law. The search for a faulty party on whom damages must rest can seriously undermine the market control system I have described. For this and other reasons, fault may well be on its way out. This is especially true since too many people have come to realize that frequently the search for a faulty party in an accident is either a sham or a fraud. When people still believed otherwise, however, the semblance of a search for a faulty party served, like consent, to reinforce the belief that the level of accidents was a matter of individual choice and not something society determined.

Finally, the temporal juxtaposition of decisions to avoid accidents and lives taken serves to make "accidental" takings of lives seem less blatant. At the time a decision to adopt a safety device is to be made, the cost of the device is both present and real; the accident costs to be saved may also be statistically known; but the lives themselves are in the future and seem conjectural. Once again, if the decision is made against the device, even the individual making the decision—let alone society—does not seem to be choosing "certainly" to destroy lives.

In medical experiments, much of this process seems reversed. It is the lives to be saved by the experiment that seem future and conjectural, while the life to be risked or taken is both present and real. Most of the elements of fault are absent—the victim usually is sick through no choice or fault of his own. As a result, only the possible presence of consent seems left to lessen the blatantness of the choice to risk a life. But consent can no more do the whole job here than it can in accidents. Totally free consent is simply too rare an animal. The usual semi-free consent serves in accident situations because it reinforces an adequate system of control governing more generally when lives are to be taken, but without seeming to infringe on our basic commitment to human life. Just such a system of control is needed in medical experimentation.

Perhaps, however, we have accepted the analogy between medical experiments and accidents too quickly. It may be that the taking of lives that happens in accident situations is different in substance from the taking that occurs in medical experiments, or would occur were we to let the man trapped in a coal mine die. If there is a difference that goes beyond the matter of appearances, beyond the existence in accidents of a complex self-operating system of control, then the problem of medical experiments cannot be solved simply by devising complex, indirect control mechanisms to balance society's interest in present as against future lives.

The nub of the argument is this: The notion is incorrect that we in some sense choose the number of people who will be killed in automobile accidents by choosing a market system that will determine how much safety is worth. The notion is only made plausible by a verbal trick—by using the words "we choose" to describe both the effects of the social system in which we live and which we tolerate, but which we cannot in fact be said to choose, and events as to which we can be said to exercise purposive choice. "We" do not choose automobile accidents, the argument runs, any more than "we" choose a world in which hundreds of thousands of Indians die young of disease and lack of food. We do not choose this because the alternative is never presented in a realistic enough fashion; it is never presented so that the costs of saving the Indians are clear. The costs of saving the Indians, like the costs of avoiding automobile accidents, are the costs of moving from an existing social system to a new one. As such, they are unknown and involve a substantial risk that, whatever pattern of life the new system brings, *more* lives will be taken than in the old system. How different, the argument concludes, is this passive tolerance of the world as it is from the active choice to let someone caught in a coal mine die, or from the decision to risk an individual human life in a medical experiment.[1]

I do not believe that this argument destroys the usefulness of the analogy between medical experiments and automobile accidents. In a way, it is no more than a mixture of two quite different points. First, a choice to save a life at the price of paying readily ascertainable costs is very different from a choice to save lives when the saving would be accomplished only by a radical restructuring of society entailing unknown costs. This point is certainly true, but does not distinguish many accident situations from medical experiments. Second, there is a genuine difference between a positive choice to subject someone to a risk or to take his life and a passive acquiescence in a system that results in lives being taken when they could be saved at ascertainable costs. This second is a distinction which, I claim, has only psychological significance. Because the choice to take lives is less obvious, it is less destructive of the essential myth that human life is a pearl beyond price.

There are, to be sure, accident situations where lives could be saved only by restructuring our whole social system. Giving up the automobile altogether might be an example. It is hard to know what the full costs of that decision would be, or whether in the end the change would save or cost more lives. As such, it is fair to say that we do not choose to take lives by having automobiles in the same sense as we choose to let the man in the mine die if we fail to rescue him. But there are other situations where lives can be saved without such a radical change. Abolition of grade crossings, differently made automobiles, and more safely constructed highways—all would save lives in exchange for readily determinable costs. We can (but do not) require these. We allow their establishment to be controlled by the market. What is more, we readily observe the results of market control. We then discuss in Congress whether intervention is justified, and we often decide not to intervene. In our passivity, we are choosing to let the indirect market control method make the choice between lives and costs, and no amount of talk about merely tolerating an existing social system can change that.

But this second point may be more subtle. It may center on the fact that there is no one who can clearly be identified with the "we" in the last paragraph. No one has purposefully chosen the market method of controlling accidents, and no one, in our society, has the clear responsibility for making radical changes in the method. These facts happily leave us with the feeling that no one is directly responsible for any specific life taken and that neither as individuals nor as a society do we choose against lives in order to save money. Yet it remains true that we are unlikely to want to scrap the system of control that luckily has come into being. And to say this is precisely to say that a method which gives *satisfactory* control of the choice between lives and cost is operating without anyone bearing the onus of having purposefully chosen the method, let alone the onus of seeming to destroy individual lives for the sake of money. Since no adequate control system over medical experiments has arisen by itself, we cannot avoid the onus of working purposefully toward establishing a control system. This indicates that we will not end with so psychologically satisfactory a result as we have in the field of accidents. But, if anything, this fact heightens the need for establishing a system in which the actual choice over the taking of lives is as diffuse as possible.

Thus, the question remains as to whether or not we can find a control system in the medical experiment field that affords an adequate balancing of present against future lives and is still sufficiently indirect and self-enforcing as to avoid clear and purposive choices to kill individuals for the collective good. It is not my purpose in this article to suggest any complete control system for medical experiments. That task—even if feasible—would require an intimate knowledge of medicine. A few of the problems involved in establishing a control system and a few suggestions leading toward such a system can, however, be mentioned.

In the first place, a direct collective societal control—like approval of research plans by a qualified government agency—is not the answer. Not only is such a device likely to be too cumbersome but, perhaps more importantly, it seems to place the whole society in the position of openly approving the taking of individual lives. Analogy to accident law suggests that this situation is to be avoided if possible, and that the best role for the government is that of watchdog to step in and demand higher standards in specific situations where a general control system, independent of the government, has failed to work adequately.

Leaving the choice to the individual doctor might be all right were there some way to insure that such a choice would tend to coincide with the choice between present and future lives that society wants. No exact correspondence is needed (any more than we require the market to bring about a perfect correspondence between accidents and costs of avoiding them). But there must be the assurance that, on the whole, the individual choice will approach what society would choose. Unfortunately, there is no such assurance today. Some doctors will be too concerned with the individual patient and thereby sacrifice too many future lives by cutting off an experiment too soon. Others will be too concerned with the unassailability of their results and, therefore, continue an experiment beyond the point at which society's interest in future lives is met. We cannot, moreover, rely on individual consciences to reduce these errors, because individual doctors do not and cannot know the degree to which our society wants present risks to be taken for future benefits. And the best a conscience can do is make individuals adhere to society's wants as these are made known by society. In contrast, the beauty of the accident system, with all its faults, is that through the market it conveys to individual deciders what society more or less wants without requiring an identifiable societal statement. (Furthermore it relies on self-interest rather than conscience to effectuate even this decision.)

It may be that no analogous system can be established for medical experiments that would control the degree to which present lives are to be risked for future benefits and yet put no one in the position of making the moral choice. I, certainly, am not going to propose such a system here. I will, however, suggest how a market device might be used to supplement other systems of control. I do not at this stage suggest that the market device I am setting out is desirable, or even worth its administrative costs. I set it out in the hope that examination of the use of similar devices will be stimulated.

The basic device would be a compensation fund for subjects injured in unsuccessful experiments.[2] A separate fund would exist at each medical center where experiments on humans were being undertaken. Moneys for the fund could come from two sources—income from successful results of previous experiments, such as new marketable drugs, and grants from government or foundations based on the expectation that the researches undertaken would be more than worth the moneys used to compensate those subjects who were injured. The effect of such a fund—apart from compensating the victims, which may be desirable in itself—would be to stimulate greater analysis within each medical center of the possible benefits and risks a given experiment entails.

There are five principal difficulties with using such a fund in helping to control medical experiments. First, any compensation system is bound to be unacceptable if it directly or indirectly suggests that a doctor is at "fault" when a properly structured experiment fails. Second, often experiments may in a sense be successful, and yet the subject will nonetheless die or fail to recover completely. (He may have lived longer or as long as he would have had he been in the control group, and yet it may be difficult to show that his death was not due to the experiment.) Third, it may be hard to distinguish a subject in a medical experiment from the ordinary patient who, presumably, would not be compensated simply because the treatment chosen for him failed. Fourth, the institutions in which medical experiments are undertaken are typically charitable and, hence, not subject to market pressures in the usual sense. Fifth, the system may unduly hamper research in new or small medical centers. All of these difficulties are serious, but none is insurmountable.

The first three are best treated together since they all pertain to the fact-finding and administration needed to award compensation. A judicial system for deciding the issues seems totally inappropriate. It smacks too much of finding mistakes or wrongdoing and, as such, would be unacceptable. Accordingly, the best way of handling the issues would be for medical centers to institute such funds voluntarily and establish administrative boards to resolve questions of fact arising under the fund. It is to be hoped that the boards would be regional (so that no center could chisel on its own unlucky experiments) and staffed primarily by scientists. Since payments would, at least initially, be a matter of practice rather than contract, the findings of such panels would come to be regarded as final. (Ultimately, this practice would be likely to change as subjects came to expect payment, but by then the tradition and function of the panels would have been established and judicial review would probably not be harmful.) The boards would determine, first, whether the injured party was, in fact, a subject in an experiment or a member of a control group for such an experiment; and, second, whether he had suffered damage as a result of being a subject; and, finally, what the appropriate compensation would be under established schedules of damages.

Determination of whether the injured party was a "subject" could be made on the basis of something like the following criterion: Would the "subject's" own personal physician (responsible only for his patient's welfare and not for the advancement of knowledge) have recommended such a course of treatment—not only at the start, but throughout the course of the "experiment" —if he had available to him the information that the experimenters had (or would have had but for use of a double-blind experimental format)? It may be readily seen that this criterion may provide compensation for members of control groups as well as actual subjects. It also considers that a person may become a "subject"—that is, be treated in a fashion based on society's best interest rather than his own—not just at the beginning of an experiment, but anywhere along its course. For this reason, and to protect the possibility of double-blind experiments, the criterion deems relevant any knowledge that the experimenters would have had, but for the experimental format chosen.

Determination of damages would be difficult for the boards. But the issues are, in fact, no harder than those faced in establishing damages before non-expert groups, as is done throughout accident law. As such, there is no reason to discuss them here.

The problem of avoiding the stigma of fault or wrongdoing also does not come up in the hypothetical system described. I do not suggest that such funds be used in place of other controls over medical experiments on humans, but only as additional controls. It follows that all the experiments I am considering will have successfully gone through whatever procedures are established for examining and approving, in plan and design, any experiment involving human beings. Failure to carry out the experiment in accordance with the approved plan and negligence in carrying out the plan would not be issues to be decided by the panels set up to administer the compensation fund. The first would be subject to whatever sanctions were made part of the pre-experiment approval procedures. The second would remain, as it is now, a part of the law of malpractice. In neither case would such determinations be needed or even useful in deciding the issue of compensation from the fund.

The fourth difficulty in using a compensation fund as an added control on medical experiments in humans arises because such experiments are usually carried out in charitable institutions. Accordingly, it may be questioned whether financial pressures have the same effect on such institutions as they are said to have in competitive industries. Would the need to pay compensation for experiments that fail cause greater care within each institution in selecting experiments and experimenters, or would it simply put pressure on the institution to try only those experiments that have the greatest potential market payoff, regardless of the scientific importance of the results? There is no doubt that some pressure for marketable results would come from such a system. But the market is not the primary or even the secondary source of funds for such institutions. These sources are the government and charitable contributions, which would continue to give according to their judgment of the reputation of the institution and researcher involved. And reputations are based largely on past successful researches—quite apart from whether the past research got financial recognition in the market or only acclaim in the scientific community. It seems unlikely, therefore, that basic research of real promise would suffer from the existence of a compensation fund.

In fact, if one views research institutions as industries that have two possible markets for their products (one the industrial market, the other the scientific community), both of which reward successes handsomely in straight financial terms, the analogy to normal market control situations becomes quite striking. In each case, the payoff for success is notable, and the point of market control is to bring the real costs involved in trying something new to the attention of those who will decide whether the attempt is worth the risks.

The fifth problem with employing a compensation fund is the danger that research in new or small medical centers will be hampered. There is no doubt that it will. A new or small medical center must find an angel. It must convince someone that what it proposes to try is important enough to justify the potential compensation-liability as well as the cost of doing the experiment itself. But, I would suggest, this is precisely the point of the market control system. Not all medical research that involves risks to humans can be justified. One way of determining if it is justified is by seeing whether there is enough confidence in the proposed experiment or in the research center where the experiment would be carried out to fund payment not only for the test tubes and animals used, but also for the human beings who may suffer injury in the experiment. If there is not, it is a fair sign that the particular experiment is too risky (in relation to its possible beneficial results) to be tried by the particular research team or center. Professor Everett Mendelsohn of Harvard has suggested on various occasions that most significant pioneering research is, in fact, carried out by a very few people in a very few places. If this is so, requiring research centers to meet the full cost of experiments (including the cost of injuries to subjects) may be one of the least invidious ways of concentrating risky research among those who can do it best.

One may summarize the use of a compensation fund in the following way. Requiring compensation of injured subjects causes the full cost of research in humans to be placed on the research center. Accordingly, approval by the center of a particular experiment will require conscious consideration not only of the possible payoff (either in market or scientific terms), but also of the risks, converted to money, that the project entails. This may not deter many experiments, but it may cause those involved in the most risky or least useful ones to consider carefully whether the experiment is worth it, whether it is best done by those who propose to do it, and whether there is an alternative, and safer, way of obtaining approximately the same results. It may well be that all these considerations are already firmly in the minds of the experimenters. If so, nothing is changed by requiring compensation. But if researchers—like auto makers, coal-mine owners, and the rest of mankind—tend to consider costs and benefits a bit more carefully when money is involved, a useful added control device will have been imposed.

I should again make clear that I am not proposing the compensation fund as the best way of introducing market controls in the area of medical experiments. I have described the fund at some length primarily to indicate that very little work has gone into the search for complex control devices that would balance present against future lives and still put no one in the position of clearly deciding against individual lives. Examination and refinement of devices like the compensation fund by people who are involved in medical research seem, to me, to offer considerably more promise than further elaborations on the infinite varieties of consent that are currently the mainstay of symposia on human experimentation.

I do not believe, however, that market controls, no matter how well studied, can ever do most of the job of balancing present and future lives in medical experiments. At best, they can just add another dimension to existing or proposed controls. In this way, they can make the total control system more indirect and hence reduce the appearance that any given individual or government agency is deciding to take individual lives for the collective good. Any other control devices used must also represent both the individual's interests and those of society and yet not be governmental, since to introduce the government too directly in the process is to place the whole of society in the position of deciding against the individual.

Given this fact, perhaps the best general system of control would be the oft-suggested establishment of groups (hospital committees, say) that are sufficiently broadly based so that their judgment can reflect society's unspoken choice between present and future risks, and yet unofficial enough so that they do not seem to represent the government choosing to sacrifice the individual for the good of the collective. Society, in the form of the government, could retain its position as the protector of individual lives and step in mainly to establish stricter rules in areas where the unofficial groups had erred and allowed lives to be taken too blatantly or in a way that undermined our commitment to human dignity.

If hospital committees are to bear the main burden of overseeing experiments and experimental plans, if they are to be the principal instruments for balancing risks to present lives against future benefits, ways must be found of increasing the information that is available to these committees. It is not enough that they be made up of people of good will; their members must also be people who have available to them some sense of the balance that society desires between present and future lives. The difficulty here, of course, is that this sense cannot be given by government decrees, since that would involve society too clearly in the process of choosing against individuals. The sense of society's wishes must, instead, be brought to the committees through as many varied inputs as possible. In effect, the more the inputs of information and value judgments to the committees are broadened, the more the committees will seem to be doing no more than ratifying broad judgments inherent in the social system. In this way, the directness—the playing God by any single group—is reduced. This would be especially true if, in addition to the committees, there was not only some kind of market test (of the type I described) to be met, but also government intervention from time to time to protect individual lives by requiring more care than either the market or the committees deemed necessary.

The most obvious—but probably least important—method of broadening the input to the committees is by broadening the committees themselves. Many of these are now made up primarily of scientists from the very medical center where the research to be approved is to take place. The presence of scientists from other research centers and the presence of non-scientific members would certainly give the committees a greater sense of where the crucial balance is to be struck. My own guess is that while scientists from other medical centers would on occasion be stricter than local scientists in approving particular experiments, non-scientists on the committees would tend, on the whole, to approve some experiments that would not now be passed. This is especially true where the potential gains from an experiment are great, but the risks involved are also great. In such areas, I suggest, doctors are perhaps unduly hampered by fear of lawsuits (incidentally, the reduction of fear of such suits might be a side benefit of the kind of market compensation system I have described) and by the worthy tradition that, after all, the individual patient is in their care. Laymen, I believe, are less likely to be so emotionally concerned with either of these two factors and, hence, are more likely to give greater weight to society's long-run interest.

All this is conjecture, however. The best way of testing lay reaction to particular experiments—indeed, the best way of broadening the inputs to the committees—lies in another device: publication of the cases decided by the committees. Such cases could well be anonymous (at least at first). They could be collected and published in much the same way that decisions of courts are collected. The reports on any case could include, first, a factual part describing, among other things, the experience of the experimenter, the antecedent tests in non-human subjects, the major risks perceived, the scientific gains perceived possible, the availability of subsequent controls to limit the risks, the origin and life expectancy of the subjects, and the nature of the consent and the manner in which it was obtained; and, second, a jurisprudential section containing the decision of the committee (whether favorable or unfavorable), together with the principal arguments made for and against the decision reached.

Such published cases would soon become the subject of intense study both inside and outside the medical profession. Analyses in learned journals by lawyers, doctors, and historians of science would inevitably follow. These would undoubtedly re-argue the more important or path-breaking cases. If law cases are any guide, the analyses would sometimes conclude that the cases were wrongly decided, but frequently that they were rightly decided, and perhaps more frequently that they were rightly decided but for the wrong reasons. To the extent that Law Reviews consider themselves courts of last appeal beyond the highest courts in the land, so would the learned journals in which this *giurisprudenza* would be dissected. From all this, a sense of what society at large deems proper in medical experiments might well arise. This sense would, in turn, guide the committees and make their decisions more sophisticated. The result would not only be better thought out decisions, but also a more complex system of controls, which, in effect, took into account much broader sources of information as to societal values. In addition, the very existence of open criticism through published cases would reduce the finality of the judgment of any given committee. They might decide one case improperly, but the community would have the feeling that over time its judgments as to the proper balance of present risks against future gains would make itself felt. Moreover, this method of introducing community views would, at least in part, avoid the dangers of governmental rule-making, for at no given time would the community as such seem to be choosing to take an individual life for the general good. (Of course, the presence of published cases— even if anonymous—might make information available that could lead to lawsuits; one advantage of the compensation fund described earlier is that, since compensation would already be given to the injured subject, no lawsuits and hence no attribution of fault would occur.)

Three practical objections can be made to the publication of hospital committee decisions. The first is that such publication would destroy the confidentiality of research and might result in the pirating of good ideas. The second is that hospital committees do not now ask for any very definite indication of the possible scientific benefits perceived in an experiment, but concentrate only on the risks to the subjects and the experience and reputation of the experimenter. As a result, it is argued, publication would be of little use in establishing the balance between risks and benefits that the public at large desires. The third objection is that published hospital committee decisions would not reflect the actual facts before the committee. Committees, to protect themselves, would so emphasize those facts that favored their decision that the results reached would seem to be obvious in every case.

The first objection, if valid, can easily be met by providing for delay in publication until after the experiment itself is completed and published. Since the aim of publication is not to pass judgment on the particular experiment, but to encourage debate (for the guidance of future committees) on which experiments are desirable and which are not, delay in publication causes no particular problems. The important point is that real cases be examined; whether the examination takes place immediately or two years after an experiment is approved or forbidden matters relatively little.

The second objection is, I believe, misplaced. It may well be that most experiments involve sufficiently small risks so that, given the reputation of the experimenter and the type of consent obtained, no specific indication of benefits foreseen is needed to justify approving the experiment. In every case where this was so, the published opinion of the committee should indicate that. And I would expect that such judgments based on low risk and high reputation would find support among most commentators. If, however, a very high-risk experiment were either approved or turned down without an attempt to learn why the experiment seemed to the investigator to be worth doing, I would expect that there would be substantial criticism. Such criticism might well bring about a change in current practice and enable some experiments that would now be turned down, absent consideration of the possible benefits of the experiment, to take place. Conversely, other experiments that involved substantial risks might not be deemed worthwhile given their small possible benefits. Either response to societal desires made known through publication and criticism would be more desirable than blind approval or rejection of a dangerous experiment.

The final objection—that written committee decisions would not represent the true facts on which the decisions were based—would seem more damaging if a similar criticism could not be made of many court decisions; yet the usefulness of publishing legal opinions remains enormous. Commentators would soon become as adept at divining the issues involved in a hospital committee decision as are legal commentators at analyzing a judicial opinion. The informed criticism of both negative and positive decisions that would follow would, I venture to predict, lose no more from the fact that the opinions would, to some extent, be artificial and stylized than does the analogous legal criticism lose from the same defect in court opinions. Thus, publication, even if the opinions were to some extent artificial, would remain a highly significant device for broadening hospital committee deliberations and thereby increasing and diversifying societal control of medical experiments.

It should be emphasized that a device like hospital committees, even if broadened in the ways described, is still fairly direct in comparison to the system of accident control. This directness will affect not only the degree of satisfaction with the device and the frequency of governmental intervention to cure results too damaging to individual lives, but also the very balance to be struck between present and future lives. Society's best choice between future and present lives itself depends on the adequacy of the control device adopted. Thus, if the control device is fairly direct, we can expect that this directness will be counterbalanced by giving a greater weight to present lives than would be the case were a more subtle and indirect control system found.

Once an adequate system of control is established, consent can play a significant role. Although we do not trust "consent" to be the "control" element determining when experiments are in society's interest, we are quite willing to use the presence of some form of consent to justify the taking of lives if other forms of control are present. The more the choice for taking lives is direct or official, however, the more crucial the consent element becomes, and the more real the consent must be. In such circumstances, only consent or its semblance keeps us from blatantly destroying the fabric of our commitment to human dignity. If instead the choice is indirect, unclear, or uncertain—for example, where the risk to the individual is minute or where no group is choosing a given individual as a victim—then we probably can allow forms of consent that could not carry the weight of a more obvious or more official choice. This is, of course, what happens in the field of accidents and what might happen in medical experiments as more adequate and complex controls are developed.

I do not wish to appear to be undercutting consent. My own feeling is that some form of consent should always be required. I feel it is the minimum that our society requires in striking the balance between present and future lives. But consent by itself is not enough. We do not, after all, allow a murderer to murder simply because he can find a victim willing to be murdered. Nor are we willing to have a completely volunteer army in time of war. In practice, the extent to which we allow people to consent to risks is a product of many factors. These include the degree of information available to the consenter, the extent to which he can psychologically comprehend the risk involved, and the types of pressures (both financial and moral) on him to go along. But they also include not only the benefits to society that might occur from his consenting, but also the controls available both over the way his consent is obtained and over the activities that involve risks to the consenter in exchange for possible good to society. The type of consent that is enough for one situation is not adequate in another. And just as the type of consent given becomes a factor in deciding whether a particular experiment is acceptable, so the types of other controls available become factors in determining what kind of consent is sufficient to justify a given experiment.

The crucial aim in all this remains the same, however. On the one hand, we want decisions that reflect societal choices and societal control when victims are taken for the common good. On the other hand, we do not want society to lose its role of protector of individual lives. These desires conflict, but both are essential to a decent society. Areas other than medical experimentation have managed more or less adequately to accommodate these conflicting needs. So far, medical experimentation has hardly tried. Consent, though useful in preserving the ideal that society hardly ever condones the sacrifice of an individual against his will, is unlikely to suffice where a too obvious societal choice to take victims is involved. Even more important, consent cannot serve as the general control system determining when the future good requires the taking of present lives. Accordingly, scholars seriously concerned with the problem of saving future lives and at the same time not undermining our commitment to the sanctity of individual present lives ought to be devoting themselves to the development of a workable but not too obvious control system, rather than to the spinning-out of theories of consent.

REFERENCES

1. This point was powerfully made by Professor Erving Goffman of the University of California, Berkeley, at the November, 1967, *Dædalus* conference on experimentation on human subjects.

2. The idea of a compensation fund is in no sense original. It has, however, usually been suggested as a device for easing the plight of the victim. I am not here suggesting it for that purpose (worthy though it may be), but rather as a way of introducing an additional control element over when a medical experiment is considered worthwhile.

LOUIS L. JAFFE

Law as a System of Control

I WOULD start with a truism. There is today in this country an enormous dynamic of human experimentation to which not only the medical profession but also the general public is heavily committed. This is concretely manifested by the enormous grants for medical research made by government and by the great foundations. Arguably the public's concern for physical well-being is excessive and possibly self-defeating. It may increase anxiety and create some of the problems medicine seeks to solve. If this is true, we might discount the exigent claims made for experimentation. No doubt those who aspire to moral leadership should temper popular excess. If obsession with health leads to disregard of spiritual values, it is our business to right the balance. But what we are seeking here is an institutional morality; and unless it is based on a realistic estimate of the forces at work, it will be more honored in the breach than the acceptance. Medical men want to experiment, and the public approves of experimentation. An occasional catastrophe will touch off a public outcry with consequent overreaction, but on the whole the public continues to finance and to applaud medical experimentation and discovery.

The objective of our quest is a system of concepts, standards, and rules governing human experimentation that gives due recognition to the various interests entitled to protection. These interests are threefold: the interest of the individual subject of experimentation in the integrity of his personality and physical well-being; the interest of the experimenter in pursuing his vocation; and the interest of the collectivity in increasing knowledge, particularly knowledge bearing upon public and individual health.

It is customarily argued that the ethics of human experimentation is governed by the proposition that the individual is an end in himself and must not figure as a means to an end beyond his own interest. This proposition is said to derive from our Judaic-

197

Christian tradition. According to this thesis, the absolute priority of each individual is central to our public philosophy. I question this thesis both as history and as a reading of our present public philosophy. Although we do not exalt the state above the individual, although we hold that the state exists for its citizenry, the individual is constantly compelled to sacrifice his interests to those of the collectivity, even as with conscription when it may mean loss of life or limb. Professor Calabresi makes the point that the law often approves of institutional and personal conduct that, statistically considered, creates threats to life or limb. But in most of the cases of which he is speaking—though not all—the threat is to persons unidentified at the time the risk is created. Because a selected individual is threatened more immediately in human experimentation, it implicates the interest of a given individual and thus symbolizes more concretely his claim to consideration. Nevertheless, the difference is one of degree and, we might say, more psychological than logical.

I hasten to give reassurance that these remarks are not the ominous prolegomenon to a program for conscripting human guinea pigs. Their intention is to suggest a more flexible, less obsessive application of the general propositions that we all accept. I have the impression that some experiments conducted in complete good faith—that is, in the belief that they are consistent with both professional and public morality—are blown up into problems by a too fastidious parsing of accepted ethical propositions.

The Mechanisms

How should the institutions of the law figure in furthering and protecting the interests implicated in human experimentation? The law as we know it is a system of decisional organs and their formal and informal products: the legislature (statutes), the executive-administrative (regulations and adjudication), and the courts (adjudication). Any of these in varying combinations can make law governing the conduct of the experimenter and the rights of the subject. There is not as yet much law explicitly dealing with human experimentation, but the common law (by which we mean the law devised and administered by the courts) has developed and continues to develop doctrines that are applicable. The physical touching of an individual without his consent may be actionable as an assault and battery even though there is no physical injury; physical touching of a subject or the manipulation of his conduct by misrepresentation or breach of a fiduciary relation is actionable as fraud; and the careless conduct of an experiment is actionable as negligence if the subject has suffered injury. These doctrines can be developed and applied by the judges with considerable flexibility so as to accommodate the interests of subject, experimenter, and collectivity. This is particularly true of the concept of consent and its close relative, the fiduciary obligation to disclose risks—particularly in the patient-physician relation—or to avoid the unnecessary taking of risks.

The advantage of common law judicial control is its flexibility—a characteristic consonant with the presently fluid condition of ethical attitudes toward experimentation. *Ad hoc* judicial decisions, it is true, may mean a stiff judgment for damages against an individual who learns only after the event the precise application of the rules governing his conduct. The individual experimenter may be protected by liability insurance, normally purchased by the institution which sponsored the experiment out of general funds or the funds supporting the project. The danger of insurance is that it may encourage experimenters to take too lightly the rules designed to control their activities. This may be a real danger if, as is alleged, experimenters resent and resist rules that limit action they are eager to undertake. As a counterweight to this possibility, the professional experimenter may feel that a judgment against him is a blot upon his professional honor.

There have been, as a matter of fact, few lawsuits concerning the legality of experiment. Though the ethics of many experiments have been challenged by professional and lay critics, in many of these there has been no detectable damage. Actions for assault and battery (unconsented touchings or touchings procured by misrepresentation or failure to disclose risk) can be brought though there has been no damage. But in the absence of damage, the individual will rarely be disposed to vindicate the integrity of his person by bringing an expensive lawsuit. Furthermore, the uninjured victim may, as would be the case with many of us, himself be caught in the dynamic of medical research and be indisposed to harass the experimenter by a lawsuit. A further reason for the paucity of lawsuits is the fact that the subject is normally not aware nor in possession of the evidence to demonstrate that his interests have not been properly protected. The medical profession resentfully clams up when one of its members is attacked and is not easily persuaded to testify against him.

If there are few lawsuits, one might conclude that we cannot look to the common law to develop in detail the applicable concepts. What then are the alternatives? The most obvious, and the prevalent one today, is that the experimenting professions must and do develop their own controls and thereby work out their own interpretation of the relevant common law principles, supplemented to a greater or lesser degree by statutory and administrative controls. The support of experimentation by public money, public health institutions, and foundation grants is highly conducive to the development of these controls by the profession. Because of this, experimentation is operating today under conditions of increased visibility. The sponsor is under pressure to justify the grant and demands, in turn, that the project be carried out under considered and considerate standards.

It has been evident for some time that the system of controls will develop in this fashion. The impressive series of declarations by national and international professional bodies attests to this. The medical profession, or at least those most caught up in experimentation, will prefer to devise and operate their own internal controls. There will be the occasional intervention of the courts where the experiment has produced serious injuries or where its conduct has been so notoriously unsound as to alert experimental subjects to seek legal advice.

These professional controls are of two kinds, those which the experimenter imposes on himself—the internalized controls of conscience and the acceptance of socially required limitations on his conduct—and institutional committees whose approval must be secured before the experiment goes forward. Some medical men, Dr. Walsh McDermott is one of the most explicit of this group, testify from their experience that neither of these will control experimental zeal to the degree desired by some critics of existing practices. The experimenter may identify his quest with the sanctified search for pure truth. He has convinced himself of the value of his experiment and will present it to the experimental subject in a way that will least alert the subject to features of the experiment that might alarm him. Thus, in the unhappy Jewish Chronic Disease Hospital case the experimental subjects were not told that the tissues they were to receive subcutaneously were cancerous. In the view of Dr. McDermott, because the committees are reluctant to veto experimentation, they will often fail to exercise an independent judgment. He has put these conclusions with brutal frankness:

These mechanisms are self-selected groups; they do not have the sanction of any constituency in society; there is no adversary proceeding. . . . The physician is probably the one educated person today who does not believe probability theory or rather operates against probability theory at all times. . . . Moreover, these juries are [composed of] senior men. They got to be senior by cutting and slashing their way through the ethics of clinical investigations, and they are then suddenly supposed to tell young men that they cannot do the same thing. . . . [These juries] are a superficial, veneer-like approach.

And he then adds in a surprising double-take:

I have no objection to their being so, as long as we do not kid ourselves into thinking that they are letting the investigator off the ethical hook.

Dr. Francis Moore said in reply to Professor Alexander Bickel's demand that a patient always be advised that he is implicated in an experimental situation:

Patients who are sophisticated enough to appreciate a properly designed random study are appraised of what is being done.

The negative implications of Dr. Moore's statement reinforce Dr. McDermott's frank estimate that the present system favors the experimenter over the individual patient or subject. Dr. Moore is happy with the present setup. Dr. McDermott is obviously uneasy, yet he does not, it seems, condemn it. If it be granted that the patient-subject today is a victim of excessive experimental zeal, the remedy in Dr. McDermott's view is to educate the experimenter and the future medical student so as to make them aware of and responsive to the interest of the subject. We must agree with Dr. McDermott that the informed conscience of the experimenter is the first and the most crucial guarantee. Whatever other and later safeguards there may be—whether committee scrutiny or lawsuit— the experimenter is the strategic center of responsibility. He not only prepares the protocol, but administers it. Moreover, when the experiment is put into effect, he may blunt the effective impact of the protections written into the protocol. That being so, it is the task of the public and of the medical schools to develop standards insofar as possible and to inculcate attitudes of concern for interests that the experimenter is tempted to minimize. The requirement of drafting a protocol in terms of the protection of the subject is itself a control. The protocols and the action taken under them should be published. In the present alerted state of public opinion, this would be a further sanction. In addition to its backward effect on the experimenter, it will make possible the study of the committee system.

In the last analysis, it may still be true that high-level committees—on which sit non-professionals (who will be busy men with little time to study these intricate proposals) as well as members of the institution's staff—will not be in a position or will not desire to impose too tight a rein on the zealous experimenter, particularly if the experiment itself seems promising and important. Insofar as this is true, the committee device may be, again to quote the epithet of Dr. McDermott, something of an "hypocrisy," but a benign hypocrisy that allows potentially useful research to go ahead where the conscience of the experimenter—in Dr. McDermott's view, the primary control—is satisfied. In his opinion, the *Helsinki Declaration,* the FDA regulations, and similar pronouncements are "honest reflections of our culture complete with all its hypocrisies" and to follow them "to the letter . . . would produce the curious situation in which the only stated public interest is that of the individual. The future interest of society and its sometime conflict with the interest of the individual, in effect, are ignored. . . . It has been most unwise to try to extend the principle of 'a government of laws not men' into areas of such great ethical subtlety as clinical investigation."

I find myself somewhat but not wholly persuaded by Dr. Mc-Dermott's evaluation of the system of internalized controls. They can be—and, I would venture to say, are to a certain extent—somewhat more efficacious *qua* control than Dr. McDermott would allow. The very requirement of formulating a protocol and thus exposing one's project to the light of day has some prophylactic effect. It will mean that some projects will not come up to the committee and that those projects will be vetoed which are flagrantly lacking in merit or which strikingly violate the standards for protection of the subject. The committee system, I gather, has developed a great deal in the last few years as a result of demands for control by the public and by the institutions that grant the funds for research. Whatever the committee's predispositions, it must to some degree respond to the demand for independent judgment. If the outsiders and nonprofessionals on the committee are not in a position to analyze the project deeply, professionals whose basic orientation is therapeutic may sit on the committee. I should think it is an exaggeration to insist, as Dr. McDermott has, that these committees do not have "the sanction of any constituency in society." Insofar as the system approves projects that do not strike the committee as flagrant in one or another respect, it *does* allow leeway to the interest of the experimenter and general public. It will mean that projects, such as those which in the past paid great dividends in the advancement of therapeutics but which would not satisfy "the letter" of latter-day official pronouncements, can proceed as they did in the past.

The committee system is today part of a system of self-regulation, but it could and probably should become part of the legal system of control either generally or on a selective basis. This change could come about by statute, by administrative fiat, or by judicial decision. It would be going too far to require that there be a committee procedure in every experiment. Every medical intervention is to some degree experimental, and the physician in his practice is constantly faced with the challenge to use new drugs or new procedures. If he is a specialist, his interest in these will not be limited to their effect in the particular case: He will be looking for guidance in the future. A general statutory requirement requiring institutional committees in any "experiment" would raise monstrous problems of interpretation, would unduly complicate medical practice, and would add unnecessary steps to experiments where the risks to the subject or patient are trivial. But as has been the practice with grants from the NIH, a governmental authority or a foundation might in specified instances require committee procedure for experiments funded by the grant.

Finally, a court exercising its common-law jurisdiction in a suit for damages could condemn experiments of high risk if there had been no committee approval of the protocol. To reach this result, the most likely recourse would be to the concept of negligence, which subjects the injury-producing action of an individual or corporate body to the test of "due care." It is particularly relevant that "due care" is a continually evolving concept. What was "due care" yesterday may not suffice today. In the famous case of the *T. J. Hooper*, 60 F.2d 737 (1932), Judge Learned Hand held that a vessel had violated the standard of due care because it was not equipped with a radio that would have given warning of approaching storms. It was no answer, said the judge, that radios had not been generally adopted. "Courts must in the end say what is required; there are precautions so imperative that even their universal disregard will not excuse their omission." Absorbed into the law in this way the committees and the procedures that they develop become a functioning part of the legal system of control.

Statutes or administrative bodies may require such procedures, but they may go further and establish standards of control. The most important example—and there are few others—is the requirement of §505(i) of the Federal Food, Drug and Cosmetic Act that before administering an "investigational drug" to a human being, the person must be informed that the drug is being tested for investigational purposes and must give his consent, except where it is not feasible or contrary to his best interests. The Food and Drug Administration has elaborated the requirements of consent in considerable detail. In its original form, the regulation defined "consent" or (using a qualifier not in the statute) "*informed* consent." In its present form, the regulation no longer purports to define "informed" consent, but the character of the regulation remains the same. It provides that the subject must be given "a fair explanation of pertinent information concerning" the drug, his possible use as a control, and—taking into consideration the person's "well-being and ability to understand"—the nature, expected duration, and purpose of the investigation, the hazards involved, the existence of alternate therapy, and the likely benefits of the drug. Ordinarily, the consent must be secured in writing. In the view of some physicians, the emphasis on risk and on alternative forms of treatment confuses and distracts the patient at the same time that it gives him a false sense of enlightenment since the hazards are as yet unknown. This criticism concludes that in the end the patient, the doctors, and the general public are all adversely affected by the too great specificity of this regulation. The objection, I take it, is not to the requirement of "consent" or to a statement of general considerations, such as is found in the *Declaration of Helsinki*:

If at all possible, consistent with patient psychology, the doctor should obtain the patient's freely given consent after the patient has been given a full explanation.

If this criticism of the FDA regulation is well-taken, as I believe it is, it suggests that detailed legal prescription of the physician's or experimenter's conduct is ill-advised. To be sure, there are no prescribed penalties—except the displeasure of the FDA—against the physician or experimenter who does not follow this procedure. Nevertheless, it is unwise to establish by law a situation in which the responsible actor is either hindered in the application of his expertise or is required to forswear himself. As a matter of fact, the "displeasure of the FDA" can be severe: the "disbarment" of the investigation, forbidding the experimenter to receive investigational drugs. If a false statement is made as to consent in reporting to the sponsor of the investigation, this can be ground for such action even if unintentional (if proposed regulations are adopted) and a federal felony if intentional.

The generalization I would derive from this criticism is that the system of legal controls should be based for the most part not on detailed statutory or administrative rules applicable to all experiments, but on standards allowing leeway for the exercise of judgment, whether the instrumentality be the experimenter, a control committee, a funding organization, an administrative body, or a court.

Finally, then, the law as a system of control is not in any realistic, creative sense distinct from private and semipublic centers and organs of control. Ethical and professional compulsions operate directly on the actors in the experimental enterprise. There is or should be a fusion, one might even say a fruitful *con-fusion*, of legal and extralegal norms and of legal and extralegal mechanisms. It was clear to Dr. McDermott that the most effective—he thought the only effective—control center is the personal and professional conscience of the experimenter himself. In his opinion, the experimenter's personal and professional conscience is also potentially the most relevant control, since external controls are apt to overprotect or overdefine the interest of the experimental subject. But if we are to rely on professional conscience, it must be a conscience informed by training and self-examination—in short, by education. It follows that no part of the program of ethical formulation is more important than the examination of the ethical problem in the educational process. It is encouraging to learn that the medical student today is much concerned with ethical questions.

The Principles

Upon what principles will the experimenter govern his conscience, the committees exercise their sanctioning function, the administrative authorities establish the conditions of experimentation, and finally the courts test the validity of experimental intervention? We need not assume that the principles will be the same at all four levels, though they will rest on a common base. In fashioning the common law, the judges will ordinarily allow a considerable latitude for the exercise of conscience and skill. A committee may demand safeguards that the law does not require. It may, for example, require experiments to be performed by a group or demand that the therapeutic and experimental functions be kept separate and be performed by different personnel. A court, on the other hand, would probably not impose such conditions even though it believed them to be wise. A committee might veto a project on the ground that it did not hold sufficient promise of fruitful results. It is unlikely that a court would feel qualified to make such a judgment, and if the experimental subject had been fairly treated, it would not condemn the experiment. Thus, there is a significant area of discretion within which conscience and technical judgment are to be exercised.

Though there is almost no judge-made law dealing specifically with experimentation in the modern sense, it is nevertheless justifiable, indeed necessary, to extrapolate a common law based on the application of relevant legal concepts. There have been few lawsuits directly raising questions of the legality of experimentation and even now, with the vast amount of experimentation, resort to the courts is spasmodic. Thus, we cannot look to the common law judges for detailed prescriptions and proscriptions. Nevertheless, we must posit a common law as the ultimate legal guardian of the interests involved in experimentation. Where there is serious debate concerning the propriety or the necessity of certain procedures, where there is a real conflict of interests, an appeal to putatively relevant concepts of the common law provides authoritative standards for judgment.

Though there are few decisions dealing specifically with experimentation, it has been stated again and again that under the common law a physician experiments at his own risk or, at the very least, he does so if he uses a novel procedure where a traditional one exists. This view—if it had, in fact, governed conduct in the past—would have blocked a substantial amount of medical progress. It has not, of course, had that effect. Are we thus to suppose that much of what we know as medical progress has been the consequence of actions that would have been held contrary to law had they been tested? I think not. This so-called standard attitude of the law rests on a few early cases that arose at a time when experimentation was conducted in a haphazard and unrationalized fashion. The earliest case was *Slater* v. *Baker*, 2 Wils. K.B. 359, 95 Eng. Rep. 860 (1767), where a novel procedure was used without the consent of the patient. The question as framed by the parties and the Court was whether the defendant doctor had practiced his profession according to the profession's standard of care. The Court held that the proper practice of medicine required knowledge and application of accepted methods of treatment. The other most cited case is *Carpenter* v. *Blake*, 60 Barb. N. Y. 488 (1871). Once again the Court held that if there was an approved procedure, it must be used. In neither case did the physician overtly defend his conduct in terms of deliberate experimentation. Experimentation as we know it today, with its planned and controlled search for new therapeutics, did not exist. There had not been developed such currently used safeguards as the initial trial on animals, the explicit formulation of a protocol and its approval by an institutional board, and the consent of the patient.

Judges are sensitive to the ethos of the times. Our society places a high premium on scientific experimentation and the pursuit of knowledge. To a greater extent than was formerly true, judges will be conscious of the conflict of interests and will seek to give due weight to each of them in any case involving experimentation carried on pursuant to current standards of propriety. The courts, for example, have been willing to take account of the conditions of modern surgery in permitting a further operation without consent where unexpected and serious pathology turns up in the course of an operation performed under anesthesia. We should proceed on the hypothesis, therefore, that in framing our ethical principles the common law will be hospitable to procedures that recognize the social value of human experimentation without sacrificing the interests of patients and subjects.

There is no single determinant of the ethical character of an experimental intervention. But the relationship between the experimenter and the subject is crucial. All commentators start from the proposition that the relation between physician and patient imposes upon the physician a paramount duty to promote the health of his patient. This duty has grown in significance and importance. Our civilization intrudes more and more upon our privacy. Government has become more and more intrusive. Religion is for many no longer a recourse in times of trouble and distress. For some people, the physician has taken the place of the priest, and the absolute devotion of the physician to his patient is a resource of great value to the beleaguered individual.

There can be no question that the physician's loyalty may be somewhat divided if he has an experimental as well as a therapeutic intention toward his patient. There is a special danger where the experiment is not for the benefit of the patient, as in transplants where the donor's death may be a necessary condition for removal of the organ. Where the patient's death seems imminent and irreversible, the therapeutic intention may yield to the experimental intention. But even where the experiment may benefit the patient, the physician-experimenter may develop an interest in the experiment which qualifies his devotion to his patient. This situation may be more likely if the patient is a charity or semicharity patient, and there has been no pre-existing personal relation between physician and patient. We do not, as a matter of fact, have adequate accounts of the physician-patient relationship in charity and semi-charity wards. What is the relation between the resident staff and the research staff? Is there a considerable mutuality of personnel? How are research projects in a great research hospital translated into therapeutic programs and policies? One could imagine that there is not a sharp differentiation between research and treatment staffs, that judgments are made on the basis of relevant classes of patients rather than by individual doctors for their individual patients. Insofar as this is so, the physician does not stand in quite the same relationship to his patient as is normally assumed and to that degree does not have the same protection.

Whether a practicing physician should be barred absolutely from experimentation has been, as we might expect, a difficult question. The Report on Human Experimentation of the Public Health Council of the Netherlands has this to say:

A practicing physician should not become an investigator on his own patient, if the experiment involves danger.

And it adds rather ambiguously, "a body of advisors should be consulted," implying that the physician may proceed with the experiment if there has been such consultation. In an earlier passage, however, the Report asserts:

A practicing physician who is also the investigator is not the person qualified to objectively judge the risk involved.

The *Declaration of Helsinki* has this to say:

The doctor can combine ethical research with professional care, the objective being the acquisition of knowledge, only to the extent that clinical research is justified by its therapeutic value for the patient.

Thus, under the *Helsinki Declaration* a practicing physician can engage in experimentation, with the patient's consent, if the experiment can be justified on therapeutic grounds. Under the Netherlands' statement, if I understand it correctly, the practicing physician cannot, even with consent, experiment if there is any "risk" involved.

The problem with an absolute prohibition is that many of the best practicing physicians have at the same time a scientific interest and, as a consequence, a strong desire to undertake clinical experimentation. The public stands to benefit from his experimentation. To forbid the practicing physician from experimentation when there is any "risk" may reduce the depth and, in the long run, the quality of therapeutic and clinical practice. This will be a loss to the general public and an unfortunate blow to persons who wish to contribute both to therapeutics and to scientific discovery. The dilemma is especially acute with respect to nonpaying patients. As we have noted, the physician in such cases may have a rather casual relation with the patient which may qualify his paramount devotion to the patient's interest. On the other hand, however, non-paying patients as a class may benefit from treatment by first-class professionals. Furthermore, as we have suggested, a separation of therapeutic and experimental staffs may become a matter of form in a hospital devoted to research. Even though an attending physician may not experiment on his own patient, he may have an interest in his hospital's activities which he cannot escape and which may color the judgment he must make as to whether to advise his patient to become a subject of the experiment.

The Netherlands' Report makes this statement:

Hospitals exist not only to treat patients but also to increase medical knowledge and skill. Animal experimentation always precedes that on humans. The public should understand that the interest of the patients requires a certain amount of experimentation.

Despite these considerations, the Netherlands' Report bars a practicing physician from experimenting if there is "danger" or "risk." The *Helsinki Declaration* does not so limit the physician, but it does require that the research be "justified by its therapeutic value for the patient." This solution is, in my opinion, the correct one. It recognizes both the legitimate interest of the physician in scientific activity as well as the interest of the public in medical progress. We must grant that there may be occasions when the patient is subjected to risks which are not in his best interest. For the most part, however, a conscientious physician's freedom to experiment will benefit the patient as well as the public. As the *Helsinki Declaration* states:

In the treatment of the sick person, the doctor must be free to use a new therapeutic measure, if in his judgment it offers hope of saving life, reestablishing health or alleviating suffering.

Indeed, the very fact that the experimenter is limited by his obligation to his patient is a source of protection for the patient in his role as subject.

It has been suggested that there be someone on the hospital staff whose function it is to represent the claims of the patient for protection. This function could be performed at two rather different stages in the process: first, at the protocol stage and, second, at the point where the decision is made to treat each patient. The former is obviously more feasible. Canvassing the interest of the patient-subject and determining what steps to take to protect him should be integral parts of the decision to do the research. There is, I think, merit in the suggestion that a physician not intimately connected with the proposed research should make an evaluation and report it to the sanctioning committee. I am somewhat less convinced of the feasibility of providing personnel independent of the operating therapeutic personnel to review the situation of each patient immediately before and during the administration of the research. Such a practice might either become just one more routine or lead to conflicts and problems out of proportion to its usefulness.

The controlled experiment intensifies the problem created by the combination of therapeutic and experimental functions. The assumption in the controlled experiment is that the value of alternative treatments is not established; and that, therefore, the physician does not know which is the better treatment. In this situation, the argument goes, the attending physician is merely guessing on the basis of hunch, or custom, or his apparent success in the past with one of the alternatives. It is concluded that it is not contrary to the patient's interest for him to become part of a controlled experiment and that it will be greatly to the interest of future patients to acquire information. Reliance on the conventional treatment may block further research. It cannot be gainsaid that the physician's therapeutic judgment may be partly determined by the experimental intention of the controlled experiment. It may turn out, for example, that a previously approved treatment is indeed the better, and that the control patient has suffered. Professor Bickel is troubled by this possibility. He has said:

This process of random selection seems to me to be entirely inconsistent with making a judgment about the individual patient, which that patient is entitled to. If you are willing to say, on the basis of your technical knowledge, that a random decision is no different from the one you make in the best of faith, having in mind only that patient's welfare, you are entitled not to disclose because you have nothing to disclose.

Dr. Moore's reply that there was, in fact, disclosure at least to "patients who are sophisticated enough to appreciate a properly designed random study" would not, I suppose, satisfy Professor Bickel. Dr. Rutstein said:

It is important for an individual to know he is in an experiment. . . . Nevertheless, if it is a situation that deserves investigation—where it is a toss-up as to whether or not what you are going to do is going to help— the investigator has little to disclose except his interest and the two alternatives.

I would conclude that if a controlled experiment is logically consistent with a therapeutic intention toward a patient, an attending physician may participate in or advise his patient to participate in such an experiment. This proposition is subject, however, to certain assumptions: *First,* the patient has been advised that he is participating and that there is an alternative which is currently used by reputable physicians; *second,* the experiment is being administered by a group; and *third,* the protocol has been approved by a properly organized committee.

Consent

It is generally understood that neither in law nor in practice is the process of consent a single, clearly defined entity. Consent is a function of the relation between experimenter and subject and is modulated by the degree of risk, the alternative treatments (in a therapeutic situation), and the value of the experiment. There is wide range of opinion as to the significance of consent. Dr. Louis Lasagna has said:

I want to take issue with Dr. [Jay] Katz's notion that consent is the pre-eminent question. Consent is primarily important in the abstract and appeals to those who are interested in civil libertarian problems.

211

The major protection of the patient, however, comes from the review of protocols by peer and non-peer groups, from the competence of the investigator, and all the ancillary facilities at his disposal, and from monitoring the performance of experiments.

Such an opinion may reflect two quite different and opposed attitudes: the angry and contemptuous attitude of the investigator who finds his project complicated by requirements of consent so elaborate that his experiment is impeded; and, on the other hand, the attitude, if you accept Dr. Lasagna's epithet, of "the civil libertarian" who is afraid that the will of the subject may be easily overborne or even disregarded, and who may take refuge from his concern in the hope that other safeguards will protect the subject.

The common law sets a high value on consent to physical invasions that threaten the health or psychic integrity of the individual. The law rightly recognizes that the body is his fortress. Nevertheless, the inviolability of the body is not absolute. In some cases, interventions are permitted even against the will of the individual. Thus, there are statutes that permit the police authorities to take a blood sample from a person recently involved in an automobile accident where there is a suspicion of intoxication. It was claimed that such a statute violated the privilege against self-incrimination. The statute was upheld by a closely divided court (5-4), *Schmerber* v. *California*, 384 U.S. 757 (1966). One of the dissenters placed his dissent on the ground that the intervention involved "violence"—overlooking, as I would think, that the law uses force to secure compliance or avoid threatened harm. Note, however, that in this case the risks to the subject are slight.

Even where consent is required (in the sense that the individual is free to refuse consent), the mere appearance of consent—a failure to protest—may suffice. Consider the case of *O'Brien* v. *The Cunard Steamship Lines*, 154 Mass. 272, 28 N.E. 266 (1891), which had to do with an immigrant who was being brought into the port of Boston. All the immigrants were lined up rather ignominiously to be vaccinated. When she passed by the vaccinating physician, Mrs. O'Brien said that she had already been vaccinated. Nevertheless, the doctor told her to hold up her arm, and she was punctured. She later claimed that she did not consent. The Court held that her actual state of mind was irrelevant; that the consent should be looked at from the point of view of the defendant. Had the plaintiff in this situation been submitting to serious risk, the Court would not have focused on the defendant alone, though as pointed out by Professor Calabresi there is a risk (though slight?) of encephalitis. There were, of course, great pressures on her to accede to vaccination that in another situation would be held to negate completely the idea of consent. (Her only alternative was to turn around and go home or perhaps into quarantine.) But given the kind of relationship, the interests of the state, the interests of getting the vaccinations done effectively and quickly, the law was prepared to take a cavalier attitude toward the claims of Mrs. O'Brien's personality. This case exemplifies the notion that in any situation, as should be true whether or not the medical personnel are public officers, the law will look at the structure of the situation to see what is demanded in terms of the interest of society, on the one hand, and the interests of the individual, on the other.

The *O'Brien* case is an example, assuming any are necessary, of the proposition that the law may require or permit the taking of certain statistically human risks because the advantages are thought to outweigh the risks. There are predictable risks of injury, including death, from the operation of automobiles. This risk, under the law as it stands, is imposed upon us without our consent. The law may compensate an injured party by requiring the automobile driver to pay if he has failed to use due care; otherwise, uncompensated injury or death must be suffered. The difference between this risk and an experimental one is that in the latter case the victims are more particularly singled out. In the automobile situation, the risk is random; it is, you might say, a function of a situation rather than the conscious determination of known individuals to subject another person to risk. Furthermore, the advantages of the automobile situation are widely distributed, at least among all those who drive or ride in automobiles or are dependent on them for goods and services. But where an individual is singled out as a risk-bearer, particularly if the risk is not taken for his immediate advantage, he should have a voice in the decision. One can imagine, however, an experimental situation in which it may be permissible to create risks for non-assenting persons, as is true of the automobile situation. There will, however, be few cases in which either the law or ethics will tolerate a total lack of consent. The function and significance of consent in the total picture vary with the relationship of experimenter and subject.

Subjects

In the search for rules as opposed to general standards, there is a disposition to conclude that certain classes of persons are not proper subjects of experimentation. Thus it may be said that children, the feeble-minded, the aged, and prisoners should never be the subjects of experimentation. These conclusions may rest—in the cases of children, the feeble-minded, or the aged—on the notion that such persons are not in a position to understand the risks involved or the nature of the experiment and thus cannot give a meaningful consent. In the case of prisoners, the objections are more obscure, but they rest, perhaps, on the notion that prisoners are under pressures to give consent which put them to unfair advantage or which are inconsistent with the aims of the criminal law. Reasoning of this sort, I would suggest, improperly makes consent an ultimate or absolute value irrespective of the interest that consent is designed to protect. A rule forbidding experimentation on a given class of persons may exclude experimentation of value to that class. Even where that is not the case, to prohibit the use of an available source of subjects may unnecessarily hobble experimentation and deprive members of a given class of an opportunity to participate that they might welcome.

Consent serves roughly two functions: First, it protects the personal integrity and dignity of the individual, and, second, it protects his health and bodily integrity except insofar as he is ready to put them at risk. In experiments where there is little or no risk—for example, in testing the efficacy of analgesics, where the risk is simply the loss of the possible reduction of pain—the prime function of consent is to protect the dignity of the individual. I would not say that small children or the feeble-minded are without any aura of dignity, but their sensibility is reduced from the normal, and the intervention involved in testing an analgesic does not, in my opinion, offend our ethic, whether looked at from their point of view or the point of view of a beholder who is concerned for them.

There appears to have crept into the thinking of some people the notion that the motivation of a consenting subject should be disinterested, that he should be acting for the benefit of mankind. There is a disposition, for example, to scrutinize closely the motivation of prisoners and to exclude their use because their presumptive motive is self-interest. This line of thinking seems to me to reflect an excessive ethical fastidiousness. (It may also possibly proceed from a subconscious impulse to glorify the enterprise—which, it is thought, might be sullied by the participation of unworthy persons.) But assuming that the experiment otherwise satisfies professional standards, the only requirement, in my opinion, is that no "undue" advantage be taken of the subject. A prisoner, even a patient, may be under pressures to consent not present in the situation of a citizen at large or a stranger. But those pressures should not be accounted an undue advantage. A prisoner, for example, may consent in order to give meaning to his life or because he hopes (though no promise has been given) to receive favorable treatment. A stranger may consent because he is paid, because he seeks excitement, or because he has a problem. Indeed, the motivation of consent is so complex, so various, and so obscure that it defies determination.

From the point of view of the experiment, the motivation of the subject is irrelevant unless his psychology is a factor in the experiment. From the subject's point of view, there is no lack of respect in allowing him to decide to participate for what seem to him to be sufficient reasons. He must be treated fairly, and the touchstone of fairness is, for the most part, what in retrospect will seem fair to him. Indeed fairness is at the heart of the whole consent problem, at least from the point of view of the subject or the patient.

It has become a cliché that the concept of consent is elusive and complex. It *is* complex whether viewed psychologically, philosophically, morally, or however. But the complexity arises, in part, from a futile attempt to give a definition that is valid for every imaginable context of law and ethics. If the definition is in terms of "fully informed" consent, it is found to be next to impossible to satisfy it in a great many situations. Consent may be relevant, for example, to the guilt of an individual who allegedly has participated or consented to the illegal course of action. Very different considerations are in question in experimentation—where what is at issue is whether an individual who has been put at risk (and who may or may not have suffered some ill effects) has been dealt with fairly. Assuming that the subject has the requisite minimum of intelligence, presumptively what he thinks is fair suffices to justify the experimental action. Both law and morals disapprove of the use of certain tactics in securing consent—such as falsification, failure to state crucial facts, and undue pressure.

What is "undue" is a function of the situation. We can decide (as, for the most part, we have) that to seek the consent of a prisoner is not undue despite the presence of pressures absent in the case of the citizen at large. He must not, however, be threatened with adverse consequences if he refuses, and for this reason his refusal should not be of record. Let us admit that problems arise in part because there are disturbing contradictions in the prison situation itself. But that statement characterizes almost any life situation, and for that reason it may be the path of wisdom to focus on the simplicities. Experimentation on prisoners offers advantages to the experimenter, to the prisoner, and to the public. It offends, I believe, only a very few persons. Similar considerations may govern the use of the aged and the derelict, persons whose interests are drastically narrowed and whose life is one of dull, inescapable monotony. To become involved in a vital experiment, to become socially useful, may provide a fillip to their lives. I would conclude with Dr. Lasagna that "the motivation for volunteering is highly complex and not easily discernible; we are all captive to certain drives. . . . I would hope that we might not be doctrinaire in our approaches toward different volunteer groups."

Finally, a word on the development of elaborately rationalized definitions of "informed consent." The most important—and it is of great significance since it may presage the future course of the ethics of experimentation—is the definition evolved by the Food and Drug Administration from §505(i) of the Food and Drug Act. The Act itself requires that where a new drug is used for investigational purposes consent must be obtained from persons to whom the drug or any control is administered. The regulation interprets this as requiring a subject to be informed that controls, whether another drug or a placebo, will be used. The statute and the regulation make exceptions if the patient's welfare requires them or "in those relatively rare cases" where it is not "feasible" to obtain consent because the patient is in a coma. The regulation is applicable to any use of drugs, even by an attending physician, if the drugs are "administered primarily for the accumulation of scientific knowledge."

Opinion differs among investigators as to whether informing a patient that placebos will be used arouses his resistance. Even if it does not, such information may complicate or skew an experiment by adding additional psychological components. The regulation takes no account of these considerations. Exceptions to the requirement of consent are limited to those made in the patient's interest. The social interest in the experiment is given no recognition, even where there is little or no risk. To my mind, this makes a fetish of informed consent. Once more I would raise the question of whether rules so rigid are a proper solution to the ethical problems involved in experimentation.

WALSH MCDERMOTT

Comment on "Law as a System of Control"

IN THE PRECEDING essay, "Law as a System of Control," Professor Jaffe sifts the ideas of a number of people and then proceeds to make a crucial contribution of his own. This key contribution is a concept I will loosely term "extrapolated common law." He shows clearly how it could serve in human experimentation to start creating a system for the institutionalizing of decisions between the interests of the individual and the interests of society. Once such a legitimatizing base was provided, the various other institutional forms, such as "ethics committees," would fall into place and acquire a reality they do not have at present. Up to the point of presenting his concept, Professor Jaffe and I have followed essentially the same analytic steps (*Annals of Internal Medicine*, Vol. 67, 1967, pp. 39, 66). I will identify these steps at the outset, therefore, the better to define the obstacle which his concept will help us to surmount.

He and I start in agreement that a convincing case exists that there is a social imperative for human experimentation in medical research and that this can lead to situations in which the interests of society and those of the individual are in conflict. We further agree in rejecting the proposition that society really holds that the individual is always, as he says, "an end in himself and must not figure as a means to an end beyond his own interest." Thus we arrive at a point where we concede the necessity at times for a decision between the interests of the individual and those of society and concede that on some such occasions it is the individual and not society that suffers harm. Understandably, because an individual might be harmed, we would like to institutionalize the process of decision, and we would like to do so with an institutional form based, in his words, "on a realistic estimate of the forces at work."

218

Comment on "Law as a System of Control"

It was from this point on that I could see no satisfactory solution.

Attempts to use the law as the institution, in my judgment, were to be avoided. While the public seems quite willing to accept that there are times in human experimentation when the interest of the individual cannot be paramount, it would probably not support the actual codification of that principle in either an administrative regulation or a statute. And these are the two forms of the law that have emerged to the forefront in this field of human experimentation. Attempts to create extralegal devices such as local committee review are likewise unsatisfactory. My objection to the committees is not that they perform no useful services, because they do provide such services of a limited sort; specifically, they serve to air the issue. But, as they are in effect self-appointed, they lack the authority to represent the interests of either the individual or society when these interests are in conflict in a particular case. For this reason they cannot be regarded as a major institutional form that meets the need; yet, they represent just about the only formal extralegal structure that exists.

Professor Jaffe also seems to have arrived at essentially these same conclusions. He appears to discard as inadequate the approach of attempting to use the law in the form of either administrative regulation or statutes. He also concedes the defects in the local committee system, although he does gently chide me for tending to exaggerate their illegitimacy.* In essence, however, he and I are in agreement concerning the various ways that have been attempted or suggested.

All of these approaches had what appeared to me to be fatal weaknesses. Thus I came to the conclusion that in medical research the problem of attempting to institutionalize the making of a judgment between the individual and society was basically unsolvable. Perhaps some day there might come to be a reasonably widespread, publicly voiced attitude on the individual vs. society issue that would permit appropriately flexible laws or administrative regulations. But until that presumably far-off day, as I saw it, we would simply have to live with the problem and handle it as best we could, by what must ultimately be arbitrary decisions. To ensure

---

* In what he refers to as my double take, I believe I am the victim of loose speech aggravated by the inevitable punctuation problems of recorded speech. The passage should read, "I have no objection to their being, so long as . . ."

that these arbitrary decisions not be capricious, I could suggest only that we rely on the cultivated conscience of the experimenter, continuously reinforced by an organized effort to increase the local visibility surrounding each decision. Indeed, this seemed to me to be the chief role served by the local committees.

Professor Jaffe has succeeded in taking us considerably further than this point. He has done so by showing clearly how the third form of law—the common law—has the degree of flexibility necessary to serve usefully in these individually complex problems involved in clinical investigation. To be sure, the common law would not give us a tribunal for deciding the propriety of a given research action in advance of the act, nor could it remove the ultimate ethical responsibility from the shoulders of the investigator. What the use of the common law would do, however, would be to grant a high degree of legal sanction to the various practices and concepts that have already been developed and will be developed still further, by the medical profession and its nonmedical consultants. These practices and concepts would thus become a body of standards that, in effect, have the formal approval of society, and it would be up to the courts to see that these standards were upheld. In Professor Jaffe's words, "Absorbed into the law in this way, the committees and the procedures that they develop become a functioning part of the legal system of control."

The "absorption" into the law would ultimately be accomplished by the accumulation of a body of judicial decisions based on such concepts as "due care." To accumulate judicial decisions can be quite a slow process. Thus, if this approach is to be used to meet our present needs, it would also be necessary, in Professor Jaffe's words, "to extrapolate a common law based on the application of relevant legal concepts." The test of "due care" would be one of these relevant concepts. The way it could be used would be in a lawsuit in which it was charged that a medical investigator had been negligent in the care of the patient. A key issue in the judicial decision would be whether the investigator had exercised "due care" in his medical acts. Proper examination of "due care" in a situation that had involved experimentation would entail a review of all precautions that had been taken. The way in which the local ethics committee functioned in that particular case would be subject to careful scrutiny, and the actual operation of such procedures as the obtaining of "informed consent" could be critically reviewed. The value of each procedure as such and some definition of the circumstances in which they could be considered appropriate would thus be subjected to a disinterested judgment in addition to the central decision as to how well the procedures had been applied in the case at hand. It seems reasonable to assume that at least some of these self-regulating practices, developed within the research establishment, would receive favorable sanction in such a review. It would be through this route that, as mentioned above, they would be absorbed into the system of legal control. Newly developed procedures would also be evaluated under due care, for one of the most valuable attributes of the concept is its capacity to adapt promptly to change in the standards of a society.

Obviously, however, the speed with which a sufficiently large body of common law is developed depends both on the frequency of lawsuits and on their issues being diverse enough so that all the main questions get covered. As lawsuits concerning human experimentation are rare, it might be years or decades before the common law could serve as the institution we are seeking. It is to meet this objection that Professor Jaffe presents the concept of extrapolated common law. By this is meant, as I understand it, that the defense counsel lacking exact precedents in the form of judge-made law would present the existence and the effectiveness of the various self-regulatory practices as relevant standards of contemporary due care that fit well within the principles of such judge-made law as does exist. He would thus *extrapolate* from this common law, using the facts of the self-regulatory mechanisms as the data that justify his doing so.

Success with this common law approach is obviously not a sure thing; the counsel could do a poor job of organizing his presentation or the judge could decide against him for reasons unrelated to the merits of the case. Incompetence or error in the judicial process represent exceptions, not the rule, however, and as avenues for their correction exist, a poor start could be corrected over time. There is certainly no reason to assume that a judge or group of judges would be any less capable to decide these issues than anyone else, for example, a local ethics committee. The best reason of all for assuming that the common law approach, speeded by extrapolation, would have reasonable prospects of success is that Professor Jaffe appears to believe it would, and he is in an excellent position to know.

Let us assume, therefore, that it will be possible to employ the common law in this way. Several quite important advances will have then been made. As outlined above, a significant portion of the problem will have been brought under legal control, and the mechanisms created for self-regulation will have acquired legal sanction. Moreover, this common law mechanism will have great flexibility in the determination of whether a particular instrument of self-regulation was a fit instrument in a particular set of circumstances, and in matters of this nature it is essential that the mechanism for decision be highly flexible. Instead of having to await a long drawn out evolutionary change throughout a whole society, sufficient to permit statutes or regulations that would face the issues squarely, it will be possible to evolve the standards flexibly and rapidly in the much smaller arena of the courts. Finally, in this connection, is the fact that the concept of extrapolation not only will serve as an accelerator, but also should act as a strong incentive to a continued scrutiny and strengthening of the self-regulating mechanisms. For, instead of being largely an exercise of professional self-discipline in public, each functioning of an instrument of self-regulation, for example, a local ethics committee, can take place with the assurance that if well done, it will be strengthening the case that can be made by extrapolation at some future date. In this way, the committee will be clearly participating in a small but real way in the slow but steady building of a legitimatized institution for decisions in human experimentation.

What are the weaknesses of this approach of looking to the common law as our instrument for decision? Or, to put it differently, assuming the common law, fortified through extrapolation, is functioning with full effectiveness, how much of the problem remains unsolved? Several points have already been mentioned: human error or malperformance; no prospective decision in a particular case; and failure to remove the ultimate ethical responsibility from the investigator. As the last-named could not be accomplished by any institution presently conceivable, and as it by no means necessarily represents a desirable goal, its absence here is hardly an institutional failure.

One area in which the common-law approach might have a weakness as our sought-for institution would be that its advocacy of the interests of society in a particular experiment might not be specific, that is, framed in terms of that experiment, but would tend to be quite general.

222

Comment on "Law as a System of Control"

For example, to what extent could the common law serve as a vigorous advocate of the best interests of society in a situation in which a powerful case for the social interest exists, yet to meet it demands the placing of an individual at an appreciable risk? One might argue that the common-law mechanism would perforce be doing this in every case, and in one sense this would be true. But in the personalized form of a lawsuit, the interest of society in the experiment itself is handled indirectly and might tend to become a side issue. By this I mean that a favorable decision based on "due care" might be very crudely paraphrased, "the physician meant well, he intended no injury, and he took due care to attempt to ensure that no injury occurred." This is clearly not quite the same as saying: "It was clearly in the best interests of society that this particular experiment be done because . . . this individual, through the hand of fate, was one of the few who would serve as a satisfactory subject; he gave his informed consent; and due care was taken to minimize the possibility of his suffering harm." I suppose that such an all-embracing decision is neither to be expected nor desired, because it would tend to get the judge into technical areas beyond his competence. Yet, its absence does mean that the common-law approach will not meet the whole need.

Another possible weakness is that extreme interpretations of due care itself could lead us into the same built-in contradictions that are present, say, in the Helsinki Declaration. For example, Professor Jaffe quotes me as stating that the physician "operates against probability theory." By this I meant, that while the physician *is* trained to weigh the probabilities of danger from off-setting risks, he is also trained to refuse to place his patient at *any* known risk *no matter how small the probability of danger* in the absence of a positive reason for doing so. Expressed differently, the fact that the probability of the occurrence of a known danger is extremely low is not in itself an ethical justification for placing the patient at risk. In an adversary proceeding involving the concept of due care, this "any known risk" principle might be invoked to establish a failure of due care.

The extent to which either of these two possible weaknesses will constitute problems cannot really be foreseen, because this approach through the common law has such a considerable degree of flexibility.

Above all, neither of these possible weaknesses, in my judgment, should obscure the very real contribution to the solution of our problem that has been provided by Professor Jaffe. For in his analysis he has shown us for the first time, so far as I know, how we can build right now major portions of the institution we are seeking—an institution I had thought was fated to remain long unbuilt.

DAVID F. CAVERS

The Legal Control of the Clinical Investigation of Drugs: Some Political, Economic, and Social Questions

THE ANALYSES of the ethical issues of human experimentation in this volume have been directed to these problems chiefly as they have arisen in our great medical and scientific centers. They are epitomized best in the bold surgical innovation and less dramatically in scientific investigation into physiological and psychological processes. Clinical investigations of drugs form a part of the behavior under consideration, but these tend to pose the ethical issues less vividly. The line between treatment and experiment is blurred, the lives of the subjects are less often at hazard, and their dignity is seldom impaired.

Yet the clinical investigation of drugs brings into play two factors absent in surgical experimentation or in the study of behavior: the regulatory authority of government and the business objectives of great industries—the pharmaceutical manufacturing industry and the industries carrying out its advertising and distribution functions. Drug experimentation involves great numbers of human subjects and a multitude of investigators—twenty-five thousand having been registered with the Food and Drug Administration (FDA) in 1967.[1] Commonly, the investigators who conduct clinical trials for drug manufacturers are not associated in this work with major scientific institutions. Moreover, the process is not cut off sharply when a new drug is approved by the Food and Drug Administration and enters the physician's armamentarium. The drug's subsequent history may reveal in unanticipated calamities the limitations of even thorough-going clinical investigation.

The clinical testing of new drugs adds political, social, and economic tensions to the tensions between the individual conscience and the need for scientific progress with which the literature of human experimentation is largely concerned. Can we in the United States continue to harness the economic objectives of industry, an elaborate system of governmental surveillance, and the creativity of biomedical science to a process of drug development that depends on human experimentation? Can we provide through the intervention of the state sufficient assurance both of the well-being of the subjects of experimentation and of the adequacy of the experiments as well as the reliable communication of their results? In the effort to achieve these ends, are we likely to impair our ability to attain the basic purpose that has called the system into being: the provision of the drugs needed for the prevention, treatment, and cure of the myriad ailments that afflict mankind?

The concerns that I suggest are not yet exigent. The adaptation of all interests involved to the drastic extension, since 1962, of government authority over an already explosive expansion in the discovery and use of drugs has been surprisingly successful. But tensions appear to be building up. They may affect the present allocation of responsibility for the clinical investigation of drugs in several directions. It is too early for prophecy, but some questions may not be premature:

1. As the government control over the investigation, approval, and promotion of new drugs grows more rigorous, will this in time produce reactions, especially on the part of the pharmaceutical industry, compelling an assumption of greater responsibility for the development of new drugs by scientific institutions and medical centers?

2. Does the present system compel a wastefully large volume of human experimentation and would a consequence of major reductions in the duplication of pharmacological and clinical testing be to accelerate the shifting of responsibility suggested in the preceding question?

3. Will the tying of new drug approvals and promotions strictly to the results of clinical investigations operate to restrict deviations in therapy from the limits thereby established if only because of the threat of damage suits by patients injured by the backfiring of experiments in treatment?

The Clinical Investigation as the Basis of the FDA's New Drug Control

In discharging its statutory responsibility to approve or disapprove new drug applications (NDA's), the FDA's most difficult task is frequently not in deciding whether to grant approval to the drug, but rather in passing upon its proposed labeling.[2] "Labeling" is defined by the Food, Drug and Cosmetic Act to include "all labels and other written, printed or graphic matter (1) upon any article or any of its containers or wrappers, or (2) accompanying such article."[3] The courts have given this definition a broad interpretation.[4] A drug's labeling must contain not only the drug's formula but also its intended uses, adequate information as to indications, dosages, and methods of use, hazards of use, contraindications, side effects, and precautions.[5] This information must be conveyed "in brief summary" and with "fair balance" in any advertisement of the drug.[6] If, either in any effort to heighten an advertisement's appeal or in summarizing the information required in the labeling, the drug manufacturer fails to convey substantially the same information, it can be charged with violation of the Act.[7] To escape seizure of its drugs or criminal prosecution, it must confess error in a "Dear Doctor" letter satisfactory to the FDA and then mail this, at a cost of approximately $40,000, to the practicing physicians of the United States, a sanction that is the product of resourceful administration rather than statutory law.[8]

The "package insert" serves the FDA as a repository of the information bearing its imprimatur (much, incidentally, as a security's prospectus serves the Securities and Exchange Commission). The "package insert" must be sent to pharmacists, inserted in the package in which the prescription drugs they dispense are shipped. It must also be sent by the drug manufacturer to any physician who writes for it, and "full disclosure" regulations further require the inclusion of the same information in mailings of samples or other promotional matter to the profession.[9] The humble package inserts, therefore, constitute the authoritative legal sources of information concerning all the prescription drugs that the FDA has approved under the 1962 amendments.

In passing upon a drug's labeling, the FDA relies for most of its knowledge on the reports of the pharmacological and clinical testing of the drug in investigations conducted in accordance with a plan submitted to the FDA in the drug sponsor's claim for an investigational drug exemption (IND).[10] Without this exemption, the unapproved drug could not lawfully be sent across state lines for testing.[11] On examining the plan of investigation in the sponsor's IND, the FDA may find that the plan does not conform to its regulations or that the plan exposes the subjects of the testing process to undue danger. It might, for example, fail to provide for adequate animal pharmacological studies previous to the tests on human beings. The FDA should then terminate the exemption.[12] If an IND exemption survives, but its fruits are found inadequate, the sponsor's new drug application may be rejected as incomplete —the fate of three NDA's in four in 1967.[13]

If an NDA is not disposed of on this ground, the FDA staff must evaluate its claims and admissions not merely on the basis of the clinical evidence submitted in the NDA, but in the light of other NDA's in the FDA's files reporting clinical trials of similar drugs—perhaps even the same drug. The FDA will also consult the relevant literature, a full listing of which is required to be included in the NDA. As has been noted, this evaluation does not call for simply a "yes" or "no" judgment. One dosage level may be safe, another questionable, but the safer dosage level may be of doubtful efficacy. A satisfactory answer may lie in between. Negotiation follows. The reports of clinical trials may include some evidence of hazard, but was the reported condition the consequence of the drug's administration or of other factors? There may have been side effects disclosed in the trials, but ought these merely to be listed as such or was their association with a given condition such as to require its listing in the labeling as a contraindication? The FDA must evaluate the sponsor's statistical work; it may have to decide whether a sponsor was justified in downgrading a side effect as "rare" or "infrequent."

The process culminating in the approval of an NDA, including its proposed labeling, is a protracted one, though most of the time required is antecedent to the NDA's submission. Estimates indicate that from the date of a drug's discovery to the NDA's approval, a period of from five to seven years will ordinarily elapse.[14] Obviously the expense is great, but the returns financially to the drug's sponsor and in improved health to the drug's users can be high. The expense of short cuts can be even higher.

The Drug Industry's Reaction to Tightening Controls

The FDA's standards for the acceptance of IND's and the approval of NDA's are likely to grow progressively more rigorous to be "consistent with the objective of being as critical and comprehensive as possible," to quote the Deputy Director of the Office of New Drugs in the FDA's Bureau of Medicine, Dr. E. I. Goldenthal, a pharmacologist.[15] "We have taken some steps to help industry improve the quality of its NDA submissions," Commissioner God-dard testified in August 1967,[16] adding that "it seems that still more steps are necessary. The high percentage of poor applications must be greatly reduced." In April 1968, he declared to a medical audience: "We are insisting upon carefully controlled, carefully managed studies."[17]

Evidence of these efforts to improve drug testing appears in a popular article in the *FDA Papers* by Dr. Goldenthal.[18] The FDA has prepared "guidelines," he reports, to "describe in general the type of preclinical studies to be used in support of the several phases of clinical investigations." Noting that the "duration of chronic toxicity studies" is now "a subject of considerable contro-versy among toxicologists," Dr. Goldenthal discloses the FDA's con-servative position on a number of the issues. Carcinogenesis studies should be lengthened; studies should be commenced to last up to seven years in the dog and ten in the monkey when a large-scale clinical trial of an oral contraceptive is beginning; like periods are specified for new estrogens or progestogens intended for unlimited human administration. Reproduction and teratology studies are re-quested on most new drugs. Comparative drug metabolism "should be the cornerstone of toxicological evaluation." Fortunately, "tech-nical difficulties and the expense" are no longer the "hindrance to progress" they once were. After July 1969, the FDA will expect metabolic data to be submitted before NDA approval. Enzyme induction should be considered in metabolic studies and in the interaction of drugs administered concomitantly.

Turning to clinical studies, Dr. Goldenthal again calls for eval-uation of the question of drug interaction. Recent findings call for complete ophthalmological surveys in many instances in patients re-ceiving investigational drugs. When preclinical and adult studies indicate safety, "the cautious use of the drug for the treatment of a diseased condition in children (i.e., Phase II) would appear justi-fiable," but its use "in normal infants and children (i.e., Phase I) does not seem defensible."

In the case of pregnant women, the package insert must warn that "the safety of the drug in pregnancy has not been established" unless specific data on the drug's effects in pregnancy have been provided. For the studies to this end, Dr. Goldenthal recommends that "a minimum of 250 patients be studied in both the first and the last trimester of pregnancy with a control group of the same size. These groups should consist only of individuals who are being treated for a specific disease entity. We recognize the risk to be taken by these small groups," he concludes, "but we must consider the safety of the total population which may receive the drug."

Something of the scale of drug investigations can be sensed by the author's use of "small" in describing a group of 250 women, and one wonders whether they share the sacrificial resignation displayed by Dr. Goldenthal. But our concern at this point is not with the ladies or Dr. Goldenthal, but with the attitude of the industry. Pressed by increasing costs of drug investigation, concurrently subjected to increasing uncertainty as to the acceptability of the results, and compelled to make full disclosure to the profession of every risk and shortcoming revealed in its products, will the drug industry and its industrial allies long remain acquiescent?

Before some of the options that are open to them are canvassed, it should be noted that the increased costs do not jeopardize the financial stability of the major components of one of the nation's most profitable industries.[19] But added expenses do trouble the economic man, and their imposition by governmental order irritates the natural one. Moreover, the industry is not confined to giants; its two thousand members include many relatively small concerns, among them producers of drugs for the over-the-counter market whose effectiveness may be called in question though their (relative) safety is admitted.[20] Even cosmetic firms may be required to pursue the IND-NDA route when an ingredient in a new hair tonic or a lotion is "intended to affect the structure or any function of the body" and so converts the product into a drug.[21] Given these circumstances, a canvass of options to which some or all of the industry's constituents may resort is not an imputation of hypochondria.

The most obvious of these options is for the industry to seek political succor. A few amendments declaratory of the way industry counsel read the existing law might be sought, as well as an appropriation rider laying the menace of a governmentally financed drug compendium designed to facilitate the prescription of drugs by generic name. More important perhaps would be to obtain attentive, sympathetic ears in the Executive Branch and a friendly spirit in the Congress, with its power of the purse. The FDA was kept on short rations for its first fifty years and the comparative liberality in its budget (now about $69 million) goes back only about a decade.[22]

Given the new Administration and an altered Congress, the

Pharmaceutical Manufacturers Association (PMA) does not seem unmindful of the importance of public opinion. It is investing $1,200,000 in four inserts to be published in *The Reader's Digest* in 1969.[23] It looks to a future, to quote C. Joseph Stetler, its outspoken lawyer-president, "unfettered by stultifying and arbitrary government controls."[24]

An alternative having fewer disruptive potentialities would be for the industry to shift an increasing volume of drug R & D to foreign parts, especially to Britain, France, Germany, and Italy. Costs are lower there, and controls less restrictive. Once a drug has been accepted abroad and tested in clinical experience, the process of satisfying the FDA requirements is not only easier but more certain.[25] Recourse to European subsidiaries and licensees may provide some revenue while the drug is being cleared for the American market. If American consumers were to complain of having to wait several years for drugs available abroad, no doubt the American firms could remind them that the foreigners must run the gantlet of clinical trials. If this failed to assuage the complainants, the companies could suggest that their patrons demand that Congress lower the barriers to speedier, less expensive drug testing in this country.

Actually, the development of drugs abroad by American firms is not uncommon. In a compilation of the new chemical entities approved for marketing in the United States in the first half of 1968, five of the total of nine drugs were declared by the compiler to be "outstanding."[26] Three of these five were developed abroad. In the four European countries noted above, thirty-seven new chemical entities were introduced in the same period, and of these thirty-seven, nine originated in the United States. (It is not clear whether any had been marketed here.) Incidentally, the same source revealed the continuing ill-favor with which combinations of drugs are viewed; twenty-three were approved during the period as against seventy-one in 1964 and 108 in 1961.

Another solution open to firms in which the development and marketing of new drugs represents a small and divisible portion of their business is for them to close out this activity or to sell it to a large competitor. Selling out may be the sole remedy for the small firm that is dependent upon new drug development. Perhaps it can entice a hungry conglomerate to gobble it up. FDA Assistant Commissioner Theodore Cron is reported by *Fortune* as foreseeing the withdrawal of many firms from "the ethical drug" field in the next few years; he is quoted as predicting that "the attrition will be terrific."[27]

A more serious and not unlikely policy for drug firms more concerned with maximizing their profits than with embellishing their scientific reputations would be to concentrate R & D within a relatively limited range of drugs designed for use under conditions assuring large markets for useful, effectively promoted products. They would emulate those publishers who strive for positions in mass markets and eschew prestige items. They would leave to other enterprises the risks of pioneering the more esoteric and hazardous drugs.

If any of these alternatives were pursued on a considerable scale, socially desirable progress in drug therapy would tend to be held back. It is not enough, however, to exhort the drug industry to avoid these paths. As economic enterprises, they are entitled to reach economic judgments on economic grounds. Even if these criteria were admixed with politics, their spokesmen would doubtless be convinced that what was good for the PMA would be good for the country.

Were the pharmaceutical industry or a substantial segment of it to adopt the options outlined above, their course would compel consideration of this question: Is the nation's dependence on private enterprise for the production of essential drugs compatible with due vigilance in protecting both the sick people who are the subjects of clinical investigations and the sick people whose attending physicians must depend on the reliable communication of the results of those investigations? If meeting ever increasing standards for the testing, evaluation, and publicizing of new drugs is not profitable for the industry except within a limited product range, must not the leaders of the medical profession and the biomedical sciences join with the federal government in creating institutions to assume the responsibility for developing new drugs now shouldered by industry, at least in those product areas to which the industry no longer wished to devote substantial resources? Obviously any such move would present problems. Manufacturing and distribution, for example, would presumably remain in private hands. No doubt, the trend would be deplored by the American Medical Association (AMA). But existing trends toward the subsidization of other costs of medical care might render tolerable the prospect of entrusting this segment of drug development to other hands than those that now engage in it.

Is the Volume of Human Experimentation in Drugs Needlessly Large?

Human experimentation—the exposure of human beings to risks of physical or psychic injury in order to enlarge useful knowledge —would be an evil but for its purpose. If it is pursued under conditions making that purpose unlikely or impossible of realization, the element of evil will remain without the offsetting excuse; even the most ardent advocate of serendipity would hesitate to defend such experimentation.

This proposition, if accepted, carries with it an obligation on the part of those who authorize, require, or carry out human experimentation. There should be a reasonable prospect that the sacrifices thereby entailed will not be wasted or, at the least, that such wastage as occurs is inseparable from the realization of benefits and so must be endured if the benefits are to be obtained. There is ample evidence that much of the human experimentation involved in drug testing is wasted. To what extent the wastage is inescapable is a matter that deserves much more consideration than it can receive in this paper.

Two bodies of clinical investigations of new drugs should be scrutinized for avoidable waste. One is the large volume of investigations carried out under IND's that never eventuate in NDA's. The other is the substantial volume of IND's filed by pharmaceutical manufacturers who propose to produce the same or virtually the same drug that has already been approved by the FDA for another manufacturer as being safe and effective on the basis of pharmacological and clinical investigations that the FDA found to be adequate.

Experiments That Never Lead to NDA's

In the light of the hazard that manufacturers might withdraw from part or all of the new drug field, the fear that far too much drug testing is being done may seem paradoxical. But the process of withdrawal reflects a gloomy look toward the future, while the overproduction of IND's represents a gloomy look toward the past. Clear evidence is lacking that the process of withdrawal has begun, but clear evidence is at hand that wasteful indulgence in clinical testing is continuing.

A well-informed witness who has testified in support of the latter proposition is Dr. James L. Goddard. Speaking before the

American Society of Clinical Oncology on April 10, 1968, Dr. Goddard, while still Commissioner of the Food and Drug Administration, declared:

> We are exposing study populations to varying degrees of risk in clinical trials of many drugs that never even reach the new drug application (NDA) stage [and are doing so] at an exposure ratio of 6 to 1. Clinical investigations will begin on about 5,000 drugs over the next five years with perhaps 500 of the products eventually being cleared for marketing. . . .
>
> We estimate that [in this period] more than 1.4 million persons could be involved in clinical trials of drugs which will never reach the market . . . close to a million of these would be subjects in Phase III trials.
>
> Close to 300,000 persons a year may be exposed to drugs which will never reach the NDA stage.[28]

Dr. Goddard recognized at the same time the existence of "strong economic motives" for drug companies to adopt "largely uncontrolled studies" with relatively large patient populations, even though such studies yield "usually equivocal" results. In an address the following day, he pointed to another problem directly related to the wasteful use of clinical investigation—namely, a "shortage of clinical investigators."[29]

Dr. Goddard had little to propose for remedying this disturbing overuse of the experimentation privilege. He urged his hearers to "consider devising some means to give priority attention to those drugs which promise a major advance in therapy." Desirable as this proposal would be in protecting new drugs of promise from being lost or delayed in the shuffle of unworthy contemporaries, it is doubtful that this mechanism would reduce the total number of drug investigations.

The phenomenon that Dr. Goddard was pointing out has its analogue in the oil industry. Many dry holes seem to be the inevitable accompaniment of success in well-drilling. But the day of the wildcatter who played his hunches is well nigh over. To minimize dry-hole losses, a well-drilling venture today is replete with Ph.D.'s and the latest electronic gear. In drug testing, better basic research, better research designs, better personnel, and higher standards of testing would mean fewer human beings exposed to clinical trials. But how is this to be brought about? It might, of course, be coerced by closer surveillance of IND's, but this would entail official contraception for ideas that the FDA staff does not find promising, with all the risks of censorship that preclearance of investigation invites. Yet institutional review boards discharge this responsibility daily. Perhaps for those IND's that would not be scrutinized by such boards in normal course and might threaten danger to the subjects of the investigations while offering limited prospects of success, the FDA should have on call an array of advisory review boards expert in various fields to whom it could turn when doubtful IND's came to the attention of its staff.

The Testing of "Me-Too" Drugs

The second area of waste in the resort to human experimentation doubtless involves fewer people and subjects them to fewer risks than does the first, but its economic and social implications reach much further. The problem springs from the FDA's requirement, viewed by it as imposed by law, that NDA's be kept secret, even after a new drug's approval.[30] As a consequence, when manufacturer B wants to reproduce A's approved drug—to bring forth a "me-too" drug in the trade's jargon—manufacturer B must begin from scratch, as manufacturer A had done. B must provide the FDA with the same pharmacological and clinical evidence as would be required in the case of a wholly new product. To be sure, in passing upon this evidence, the FDA will have the benefit of its secret knowledge of the experience A reported and such studies and reports of experience as may have appeared since the approval. Of course, this information will improve B's chance of success.

It is reassuring that the clinical population on which B's trials will be conducted will be getting much the same drug under much the same conditions as the patients to whom A's approved drug is being administered. But the benefits are not fully shared. The processing of the two drugs may not have been identical and this may sometimes have clinical consequences. Moreover, B's clinical investigators will be denied knowledge of problems encountered in A's testing that are not disclosed in A's labeling. Finally, the choice of drug therapy for the patients used in B's studies may have been influenced by the investigators' need for subjects for testing. Perhaps most serious in terms of the social cost is the involvement of that scarce resource, clinical investigators, in an activity whose principal value is the protection of A's economic position.

One reaction to B's position is that the FDA's requirement provides additional information concerning the drug's merits and demerits, and thus is worthwhile, however burdensome to B. But that contribution is not exacted of A's licensees, C, D, and E. If

235

they obtain A's drug or the privilege of producing it, the FDA will allow them, with A's consent, to incorporate in their NDA's the data from A's own animal toxicity studies and A's clinical testing on humans. The licensees must establish in their NDA's that their manufacturing processes (for example, for encapsulating the drug) are good, and they must have their labeling approved. Nevertheless, their route bypasses most of the long years that B must travel to an approved NDA.

This process may seem a reasonable way of allowing A to enjoy the economic advantage of having been the first to discover, develop, and market the drug. But the federal government has provided a method whereby a discoverer can secure legal protection for his discoveries: the patent system. If A has patented his drug, he will have patent protection for seventeen years, and by the end of that period the drug may well have become "generally recognized as safe and effective" and hence no longer a "new drug." The secrecy of the NDA allows the practical equivalent of patent protection for a period of five years or more, during which time A can often get a firm grip on the market for the drug bearing its brand and trade names. When Dr. Goddard was testifying before the Subcommittee on Monopoly of the Senate's Select Committee on Small Business, Senator Nelson remarked: "So we are in the most unusual position where a private company has more authority to delegate the right to manufacture a drug than if exercised by the FDA?" When Dr. Goddard replied, "Yes, sir, in a sense," Senator Nelson observed, "That is an incredible situation." When, in the same interchange, he expressed the view that an NDA is "almost better than a patent," Dr. Goddard's response was, "That is what I am told, Senator."[31] It should be noted that Dr. Goddard reported in the same hearing an FDA estimate that about half the NDA's were for patentable products, but he pleaded ignorance when asked how many drugs in that half had actually been patented.[32]

The success of a patented drug stimulates competitors to acquire a share of its market by developing, by means of "molecular manipulation," non-infringing drugs that will have many of the same uses as the patented drug while permitting some product differentiation.[33] Disclosure of the patented drug's NDA would doubtless cut down the time between conception and FDA approval of this type of "me-too" drug, even though the significance of its distinctive characteristics would have to be ascertained by clinical testing.

Legal Control of the Clinical Investigation of Drugs

This problem has special relevance to the issue of human experimentation not simply because of the duplication of testing that is required of B and all the other non-licensed companies that wish to produce "me-too" drugs. It is also critical because of the impact that the removal of the secrecy now conferred on animal studies and clinical testing would have on the economic position of the industry and its readiness to pursue drug research and development. Would the ability of competitors to enter the market before the firstcomer A firmly established its position mean the breakdown of the extraordinary price structures that the major pharmaceutical firms have been able to maintain? Here is a menace to profitability that, if realized, would be far greater than the increased expenses involved in raising research standards, a cost increase that might well be converted in time to a saving.

The removal of secrecy would, moreover, give great impetus to the "generic name" drug, and this at a time when the soaring costs of medical care have produced in the federal, state, and local agencies that subsidize medical care a lively interest in the prospect of reduced costs through either the purchasing of generic name drugs or the use of their prices to set ceilings on reimbursable drug expenditures.

Into this cauldron of contention over which the Congress and a number of state legislatures have been hovering, the issue of "therapeutic equivalency" has been injected and is now being vigorously pressed by the PMA.[34] Even though several makers' drugs are the same in that all satisfy the generic specifications of official compendia, this does not insure that they will all have the same therapeutic effects. Differences in manufacturing processes or in "inactive" ingredients may account for the variations. Thus, in October 1967, the FDA had to suspend its certification from all the producers of chloramphemicol (a potent antibiotic) save Parke-Davis, its originator, because only batches produced by Parke-Davis were yielding the needed therapeutic effects.[35]

How widespread the differences are among "identical" drugs is a matter in controversy. In August 1967, Dr. Goddard testified that he knew about two dozen examples of demonstrated lack of therapeutic equivalency, but he characterized them as "only isolated instances."[36] The FDA is, however, reported to be seeking an additional one million dollars in its next appropriation for research and clinical trials directed primarily to this problem.[37]

The FDA has prudently avoided taking a position on the

desirability of withdrawing the secrecy rule, shielded by Department of Justice advice that it lacks legal power to do so. When asked by Senator Scott at the Small Business hearings as to whether placing "clinical data furnished by an individual company in the public domain" would "encourage or discourage more research in private industry," Dr. Goddard replied:

Senator, I am hard put to answer you on that. Some people have the opinion that it would discourage it. I tend to think that it would not, because the firm that gets into the market place first . . . has the marketing advantage in terms of intensive advertising [and] does tend, the record shows, to hold a competitive advantage in the continuing sale of that product through prescriptions written by physicians.[38]

But the record to which Dr. Goddard alludes was not based on laws that would permit "me-too" manufacturers to incorporate their predecessors' animals studies and clinical studies in their own NDA's. It did not reflect the consequences of growing pressures by public health and welfare agencies to follow generic name purchasing and pricing policies. These will be stepped up greatly if government medical benefits are extended to cover out-patient prescriptions, with the result that the volume of prescription drug purchases subsidized by government would, it has been estimated, rise to nearly 45 per cent from the current 13 per cent.[39] It is surely within the bounds of possibility that these pressures will drastically alter the pharmaceutical drug industry as we know it today and will significantly reduce the amount of clinical research pursued by its constituent firms. If so, in the ensuing vacuum, a substantial part of the burden of new drug research and development would have to become the responsibility of non-profit and governmental medical and scientific institutions.

The Effect of Approved Labeling on Experiments Deviating from Its Directions

The emphasis on the need for obtaining the patient's consent before exposing him to experimentation that has resulted from the 1962 amendments, the FDA's 1967 consent regulations, and the NIH requirements for institutional review has brought the problem of consent into sharp relief. Thus cases will probably be infrequent in which clinical investigations of new drugs will be begun before consents have been obtained from the subjects or at least before a good faith determination has been made that to obtain consent is not feasible or in the best interests of the patients. But drug experimentation does not stop with the approval of a new drug. While a manufacturer must seek to amend its NDA if it wishes to enlarge its claims for an approved product or to change the dosage or mode of administration, the federal law imposes no legal inhibition against experimentation by physicians who obtain an approved drug in the local market and use it experimentally within their own states.[40] Moreover, an "experiment" may occur in the eyes of the law when a patient is given a treatment that departs from accepted norms— though how far that departure may be carried before the physician is exposed to the risk of liability for a resulting injury is a much-mooted matter today.

In both these situations, which have not been formalized by IND's, the risk that consents will not be sought is surely greater than where IND's have been filed. Moreover, the obtaining of consent should not be viewed as a sure safeguard against liability. A consent is no better than the adequacy of the information given the subject as to the nature and hazards of the experiment. This adequacy is not revealed by the consent forms in general use. Hence, when the patient's memory of what he was told concerning the risks he was to run differs significantly from the physician's recollection of what he had told his patient, the plaintiff has a question of fact which he can insist a jury should resolve. Accordingly, where the risks of an experiment or of a novel treatment are substantial, the cautious physician might do well to include in his consent form a checklist of the matters concerning which he intends to inform his patients so that the execution of their consents could attest the coverage of those points.

If the shield of a signed consent can be pierced, there remains the question as to whether there is a legal basis for imposing liability on the physician who has treated the plaintiff. Warnings have been voiced that if the physician knew—or should have known —of the prescribing information in the drug's approved labeling but departed therefrom, a court may view this departure as a ground of liability. Moreover, the chief legal officer of the FDA, William W. Goodrich, has suggested that not only the physician but also the author and the publisher of a textbook on which the physician relied when he exceeded an FDA-approved dosage might be held liable in damages for the resulting harm.

Mr. Goodrich's warning came in response to a question by the publisher of a medical text after a child had died from an overdosage that the text, but not the approved labeling, had permitted. News of this warning led Dr. Walter Modell, editor of *Clinical Pharmacology and Therapeutics,* to write an explosive editorial in the May-June 1967 issue of that journal, an editorial which in due course appeared in the *Congressional Record.*[41] Dr. Modell declared in part:

When the FDA announces that a drug is not only safe but effective in a given dosage range, this announcement, the FDA holds, now has official stature. The FDA indicated that it is striving for a single published source of all information on dosage, contraindications, dangers, and so forth, which will supersede all other works and to which all doctors will have to turn like Holy Writ when they seek help on drugs. When this comes to pass no writing on therapy will be more expert than that of the group of non-experts in the FDA who pass on the contents of drug package stuffers.

The implications of this unprecedented FDA program are shattering. . . .

It is held by many that it takes about five years before a definitive statement can be made about a new drug. This implies that there must be free and unrestricted expression of opinion and publication of experience with drugs already officially described and delimited if progress is to be made in therapeutics and if egregious errors, one way or the other, by the FDA, are to be promptly published and rectified.

If the medical press must keep its hands off dosage, what resources does the FDA have for the writing of its Bible?[42]

Letters by Dr. Goddard and Dr. H. L. Ley, Jr., then Director of FDA's Bureau of Medicine and now Commissioner, in the next issue of *Clinical Pharmacology and Therapeutics,* intended to reassure the militant editor, were quite unsuccessful,[43] and in the March-April 1968 issue Dr. Modell returned to his attack on FDA "censorship."[44] Before the issue went to press, however, he received for publication a copy of an address by Dr. Julius Hauser of the Office of the Associate Commissioner for Compliance, in which Dr. Hauser expressly disclaimed on behalf of Drs. Goddard and Ley any intention to censor medical writings and explained Mr. Goodrich's letter as simply a warning to the publisher of the risk of a damage suit.[45] Dr. Ley had suggested that this risk could be removed in the future by a mere footnote reference pointing out that the views published were those of the author and that "significant details regarding usual dosage" could be found in the package insert.[46] Dr. Modell was satisfied. He retained his editorial, but added a note recording his victory.

To a lawyer-observer, it is difficult to see wherein Mr. Goodrich's letter represented censorship or the address by Dr. Hauser a "victory" for Dr. Modell. On the other hand, Dr. Modell's concern has a genuine base, regardless of the FDA's intent. The package insert is a device designed to limit "all promotion within the bounds of safety and effectiveness."[47] Moreover, as Dr. Hauser recognized, FDA's authority extends to bar drug manufacturers from disseminating reprints reporting studies that go beyond those bounds —unless, of course, the transgressing passages are removed.[48] And, as Dr. Goddard declared in his reply to Dr. Modell: "Without the insert . . . the entire process of new drug approvals is a useless gesture."[49]

Only time and more court decisions will enable lawyers to gauge how hazardous it will be for physicians, either in the course of clinical investigations not subject to IND's or in the treatment of patients, to depart from the prescribing information set forth in the package insert. If courts begin to hold this a basis for liability, then Dr. Modell's fears may begin to be realized, however circumspect the FDA may strive to be.[50]

It is becoming apparent that in the use of the approved labeling device as a mechanism for the control of drug promotion, some provision should be included for an optional, procedurally simple, authorization by the FDA of experimental deviations from its prescriptions by qualified investigators based in institutions having review boards prepared to approve the proposal. Conclusions reached in such a study could also provide a basis for the initiation of a proceeding by the FDA—or even by the investigators—requiring the drug manufacturer to show cause why its labeling should not be amended to conform to the new findings. Often, no doubt, the respondent company would gladly acquiesce in the proposed change. The substitution of a physician's drug compendium for package inserts as a medium of communication would make the adoption of some such measure all the more desirable.[51]

In Brief Summary

The foregoing elaboration of some questions suggested by governmental regulation of human experimentation in the clinical investigation of drugs may have seemed to stray far from the ethical issues so sensitively discussed by other contributors to this book of essays. But, as we have come to see in the law, questions of professional ethics fall under the broader rubric of professional responsibility, and the effort to establish effective governmental controls over new drugs may in time produce a major shift in the responsibility for carrying out drug investigations. Moreover, if those controls are now resulting in a needlessly large volume of clinical trials, this too would seem to implicate professional responsibility. A sensitive concern for the obligation of the investigator to his subject, especially when the latter is his patient, is scarcely lessened if the situation is needlessly multiplied several hundred thousand times a year. Finally, in this field of professional activity where the law's relations with medicine and science are so uneasy, all three callings will have to maintain a continuing scrutiny of the operation and effects of governmental controls if the effort to reinforce ethical obligations by legal duties is not to impair the progress of research and innovation in drug therapy.

REFERENCES

1. Testimony of FDA Commissioner James L. Goddard, "Competitive Problems in the Drug Industry," Hearings Before Subcommittee on Monopoly, Senate Select Committee on Small Business, 90th Cong., 1st Sess. (1967), pt. 2, p. 742 (hereafter cited as "Drug Industry Hearings").

2. In what follows, the term "drug" will be used to refer to those drugs which, because of their potentialities for harm in lay hands, the law allows to be sold only on prescription, although drugs sold "over the counter," if new, must also be approved by the FDA for safety and effectiveness. The statutory criteria identifying prescription drugs and subjecting them to special controls were added to the Food, Drug and Cosmetic Act (hereafter cited as "FDC Act") by the Humphrey-Durham Act of 1951. They are codified as §503(b), 21 USC §353(b). The statutory definition of "new drug" does not distinguish between prescription and over-the-counter drugs. FDC Act, §201(p), 21 USC §321(p).

3. Idem, §201(m), 21 USC §321(m).

4. Labeling, though not shipped with a drug in interstate commerce, may nevertheless be found to be "accompanying" the drug if the labeling is displayed with the drug at point of sale. United States v. Kordel, 335 U.S. 345 (1948). A book commending the drug (honey) when so displayed has been held to be labeling. United States v. 250 Jars etc. of U.S. Fancy Pure Honey, 244 F. 2d 288 (6th Cir. 1965), distinguishing United States v. 24 Bottles "Sterling Vinegar and Honey," 338 F. 2d 157 (2d Cir. 1964).

5. FDC Act, §502(f), 21 USC §352(f), requires that labeling bear "adequate directions for use" and "adequate warnings" against unsafe uses, but exemptions from these requirements may be granted by regulation. Accordingly, the FDA has exempted prescription drugs when dispensed from

most of these requirements, provided they are fully met in the labeling of the package from which the drug is to be dispensed. See 21 Code of Federal Regulations (hereafter cited as "CFR") §1.106(b).

6. The 1962 amendments gave the FDA authority to regulate advertising of prescription drugs, previously vested exclusively in the Federal Trade Commission. See FDC Act, §502(n), 21 USC §352(n). The requirement of "fair balance" is contained only in regulations; it was elaborated in amendments issued in June 1968. See 33 Fed. Reg. 9393, amending 21 CFR §1.105(e) (6), (7).

7. If the advertisement of a drug does not comply with the FDA's regulations, the "drug . . . shall be deemed to be misbranded." FDC Act, §502, 21 USC §352. A misbranded drug is subject to seizure; its introduction or receipt in interstate commerce is a crime. *Idem,* §301(a), (c), 21 USC §331(a), (c).

8. The FDC Act makes no provision for the "Dear Dr." letter. Of course, an alleged violator can refuse to send such a letter and, instead, fight prosecution or seizure in the courts. For eight examples of such letters, see Drug Industry Hearings, pt. 2, p. 808. For the cost estimate, see Sheldon Zalaznick, "Bitter Pills for the Drugmakers," *Fortune* (July, 1968), p. 148.

9. For the legal basis of the "package insert" requirement, see note 5, *supra.* The sponsor seeking approval of a "new drug" must submit specimens of its proposed labeling to the FDA. The FDA's determination of whether the drug is safe and effective is made on the basis of the conditions set forth in proposed labeling. See FDC Act, §505(b), (d), 21 USC §355(b), (d).

10. The statutory basis of the IND (that is, the "notice of claimed investigational exemption for a new drug") is FDA Act, §505(i), 21 USC §355(i). For regulations governing the IND, see 21 CFR §130.3.

11. FDC Act, §505(a), (i), 21 USC §355(a), (i).

12. The IND regulations specify eleven grounds for terminating an investigational drug's exemption. 21 CFR §130.3(d). Absent an imminent hazard, the FDA will terminate only after failure by the drug's sponsor to make an "immediate correction."

13. Testimony of FDA Commissioner James L. Goddard, Drug Industry Hearings, pt. 2, p. 762. If two groups of applications presenting special problems were included, the ratio of "incompletes" to approvals would be five to one. *Idem.*

14. *Idem,* p. 743; see also testimony of Dr. H. E. Van Riper, *idem,* pt. 6, p. 2359. Reference to the longer period seems more common.

15. Dr. Edwin I. Goldenthal, "Current Views on Safety Evaluation of Drugs," *FDA Papers,* No. 2 (May, 1968), pp. 13, 18.

16. Drug Industry Hearings, pt. 2, p. 764.

17. Address to American Society of Clinical Oncology, April 10, 1968, as reported in F-D-C Reports ("Pink Sheet"), No. 16 (April 15, 1968).

18. See Dr. Edwin I. Goldenthal, note 15, *supra*. The quotations in the three following paragraphs of text are all derived from this article.

19. In 1950-65, the drug industry's average rate of return was exceeded only by that of the automobile and cosmetic industries among fifteen major consumer industries. See Drug Industry Hearings, pt. 5, p 1842 (Part 5 contains extensive data and economic analyses on the industry's profitability.) In 1965, 77 PMA member firms spent $365 million on pharmaceutical research on ethical drugs. For six firms spending over $20 million for R&D, the average R&D/sales ratio was 11.3 per cent; for seven firms spending $10-20 million, 10.1 per cent; for eight firms spending $5-10 million, 12.3 per cent. *Idem*, pt. 6, p. 2334, Table 22.

20. Presumably, if not (relatively) safe, these drugs would be deemed prescription drugs. The number of drug manufacturers is an estimate by Commissioner James L Goddard. Drug Industry Hearings, pt. 2, p. 722. Of the 2,000, 861 are "principally manufacturers of prescription drugs." *Idem*, compare note 27, *infra*.

21. See FDC Act, §201(i) (3), 21 USC §321(i) (3).

22. For a report on the penurious state of the FDA until Fiscal Year 1959, when its appropriation reached nearly $11 million, and on the use by Congress of appropriation cuts to curb its zeal, see D F. Cavers, "The Evolution of the Contemporary System of Drug Regulation under the 1938 Act," National Library of Medicine, Conference on the History of Drug Control (1968; publication pending).

23. See F-D-C Reports, Sept. 2, 1968, T. & G. p. 2.

24. *Ibid.*

25. Some complain that the FDA gives insufficient weight to reliable foreign studies, thereby compelling needless clinical trials here In 1965, of all R&D expenditures, the percentage spent abroad by 77 PMA firms averaged only 5.9 per cent within the drug firms and 1.7 per cent outside the firms. PMA, "Ethical Pharmaceutical Industry Operations and Research and Development Trends, 1960-1966," Drug Industry Hearings, pt. 6, p. 2328. An increase was predicted for 1966. *Idem*, p. 2326.

26. F-D-C Reports, July 8, 1968, p. 8, citing the semi-annual report by Paul de Haen.

27. Zalaznick, "Bitter Pills for the Drugmakers," p. 151. PMA President C. J. Stetler estimates the number of pharmaceutical firms at 1,500. Of these, the 136 PMA members produce 95 per cent of prescription drugs. Drug Industry Hearings, pt. 4, p. 1412.

28. See note 17, *supra*.

29. Address at the Alabama Medical Center, April 11, 1968, as reported in F-D-C Reports, No. 16 (April 15, 1968). See Bernard Barber, *Drugs and Society* (New York, 1967), pp. 20-24.

30. The secrecy policy rests on two statutes: FDC Act, §301(j), 21 USC §331(k) (forbidding disclosure of any "method or process" which is a "trade secret"); *idem,* §505(j), 21 USC §355(j) (regulations must have "due regard for the professional ethics of the medical profession and the interests of patients") and the U. S. Criminal Code, 18 USC §1905 (forbidding the unauthorized disclosure by officials of "trade secrets, processes," and so forth, and "confidential statistical data" obtained from their investigations or reports). *Quaere* whether these would preclude mandatory disclosure of animal toxicity studies or, if subjects' names were withheld, Phases I, II, and III testing. See D. F. Cavers, "Administering That Ounce of Prevention: New Drugs and Nuclear Reactors," *West Virginia Law Review* (1968), pp. 233, 256-58. The 1966 Freedom of Information Act, amending §3 of the Administrative Procedure Act, 5 USC §552(b), exempts from disclosure trade secrets, "commercial or financial information" that is "privileged or confidential," and "medical files and similar files the disclosure of which would constitute a clearly unwarranted invasion of personal privacy." *Idem,* §552(b) (4), (6).

31. Drug Industry Hearings, pt. 2, p. 747.

32. *Idem,* p. 743.

33. In Fiscal Year 1967, the FDA approved NDA's for 14 new chemical entities and for 69 other drugs which Dr. Goddard declared "were what have been called 'me-too's' or molecular manipulation." The FDA later corrected the latter figure by subtracting seven new combination products. *Idem,* p. 757.

34. See, for example, testimony of C. J. Stetler, PMA President, Drug Industry Hearings, pt. 4, p. 1367.

35. These certifications were canceled in January 1968 for nine companies; a tenth, Rachelle Laboratories, submitted additional clinical data that are still under review. FDA Press Release, January 19, 1968.

36. Drug Industry Hearings, pt. 2, pp. 796-97. Later he referred to "12 isolated instances." *Idem,* pt. 4, p. 1259.

37. See F-D-C Reports, T. & G. p. 5 (August 12, 1968). The FDA hopes to develop "equivalency standards."

38. Drug Industry Hearings, pt. 2, p. 756.

39. In Fiscal 1967, direct federal purchases of prescription drugs amounted to $177.3 million, or 5.2 per cent of industry sales; "indirect" federal purchases amounted to $264.9 million, or 7.8 per cent for a total of 13 per cent of industry sales. It has been estimated that, in 1970, direct federal purchases would continue at 5.2 per cent of the total, but if prescription drugs were to be added to Medicare, the indirect federal purchases would rise to 38.5 per cent, for a total of 43.7 per cent of industry sales. Data supplied by letter from the Department of Health, Education and Welfare.

40. A violation of the "new drug" provisions of the FDC Act is effected by the drug's "introduction or delivery for introduction into interstate commerce." FDC Act, §301(d), 21 USC §331(d).

41. 113 *Congressional Record*, p. S7884 (June 8, 1967).

42. *Clinical Pharmacology and Therapeutics* (1967), pp. 359-61, reprinted in at least half a dozen medical periodicals. See *idem*, p. 752.

43. *Idem*, p. 749-54 (including two Replies and an "Answer to Dr. Goddard's Countercharges" by Dr. Modell).

44. *Idem* (1968), p. 271.

45. *Idem*, p. 275.

46. Dr. Modell considered authors and publishers of drug treatises to have been "pressured" into publishing this disclaimer (*idem*, p. 750) which Dr. Ley had suggested as one of various means of showing that "differences of opinion exist regarding use of the drug." *Idem*, p. 751.

47. "Statement of the Food and Drug Administration, James L. Goddard, M.D., Commissioner," *idem*, p. 752.

48. *Idem*, p. 275. "Literature and reprints . . . description of a drug . . . which are disseminated by or on behalf of its manufacturer" are "labeling," 21 CFR §1.105(1) (2), and so must conform to the FDA-approved package insert.

49. *Clinical Pharmacology and Therapeutics* (1968), p. 752. No doubt it was not the insert that Dr. Goddard viewed as essential but rather a set of officially approved specifications that the FDA is prepared to police.

50. The New Jersey Supreme Court has admitted a package insert in evidence to allow the jury to find from it that a dentist using a drug (Epinephrine) was on notice of a contraindication (hypertension) reported in the insert and so was negligent in failing to take adequate precautions (ascertaining whether the patient was hypertensive) before administering the drug. *Sanzari v. Rosenfeld*, 34 N.J. 128, 167 A. 2d 625 (1961). Two prior cases had admitted inserts as *prima facie* proof of the relevant standard of care; they showed the approved methods of using the drugs involved. *Julien v. Barker*, 75 Idaho 413, 272 P. 2d 718 (1954); *Salgo v. Leland Stanford, Jr., Univ. Bd. of Trustees*, 154 Cal. App. 2d 560, 317 P. 2d 170 (1957). On the significance of the *Sanzari* case, see Neil L. Chayet, "Power of the Package Insert," *New England Journal of Medicine* (1967), p. 1253.

51. The FDA has been exploring the feasibility of a compendium to serve as a vehicle to bring officially approved prescribing (and price?) information concerning prescription drugs to the practicing physician. See testimony by FDA Commissioner James L. Goddard, Drug Industry Hearings, pt. 2, pp. 766-67. A bill, S. 2944, 90th Cong., 2d Sess., to provide for a compendium financed by industry was introduced by Sen. Nelson on February 7, 1968. See 114 *Congressional Record*, pp. S1006-S1010. Somewhat earlier, C. J. Stetler, PMA President, had reported the opposition of the industry and the AMA. See Drug Industry Hearings, pt. 4, pp. 1401-1403.

IRVING LADIMER

Protection and Compensation for Injury in Human Studies

THE SECTION on "Principles for the Clinical Evaluation of Drugs," Ethical and Legal Aspects of the World Health Organization Scientific Group Report concludes with this statement:

> It is not possible under common law to absolve the investigator from liability for negligence; nor should he be so absolved. Liability for negligence remains a useful check on the incompetent or unscrupulous investigator. However, injuries or mishaps with medical consequences may occur during the course of research in which there is no question of negligence.

> There has been a failure to consider the needs of human subjects who are injured in the course of an ethically irreproachable human experiment. There is need for some process, such as an insurance system, that will pay for medical care, where necessary, and provide appropriate compensation when research subjects sustain injury or death during an investigation, regardless of possible negligence and without prejudice to liability. The cost of this protection should be considered part of the basic cost of the conduct of clinical investigation.[1]

This simple summary of a complex situation, ending with a plea that something should be done, requires immediate attention in view of the breadth and scope of clinical study of all types and the imminent possibilities of injury to the participants. Although research investigators in medicine are generally considered among the most competent and careful health practitioners, they are by no means immune from human acts of omission or commission that may constitute legal fault, negligent or not. In fact, several American cases have arisen involving harm to patient-subjects during recognized experimentation. None has so far been the subject of an appellate court decision, but a Canadian case, following Anglo-American legal principles, has clearly established liability.[2]

247

Protection of Parties

The possibilities, indeed the probabilities, that there may be adverse consequences flowing from human studies are upon us. A logical and comprehensive approach would call for prevention as well as protection of all participants. The conventional tendency to consider solely the protection of the investigator, and perhaps the sponsor, in case of suit is shortsighted and not in accord with the public interest and responsibility accorded medical investigation. The broad and proper view must first look toward the patient-subject, but must also encompass the medical team, the supporting instititutions, and, in a real sense, the general public. All have significant interests and deserve protection in the initiation and performance of any studies, legally as well as ethically, and in the event of untoward occurrences and later burdens. With this objective, a proposal for clinical research insurance was advanced as early as 1960 and published by this author in 1963.[3] In connection with a review of rights and responsibilities of those engaged in such research, this proposal was again recommended.[4]

Despite the general acceptance of the concept by investigators, chiefly physicians, who at once recognized their first professional responsibility—to care for their patients, regardless of cause—the philosophy of nonfault liability met with resistance on the familiar grounds that there should be no liability without clearly established negligence or other misfeasance, and that threat of damage suit served the salutary purpose of discouraging carelessness. Of late, however, there has been an increased disposition to acknowledge the greater social responsibility of safeguarding voluntary participants, both investigators and their partner patients, and the importance of demonstrating professional concern when research is undertaken primarily for scientific advancement.

Widespread interest at all levels demands community consideration of study goals and procedures, including advance protection. It can no longer be assumed that science, despite the great technological progress we have witnessed, may or should proceed without regard for those who make it possible. In particular, we cannot assume that research investigators and patient-subjects will accept risks and hazards without some assurance of reparation if injury, disability, or death occurs. Two protective phases are needed.

Protection and Compensation for Injury in Human Studies

First, *preventive* techniques are required that include a rational basis and need for the proposed study, proper study design, competent and qualified investigators and staff, adequate equipment and materials, a suitable research environment, and selection of individuals or groups in necessary number and type.

Second, *compensatory* measures, including health and medical care, economic recompense, and social and other reparation, must be available to those who may be harmed or injured.

It is submitted that current systems do not adequately meet these requirements. At present, we may be considered as governed by voluntary ethical codes and guidelines for proper research behavior and by standard legal liabilities. The codes and guides, such as the Declaration of Helsinki and the earlier rules set forth following the Nuremberg Trials, may be said to represent the intrinsic professional tenets of concern for the patient, individual integrity, and reasoned fair play. Many have considered these elaborations of the "Golden Rule," and further implementation, as in the American Medical Association Ethical Guidelines for Clinical Investigation, largely presents definitions of the broader Helsinki doctrines.[5] These statements are, for the most part, moral principles and, as such, do not indicate the need for a scheme of protection and contain no such specifications. The first recognition of the duty of the investigator and sponsor to make such provision, incorporated in a declaration of principle, appears in the report of the WHO Scientific Group, "Principles for the Clinical Evaluation of Drugs" cited at the outset of this paper.

Likewise, federal statute and federal policy does not include protective elements. Thus, the 1962 Amendment to the Food, Drug, and Cosmetic Act, which includes, among other things, the general requirements for consent when employing investigational new drugs, does not impose a penalty nor a stipulation for protecting patient-subjects who consent or even those whose consent is not obtained. The FDA Statement of Policy, delineating the agency's interpretation, is also silent in this respect. The Public Health Service now specifies that an institution seeking contract or grant support for research involving human subjects must submit assurances that the safety, health, and welfare of study individuals are safeguarded. Although these extramural requirements, like those for the Service's intramural programs, cover obtaining consent, evaluating risk and benefit, and reviewing, they do not refer to post-study compensation or other restoration. The subject has been broached on many occasions and administrative funds for this purpose are available, but there is no mandate for insurance or health benefits. In an extensive review and comparison of the FDA and PHS approaches, William Curran has noted the emphasis of both agencies on consent and the difference between centralized and decentralized project review and the omissions on the part of both of significant guides and protective requirements.[6]

Since these essentially voluntary controls do not impose or induce the hard protection which the ordinary person understands —as in health-and-accident policy—can we rely on the structures of institutions? By virtue of the Public Health Service policy, practically all medical schools, research centers, and teaching hospitals as well as allied agencies have review committees. These are composed of "sufficient members of varying backgrounds," and many include lawyers, social scientists, theologians, and laymen who might be more concerned and more conversant with management of liability than the medical and health professionals. No special arrangements for compensation, however, have been developed or at least widely promulgated. Instead, they have tended to rely on broad interpretation of individual professional liability (malpractice) policies and the school or hospital coverages. Under these systems, the usual mode is settlement or suit. A case must be based on a claim or charge of negligence or deliberate tort, and no reference is made, within these contexts, to the special issues of clinical investigation where adverse consequence may be the most likely result of some procedures, regardless of fault.

Clinical Research Insurance

An article in the Law and Medicine series of the American Medical Association on the subject of insurance coverage for clinical investigation raises the question of the need for special coverage quite simply:

Most physicians realize that it is unwise to engage in the practice of medicine without adequate insurance coverage for professional liability. . . . Many physicians who engage in clinical investigation, however, wonder whether the insurance they have is adequate for the risks that arise from this part of their practice.[7]

The author notes, as has previously been stated, that "there have not been, as yet, any reported court decisions involving liability of a physician for activities relating to clinical investigation." He describes such activity as including basic scientific investigation, concerned with pharmacology or physiology of a substance or procedure in relation to man; initial trials for determining safety or effectiveness of a substance or procedure; and general clinical trials for diagnosis, therapy, or prophylaxis in a statistically significant group of persons. He believes that the absence of cases so far does not mean that such activity is without risk and suggests that liability might arise from failure to obtain valid consent, observe reasonable care for the safety of the subjects or others, or for allied reasons. "Caution would indicate that insurance protection should be provided for such risks," he concludes.

Examination of existing policies and decisions interpreting the coverage clauses suggests that, although courts tend to construe the language strictly against insurance companies, the operative clauses generally refer to "malpractice" as failing to render professional services in the practice of the profession of medicine. While it is appreciated that scientific investigation of some type is doubtless associated with the customary practice of healing, whether curative or preventive, one of the essentials of clinical study is the emphasis on the problem rather than the patient. There are recognized differences in purpose, expectations, relationships, and quantitative and qualitative aspects of certain procedures, even though, in appearance, the methods used for research and for health care may be essentially the same.[8] This author has pointed out, in a review of the subject in 1955, distinctions such as these:

In research, the investigator chooses patients or subjects within his interest.
In therapy, the patient chooses the doctor because he is sick or seeks to be well.

In research, the investigator may pay the subject or limit charges for treatment.
In therapy, the patient pays for treatment or a third party assumes the costs.

In research, the exchange of information is more active and specific.
In therapy, the exchange is limited since conventional practice is assumed.

In research, expectations include new or different modes and unknown risks.
In therapy, expectations are limited to standard practice and generally known risks.

251

From a purely commercial point of view, the contemplation of the insurer, and the basis for calculation of premiums relating to standard practice and usual risk experience, research may well be excluded from the regular policy. Certainly, in so-called programmed or protocol-defined studies, there is every reason to believe that an insurance carrier would argue that the policy was not intended for such a broad and novel scope. Thus, Richard Bergen of the AMA Law Division holds the opinion that there is good reason to consider additional protection to assure that clinical investigation will be covered. He speculates on two alternatives: that premiums on all policies might be increased to cover both therapy and research risks; or, preferably, that specific personal insurance for research be written, so as not to impose additional costs on physicians who do not engage in human studies. As to the latter alternative, he believes that it is appropriate for the sponsors to assume the cost of protection as a cost of doing business.

This recommendation was offered, in implied fashion, by the present writer at the first major interdisciplinary conference analyzing these issues.[9] A definite program was later proposed[10] and later elaborated.[11] Unlike the suggestion of Richard Bergen of the AMA, noted above, which would add another clause for research coverage to the standard policy, the nonfault concept, deemed particularly applicable to this form of endeavor, was strongly advocated. Others have since come to much the same conclusion,[12] in part from considerations of possible catastrophic accidents, as in atomic-energy research and engineering,[13] and recent proposals for meeting costs of widespread "statistically likely" personal and property injuries, as in motor-vehicle accidents and failures. Albert A. Ehrenzweig, a professor of law and insurance, has developed a fuller variation for hospital accidents, following from his analyses of traffic victims on ground and in air and related hazardous products casualties.[14] These proposals have in common the replacement of the negligence or fault basis of liability and the legal adversary system with a recognition of the need for immediate recompense regardless of fault, provided under an administrative system. Although the details differ, the philosophy of prompt help to the victim is stressed.

The "Non-Fault" Concept and Doctrine

To impose liability on an individual or his supporter and sponsor without first establishing some guilt in the legal sense, such as negligence or misconduct, may appear unfair, even "un-American." We are accustomed to the principle that each one, personally or corporately, is responsible for his actions (or nonactions) which some duty requires. The corollary holds that no liability should be imposed without some legal dereliction. Morally and socially, we have recognized, no such parallelism exists or even applies, since we assume burdens of help and care for others, whether or not required.

The fact is that law also is not that stringent. Sometimes the imposition of liability is considered a miscarriage of justice, as witness the following theme by R. P. Bergen in another of the Law and Medicine series of the AMA Law Division, arguing for early action to prevent medical accidents:

The foregoing decisions [cases against physicians, residents, interns, and students] are but a sampling to show that medical accidents, with or without fault, can lead to damage suits. Even though the law theoretically imposes damages only if someone was at fault in causing injury, physicians, residents, interns, and even medical students can be subjected to litigation when a medical accident occurs, even if there is no fault. Sometimes there is a miscarriage of justice and damages are awarded in the absence of fault.[15]

Important as the army of proposals to avoid malpractice and the devices suggested to avoid liability for mishaps may be, the major consideration must be "what happens if something happens?" It has long been argued that conventional tort liability in law is not appropriate for medical action where the physician and health worker, by definition and otherwise, seek to help and heal. The surgeon's slip of the knife is not the same as the intruder's slash and the workman's cut. Rarely is there an intended harm, and often the injury results from a reasonable professional decision to aid the patient in a particular way. Despite a long and well-established series of cases holding that the doctor cannot be held for an honest mistake in judgment, Bergen has shown that it is not always easy to differentiate such an act from a negligent one or from an oversight that the prudent and experienced practioner would not have made. Also, the rule that the case will be reviewed in light of the standards of the community in which it arose is fast being eroded, so that both parties to medical liability litigation may be subjected to nonlocal practice.[16]

Most physicians would agree that, fault or not, the ethics of the profession and personal conviction place the welfare of the patient first. Idealistic as this concept is, especially in the face of acceptance of legal responsibility, many consider that liability insurance serves that purpose. Settlement out of court without the implications and indignity of litigation and without the technical concession of fault is, therefore, the most prevalent form of conclusion to malpractice allegations.

In the conventional professional liability area, there appears to be increasing dissatisfaction with the current insurance system. As stated in the 1969 Report of the American Medical Association's Board of Trustees:

> Its costs are excessively high in relation to the compensation finally received by claimants. Most important, the patient, the physician, and the insurance carrier are forced into a time-consuming and costly legal gamble on the outcome of a trial which often has no bearing on the true merits of the patient's claim. A more efficient system for the protection of both patients and physicians is long overdue.[17]

Although the Report emphasizes proof of fault as a basis for compensation, it suggests:

> Some mechanism for prepaid protection should be developed which will provide economic protection for persons injured as a consequence of medical or other accidents arising in the course of patient care.

Thus, to offset the rising curve of malpractice suits and charges and "assure equality in malpractice litigation," the AMA would be interested in dual insurance: standard professional liability coverage, matched by insurance prepaid by or on behalf of the patient. Such responsibility on the part of the patient, it is hoped, will reduce not only physician premium costs but also frivolous plaintiff allegations.

As far as research is concerned, such a plan would, of course, only be applicable to patients who may also participate in therapeutic studies and to other volunteers who recognize such potential benefits that they would also be willing to share all aspects of the risk. The proposal illustrates, however, that long-held concepts of professional responsibility are undergoing re-examination in all quarters; nonfault liability, therefore, need not be regarded as an unsupportably radical approach.

If physicians in regular practice tend to feel that protection for the patient is as important, from a legal aspect, as protection for professionals and their institutions, then *a fortiori*, clinical investigators who admit and declare a partnership with patient-subjects should endorse this philosophy. A committee of investigators supported by project grants of the National Institutes of Health, through a spokesman (Dr. George Schreiner, Georgetown Medical Center) endorsed such a measure and, recently, the Grants Division of the NIH began a study of these possibilities. At the Fourth Bethesda Conference of the American College of Cardiology on "The Relation of the Clinical Investigator to the Patient, Pharmaceutical Industry and Federal Agencies," the subcommittee concerned with the rights of patients recommended such study, and many lawyers and physician-investigators have requested full and serious inquiry along this line.[18]

Meeting Social Responsibility

Accepting the patient's participation in return for benefits deriving from biomedical research argues for social responsibility that would remove the adversary approach and proceeding, whenever potential or actual injury arises out of human studies, notably those principally for scientific advancement. The magnitude and importance of the issues gravely and forcibly affect the public interest. Although it is universally agreed that volunteers who have consented to take part in research may not be recruited or used unless all reasonable means are taken to assure their safety, there is always the possibility of adverse consequence, directly or indirectly.

Some assurances, therefore, must be provided for handling injury. These should be comprehensive, covering all aspects of participation for the patient or subject; they should also relieve the investigator of personal and economic jeopardy. In the absence of such a common-sense arrangement, there can be no proper expectation that volunteers or investigators will long engage in research projects. As more is advertised and known about experimental medicine, and as patients pay their own way (personally or otherwise) and are not considered automatic research "material," the pressures for protection of this kind will mount. It is preferable to prepare in advance, in a climate of scientific and public accord, rather than to react to another "thalidomide" incident or a publicized case of patients used without their knowledge and consent.[19]

Appropriate Protection

Since we do not now have the certainty of adequate protection, due to the present system of litigation and settlement which often results in capricious awards or losses, and in no sense do we have an equitable solution, the "umbrella type of liability insurance," even if extended, will not meet the needs of all concerned parties. It is therefore submitted that, if society accepts the benefits of research, society should accept responsibility for careful process and protective measures. No one should be inhibited from undertaking valid and approved studies because of the legal hazard alone; but no patient or subject should be placed at disadvantage for agreeing to serve. The cost of protection should, therefore, be considered a proper charge on the business of conducting research, to be assumed by the sponsor, in much the same way as other basic administrative costs are assumed by government, industry, or service institutions and agencies. It will be recognized that this is the well-known principle underpinning workmen's compensation, in which the employer bears the cost of insurance for injuries arising from authorized work performed at his request and for his advantage.

In view of the current American pattern of research efforts, entitlement to recompense for physical or mental injury or economic loss should depend on the relationship of the parties and on the causal connection of the adverse outcome to the clinical study. In short, an application of the workmen's or industrial insurance concept, rather than employer liability or malpractice, would seem proper and feasible. Solely by being a recognized patient who has suffered through an established relationship, compensation would accrue. It would not be necessary to show fault, negligence, or lack of caution. Where culpable negligence or malfeasance might exist, the patient would not necessarily lose the right to sue—an option available under some state compensation laws —but, generally, the nonfault system would apply. Of course, no one would be twice reimbursed, and no one would twice suffer. An alternative, with greater administrative difficulties and increased cost—but with perhaps some advantage in business and insurance principle—would be limited health and accident insurance for each volunteer. Under this plan, payments would be made on showing of medical need, again without regard to the reason or problem of fault. The workmen's compensation form, however, is preferable since a sponsor could carry such coverage for his entire research enterprise, without special project or patient policies, thus insuring all participants as and when they enter, with minimum administration.

The contingencies which should be covered include: first, consequences due to application of the experimental substances, procedures, or withholding of standard practice; second, incidental or accidental events associated with, but not directly related to the studies; and, third, peculiarities of the participants. The last named would encompass the idiosyncratic or "allergic" reaction, the bugaboo of plaintiffs in many malpractice cases, in which the claim of injury is countered by the defendant as a rare, if not unique, response to a generally small or limited risk. It is highly desirable to cover all of these contingencies to avoid the need for distinguishing among them, to establish good faith on the part of the profession and broad responsibility for any proximate consequence. There is no great likelihood of self-inflicted injury, contributory negligence, or defiance of the doctor or hospital, such as would rule out a plaintiff suing under a regular liability policy. It would be fair, however, to exclude situations created by the patient or subject with intent to profit under a compensation system.

Consequences

What consequences or occurrences should be compensable? In general, they would be the same as those usually included in the damages bill under any suit or settlement, namely:

1. Illness or disability: direct or immediate; subsequent or indirect; relating to physical, mental, emotional or social detriment, limited, extended or chronic.

2. Death: immediate or subsequent.

3. Income loss: immediate, subsequent, or potential.

Any one or several of these may arise during or following a study. Thus, the compensation may be due at once or later to the individual or dependent or any other person who may be entitled to damages. The most important factor—medical care and related service, such as rehabilitation or home or institutional aid—would likely begin at once, probably in the same environment and provided by the same staff. An appropriate plan would recognize that termination of a project would not necessarily terminate the need for protection since, as noted, some of the needs may arise later. This consideration argues for some type of insurance based on regular payment of premiums rather than on self-insurance, although that may be feasible for a large, permanent research agency or a government enterprise.

In sum, protection should be commensurate with the requirements and character of clinical investigation and should provide, *first*, high quality medical care and support including hospitalization and, *second*, cash compensation in appropriate measure. There should be no damages of a windfall or exemplary nature, solely the necessary award to restore the individual to a reasonable status. There should also be no speculative costs; a full or partial schedule, such as under workmen's compensation regulations, may be helpful as guidance in this respect. The program should, in effect, encourage the enlistment of patients and healthy volunteers and not serve to demean medical research or promise exorbitant returns. The protection proposed is that which is required: care and costs, not a gamble or a reliance on the uncertain and ambiguous liability suit or settlement.

It must be admitted that there are a number of problems, but two are significant. The first, accepting the principle, questions whether it is reasonably possible to define "medical research" and its consequences, so that untoward results and injuries which may be due to treatment or the natural course of disease are not improperly attributed to the study or its investigators. No one can assure that definitions and medical causation will be equivalent to their legal counterparts and thus present no problems of coverage and compensation. Naturally, guidelines and sharing of experience as well as adjudication, as developed by compensation agencies, will have to be employed. With interest in success and the application of scientific evaluation and fair review, this important problem should be capable of solution.

The second, more philosophic, question inquires whether investigators will be so relieved of personal concern, since the salutary threat of suit will not exist, that they will no longer observe optimum diligence and care. To this, one can only reply that investigators, properly chosen, have earned the respect of their co-professionals in practice as among the most competent and qualified. It is unlikely that the provision of appropriate protection will lower their standards. In individual cases, as always, other constraints and sanctions—including ineligibility for coverage—can always be imposed.

Experience

It is finally asserted that there is little experience to estimate program costs. There have been several cases, clearly within the definition (funded research under a responsible sponsor observing a protocol) in which settlements have been made. But the dearth of experience is no warrant for postponing a desirable system, especially since there are established means for meeting this issue. A simple method, applied by this author in initiating a malpractice program under similar circumstances, merely set an arbitrary but reasonable premium cost for the first two years, subject to re-evaluation, with provision for increasing or decreasing the charges based on initial and later experience.

As a comment, it is unlikely that the costs will be great, probably a small fraction of customary malpractice premiums. First, there are few compensable occurrences within responsible research institutions, where most of the studies are conducted. Second, the assumption of medical care, most likely at the sponsor's premises, will reduce such costs. Third, the adoption of such a system should tend to improve prior protection, controls, and research design; this is especially true for studies approved by research review committees. Fourth, the spirit and philosophy of this form, which should be fully explained in advance in discussions with participants, should serve to diminish rather than induce any questionable claims. Many now advocate, for example, that the protective measures be incorporated as part of the investigator-subject conversations leading to understanding and informed consent.

In view of the inherent hazards of clinical investigation, appropriate protection for all participants should be established in the public interest through a form of compensation insurance, whereby restitution may be made for any untoward result, based on the relationship of the parties and injury due to the research, rather than through adversary litigation based on fault or negligence. The costs should be borne by the sponsors as an accepted cost of the enterprise. Such an approach will provide proper and needed protection for all, without gamble, and should prove reasonably inexpensive. It accords with the nature and dignity of clinical research and demonstrates the public and social responsibility of the profession. A voluntary, organized method will accommodate all interests and also avoid the present inequities and uncertainties and the imposition of undesirable controls.

REFERENCES

1. World Health Organization, "Principles for the Clinical Evaluation of Drugs," *Technical Report Series* No. 403 (1968), p. 19.

2. Halushka *v.* University of Saskatchewan, *et. al.*, 53 D.L.R. (2d) 436 (1966).

3. I. Ladimer (editor), "Clinical Research Insurance," *Journal of Chronic Diseases,* Vol. 16 (1963), pp. 1229–35.

4. I. Ladimer, "Rights, Responsibilities and Protection of Patients in Human Studies," *Journal of Clinical Pharmacology and New Drugs,* Vol. 7 (1967), pp. 125–30.

5. American Medical Association, Declaration of Helsinki and AMA Ethical Guidelines for Clinical Investigation (pamphlet; 1967).

6. See the essay in the present book by W. J. Curran, pp. 402–454.

7. R. P. Bergen, "Insurance Coverage for Clinical Investigation," *Journal of the American Medical Association,* Vol. 201 (1967), pp. 305 and 306.

8. I. Ladimer, "Ethical and Legal Aspects of Medical Research on Human Beings," *Journal of Public Law,* Emory University, Vol. 3 (1955), pp. 467–511. Reprinted in part in Ladimer and Newman, "Clinical Investigation in Medicine," Law-Medicine Research Institute, Boston University Press (1963), pp. 179–210.

9. National Society for Medical Research, "Proceedings of the First National Conference on the Legal Environment of Medical Science" (Chicago, 1959).

10. Ladimer, "Clinical Research Insurance," *op. cit.* note 3.

11. *See,* Veterans Administration, "Medical Ethics and Research," Symposium of Research and Education Service, Department of Medicine and Surgery, (Cincinnati, 1967) Monograph 10–2 and I. Ladimer, "Social Responsibility in Clinical Investigation," *Medical Science,* Vol. 18 (October, 1967), pp. 33–41, based on "Bloomfield Lecture," Case Western Reserve School of Medicine.

12. D. L. Stickel, "Organ Transplantation in Medical and Legal Perspectives," *Law and Contemporary Problems,* Duke University, Vol. 32 (1967), pp. 596–619.

13. Atomic Energy Act, Price-Anderson Amendments, 10 U.S.C. 2354, 72 Stat. 972 (1958). Also, Columbia University Legislative Drafting Fund, "Financial Protection Against Risks of Major Harm in Government Programs," prepared for the National Security Industrial Association (March, 1963).

14. A. A. Ehrenzweig, " 'Full Aid' Insurance for the Traffic Victim" (1954). Also "Compulsory 'Hospital Accident' Insurance: A Needed First Step Toward Displacement of Liability for 'Medical Malpractice,' " *University of Chicago Law Review,* Vol. 31 (1964), pp. 279–90.

15. R. P. Bergen, "When to Start Medical Accident Prevention," *Journal of the American Medical Association,* Vol. 208 (1969), pp. 2557–8.

16. W. J. Curran, "Village Medicine versus Regional Medical Programs: New Rules in Medical Malpractice," *American Journal of Public Health,* Vol. 58 1968), pp. 1753–4.

17. American Medical Association, Report of Board of Trustees, "Medical Professional Liability" (Report: D-A-69), (1969), pp. 1487–93.

18. American College of Cardiology, Conference Report, "The Relation of the Clinical Investigator to the Patient, Pharmaceutical Industry and Federal Agencies" (August 1966); *American Journal of Cardiology,* Vol. 19 (1967), pp. 892–907. Also G. Schreiner and D. Bogdonoff, "Limbo to Limb—the Moral and Legal Entanglements of the Clinical Investigator," *Clinical Research,* Vol. 11 (1963), pp. 127–30.

19. I. Ladimer, "Current Issues in Research and Experimentation on Human Beings," Memorandum for *Dædalus* proceedings (Nov. 3 and 4, 1967), p. 5.

LOUIS LASAGNA

Special Subjects in Human Experimentation

THERE ARE strong passions in the breasts of laymen and professionals alike concerning the use of special groups of the population as experimental subjects. To certain people, there is something particularly heinous about human experimentation that involves prisoners, or children, or students, or the dying. It is the purpose of this paper to examine the reasons for these objections, to appraise their validity, and to offer some guidelines for dealing with the special problems pertaining to these subject groups.

Debates over the use of prisoners as volunteers illustrate how social attitudes about non-health and non-research matters can become tangled with the specific ethical and scientific issues of biomedical investigation. The unprivileged status of criminals was clearly taken advantage of in earlier times. The ancient Persian kings and the Egyptian pharaohs are said to have treated criminals as expendable experimental material, much as a modern laboratory researcher might order a supply of rats or rabbits. The practice was apparently still in vogue in eighteenth-century England, since Caroline, Princess of Wales, "begged the lives" of six condemned criminals for experimental smallpox vaccination before submitting her own children to the procedure. (She also procured, for further trial, "half a dozen of the charity children belonging to St. James' parish.")

During the Nuremberg trials in 1947, the German physicians cited earlier reports, from the world literature, of experiments on criminals. Early in the twentieth century, Richard P. Strong (later Professor of Tropical Medicine at Harvard) infected with plague some criminals condemned to death. Strong is said to have asked permission of the Governor of the Philippines, but not of the inmates.[1] He also produced beriberi in another group of twenty-nine Philippine convicts, two of whom died as a result of the experiments. The convicts, who were under sentence of death, were volunteers and received "an abundance of cigarettes and also cigars if they desired them" as a reward for their participation.

In 1915, Goldberger produced pellagra in twelve white Mississippi convicts in an attempt to discover a cure for the disease, but in this case formal agreements were drawn up with the convicts' lawyers, agreeing to subsequent parole or release.

In the 1940's, over four hundred convicts in Chicago were infected with malaria as part of a wartime crash program to develop new drugs for the prevention and treatment of this infection. Malaria was a major threat to Allied troops in the Pacific Theatre and had been suppressed in the past largely by quinine, but the supply of quinine had been partially shut off due to Japanese occupation of the Dutch East Indies.

These prisoner volunteers were required to sign the following document:

I . . ., No. . . ., aged . . ., hereby declare that I have read and clearly understood the above notice, as testified by my signature hereon, and I hereby apply to the University of Chicago, which is at present engaged on malarial research at the orders of the Government, for participation in the investigations of the life-cycle of the malarial parasite. I hereby accept all risks connected with the experiment and on behalf of my heirs and my personal and legal representatives I hereby absolve from such liability the University of Chicago and all the technicians and assistants taking part in the above-mentioned investigations. I similarly absolve the Government of the State of Illinois, the Director of the Department of Public Security of the State of Illinois, the warden of the State Penitentiary at Joliet-Stateville and all employees of the above institutions and Departments, from all responsibility, as well as from all claims and proceedings or Equity pleas, for any injury or malady, fatal or otherwise, which may ensue from these experiments.

I hereby certify that this offer is made voluntarily and without compulsion. I have been instructed that if my offer is accepted I shall be entitled to remuneration amounting to . . . dollars, payable as provided in the above Notice.[2]

Governor Green of Illinois appointed a special tribunal to examine the problem. The committee recommended that the subjects be informed of the possible hazards of their volunteering, that they be able to refuse to participate without fear of additional punishment or of deprivation of ordinary privileges, and that "all unnecessary injury and physical and mental suffering be avoided."

The Green Committee accepted the principle that the parole system is desirable, that reduction of prison sentence is justifiably viewed as a reward for good conduct, and that service as a subject in a medical experiment was a form of good conduct.

The committee appreciated that prisoners might be motivated by "good social consciousness," a desire for reduction in sentence, or both, but went on to say:

A reduction of sentence in prison, if excessive or drastic, can amount to undue influence. If the sole motive of the prisoner is to contribute to human welfare, any reduction in sentence would be a reward. If the sole motive of the prisoner is to obtain a reduction in sentence, an excessive reduction of sentence which would exercise undue influence in obtaining the consent of prisoners would be inconsistent with the principle of voluntary participation.[3]

As long ago as 1856 Claude Bernard condemned the use of criminals in experimentation, and as recently as 1961 the World Medical Association held that "persons retained in prison penitentiaries or reformatories, being captive groups, should not be used as the subjects of experiments."

Paul Freund of the Harvard Law School has expressed the following opinion:

I suggest here that [prison] experiments should not involve any promise of parole or of commutation of sentence; this would be what is called in the law of confessions undue influence or duress through promise of reward, which can be as effective in overbearing the will as threats of harm. Nor should there be a pressure to conform within the prison generated by the pattern of rejecting parole applications of those who do not participate. It should not be made informally a condition of parole that one go along, be a good prisoner, and subject himself to medical experimentation.[4]

While one school of thought is opposed to the use of prisoners because they represent a "category of abused persons," another objects to their use because of the fear that convicts will not pay their full measure of penance to society. This "turn-the-screw-a-little-tighter" philosophy is exemplified in a 1952 resolution adopted by the House of Delegates of the American Medical Association:

Whereas, during recent years, numerous medical and scientific experiments and research projects have been conducted partly or wholly in federal and state penal institutions; and

Whereas, volunteers among the inmates of such institutions have been permitted to participate in scientific experimental work and to submit to the administration of untested and potentially dangerous drugs; and

Whereas, some of the inmates who have so participated have not only received citations, but have in some instances been granted parole

Special Subjects in Human Experimentation

much sooner than would otherwise have occurred, including several individuals convicted of murder and sentenced to life imprisonments; and

Whereas, the Illinois State Medical Society's delegation to the American Medical Association's clinical session wholeheartedly supports research and progress in the fight against disease but does believe that persons convicted of vicious crimes should not qualify for pardon or early parole in this manner; now therefore

Resolved, that the House of Delegates of the American Medical Association express its disapproval of the participation in scientific experiments of persons convicted of murder, rape, arson, kidnapping, treason, and other heinous crimes, and also urges that individuals who have lost their citizenship by due process of law be considered ineligible for meritorious or commendatory citation; and be it further

Resolved, that copies of this resolution be transmitted to the Surgeons General of all federal services, the governors of all states, all officials of state and federal penal institutions and parole boards.

More recently, articles have begun to appear that attempt to justify the use of volunteer prisoner subjects on humane grounds rather than simply on the basis of expediency. It has been pointed out by J. C. McDonald, for example, that volunteering presents an opportunity to break the monotony of prison life, which tends to be both regimented and stereotyped: "To these inmates, life is basically a bore, and one day is quite like another." Participation in an experiment can be both refreshing and exciting (perhaps especially because it includes elements of the unknown and of personal risk).[5] It gives the prisoners something to talk about; moreover, *they* become an item of conversation for fellow prisoners. The volunteers may, for a time at least, be "the elite of their own society."

The experiment also provides an opportunity for the prisoner to maintain, or develop, a sense of personal value. Participation as a subject may involve sacrifice, perseverance, altruism—a chance for the inmate to prove to himself or to friends and relatives that he can do something worthwhile. The prisoner volunteer may also profit considerably from his contacts with the clinical investigator or technical staff, whose relation to the prisoner is likely to be a more cordial and sympathetic one than most of the relationships experienced by the convict in the past, either in or out of prison. The prisoner need not be suspicious of, or antagonistic toward, the doctor, who is not a part of the penal system and can serve as a friend or adviser.

Some prisoners also believe that they are logical choices for

265

medical experiments; they have no job and may have no family or responsibilities, no one who is not already adjusted to "doing without them." They may, therefore, be willing to accept risks for the common good that they themselves would avoid if they were not in jail.

Finally, the prisoner volunteers seem to develop, at least in some situations, an *esprit de corps,* and group satisfactions reinforce the individual satisfactions derived from participation in an experiment.

In Iowa, a specific law was finally enacted to cover an arrangement that began in 1949. Despite an occasional elopement of prisoner volunteers from the metabolic ward of the University of Iowa Medical Center, this arrangement has worked smoothly since 1949, except for a two-year period during which the legal status of the practice was in dispute. The Iowa Code now states:

The board of control may send to the hospital of the medical college of the state university inmates of the Iowa state penitentiary and the men's reformatory for medical research at the hospital. Before any inmate is sent to the medical college, he must volunteer his services in writing. An inmate may withdraw his consent at any time.

R. E. Hodges and W. B. Bean have speculated on the reasons for volunteering by prisoners in this situation.[6] Like others, they believe that the relief from monotony is an important factor for some prisoners. Monetary gain, while a possibility, seems minimized by the one-dollar per-day remuneration. These authors point out that prison volunteers are less reluctant to be visited by their children in a hospital environment, and that many may be motivated by "a longing for feminine proximity." For others, volunteering at Iowa represents a chance for escape or the hope for preferential prison treatment in the future.

These authors state that "for their participation in research activities, [prisoners] receive no reduction of their sentence nor any favoritism regarding paroles. We do, however, send a letter to the warden at the termination of each experiment expressing our appreciation for the inmate's participation in the study. It is possible that this letter in the prisoner's file may favorably influence the parole board."

What is an ethically defensible point of view toward the use of prisoners in research? The situation is extremely simple if one believes that a prison sentence is for punishment alone, and that each prisoner must not only serve his full sentence, but also live as boring and stultifying a life as possible while in jail. Pursuing this philosophy to its logical conclusion, one would not allow volunteering for *any* purpose, including ordinary job assignments within the prison that might result in reward for the prisoner, either in the form of money or parole credit. Such an attitude is not tenable, I submit, in our present intellectual climate.

If one takes the position that prison should serve, at least in part, a rehabilitative role, it is considerably more difficult to draw up a rigid set of rules. A few points, however, seem indisputable. No experiment should be performed (on *anyone*) that is brutal, inhumane, or so badly designed or executed that no useful information is likely to result. These adjectives imply value judgments, of course, but the principle is nevertheless an important one. The relevant issues should be decided by a review committee of some sort—one that involves, at the very least, a group of qualified scientists who are not directly implicated in the research and, possibly, a mixed group of laymen and scientists, including prison officials. It should be a rule of thumb in all human research that no experiment is tolerable that cannot be justified to a group of reasonably unbiased, rational, intelligent human beings.

The problem of obtaining informed consent should pose no *special* difficulties in regard to prisoners. Since almost invariably the prisoner will be a healthy, non-patient volunteer, he should be treated exactly like any other healthy volunteer. Thus, all the details of the experiment, including a full exposition of the risks, should be discussed candidly with the potential subject.

The problems of remuneration and "unreasonable incentive" (that is, a reward so great that it persuades the subject to accept risks that he otherwise would not) are also not specific to the prisoner volunteer, although they are no easier of solution in this group. *Should* a volunteer (prisoner or not) be able to risk his life for a large reward (parole in the case of the prisoner or $1,000 for a medical student who is badly in debt)? Should all volunteering be independent of reward?[7] If so, then volunteers for all experiments would have to be "signed on" without discussion of compensation. This is obviously not the case at present. A healthy volunteer is often extremely interested in the compensation. Many volunteers participate in experiments precisely *because* they will be compensated, and the amount of reward is expected to be related to the amount of discomfort or inconvenience they may suffer. Filling out questionnaires will command one level of reward, taking a drug and providing urine specimens another, being stuck in an artery or vein repeatedly for blood samples still another.

It has been argued that the prisoner is "captive" in a special sense, but is not the person in need of money a captive to poverty? Is not the guilt-laden neurotic volunteer captive to his disturbed emotions? Is not the Mennonite or Brethren volunteer a captive to his religion? Is anybody more "captive" than the twin or parent of a child dying of chronic nephritis and desperately needing a kidney transplant? All decision-making can be looked upon as a weighing of the advantages and disadvantages of various courses of action, or of the relative merits of action and non-action. Does it really "protect the rights" of a prisoner to forbid him to volunteer for a dangerous but potentially important experiment in anticipation of some reward? Is such volunteering—if it is not forced upon him by arbitrary fiat from some authority—generically different from the case of the test pilot who risks his life in return for money, excitement, or both?

Those who remain convinced that a prisoner should *not* be allowed to undergo possibly risky experimentation in the hope of shortening his sentence might consider certain methods of handling this objection. One possibility would be to allow *no* credit for volunteering. (I assume that no one would favor lengthening a prisoner's sentence because he volunteered to be a subject: That alternative seems both extreme and unrealistic.) Or one could allow the volunteer prisoner's record to show only that a day or a week was spent in "work," with the type of activity being unspecified. A day spent as a research subject would then be counted equally with a day in the prison laundry or the license-plate shop. If the records scrutinized by parole officers scrupulously avoided mention of volunteering for research, conceivably the inmate would have little incentive to believe that his prison term would be differentially affected by involvement in an experiment. (A prisoner who has heroically risked his life to save another convict who was caught in a machine should presumably have that fact entered in his record, although perhaps some would suggest that this act, too, could be construed as a calculated attempt to get extra parole benefits.) Monetary rewards can either be kept low or abolished, if remuneration represents a difficulty in regard to undue pressure to volunteer.

The dying patient provides another set of problems. It could be argued that a person with only a short time to live should not have any of his few remaining days taken away from him. There is no difficulty, in my opinion, in administering a potentially toxic drug—as are most anti-cancer chemicals, for example—to a dying patient who may benefit personally from the drug. In such cases, the ethical problems—informed consent, the original decision to perform the experiment, and so forth—do not strike me as being unique to the dying patient.

There are difficulties, however, when one plans to use seriously ill patients for research. Two objections to the use of the dying volunteer in such circumstances are scientific in nature, and not ethical. Such studies may, for example, mislead the investigator in regard to the physiologic effects or metabolism of a drug because of the serious somatic and psychologic derangements attendant on the patient's illness; they are also likely to generate spurious fears about the drug's side effects and toxicity because of the occurrence of spontaneous untoward events, including death, that are in fact not due to the drug, but may be attributed to it.

Unquestionably, there have been instances in the past where dying patients have been subjects without being aware of it, the justification being that "they were dying anyway." It is not possible to defend such an attitude, legally or ethically, and I shall not attempt to do so. But the problems here are not unique to the dying patient, and the technique of obtaining consent should, in general, not differ essentially in terminal and non-terminal patients.

But what of the use of dying patients who truly volunteer for studies unrelated to their specific illnesses? Suppose a patient who knows he is dying of cancer is asked for permission to do some metabolic studies on a new drug proposed for the lowering of blood cholesterol levels? Is there any ethical problem if such a patient understands what is planned, knows that the data obtained will not affect his own illness, but desires to participate to help people with hypercholesterolemia, or perhaps a son with this condition? I submit that there need not be.

I am concerned, however, about the use of students as volunteers in experiments conducted by their academic superiors. If a student is of age to give consent, there would seem to be no special ethical problem about volunteering in *general*. But if a student in a classroom is asked to volunteer by his instructor, there is at least the implied threat of loss of affection (and decreased academic grade) if the student fails to volunteer, which takes the situation into a nasty area of restricted choice. Furthermore, it has been the practice in some institutions actually to give extra credits for such participation, a procedure that raises the issue of infringement of the rights of those who do not volunteer or are not chosen after volunteering. Should the non-volunteers at least be allowed another means (non-experimental) of earning extra credits equal in amount to those earned by the volunteers, so as not to be academically disadvantaged? Perhaps, but the problems involved in being "fair" to all parties concerned suggest that it may be simpler, as well as more ethical, for professors to avoid soliciting volunteers from student groups whose academic standing or future employment may be in their hands. It is not enough to say that a professor will not be swayed in his marking or writing of reference letters by whether a student has volunteered; the *belief* that he will do so is enough to act as a troublesome influence on both the volunteer and the non-volunteer.

Some of the thorniest problems relate to the use of children, whose "consent" has to be obtained by proxy from a parent or guardian. In general, children who are ill and may benefit from an experimental drug or surgical procedure pose no more ethical problems than those that exist when a sick child is to be given an "approved" drug or procedure. In both instances, the consenting party must be made aware of the risks and hazards involved in action or non-action. In the experimental situation, however, there will usually be the added protection for the subject of a protocol review by a board of the investigator's peers or by a mixed layman-scientist board. This is not to say that children should be chosen as the *first* subjects to receive a new treatment. Unless the disease is uniquely pediatric, there seems to be good reason to perform the earliest experiments in adults who can *personally* consent to the procedure, rather than to utilize a subject for whom a third party must give consent.

Should children be used as experimental subjects when they are not to receive treatment that can benefit them personally? Children are often used as subjects (without *anyone's* consent) in educational surveys or psychological testing, but here the risks are presumably negligible or nil, and society is ordinarily not inclined to object. It is not so easy to justify doing early drug "dose-range-finding" studies on healthy children, since they cannot legally consent to such procedures, and it is difficult to know how much understanding they would have of the problem were their "consent" sought in an informal way.

On the other hand, ruling children out of all clinical trials that do not involve treatment of the sick could preclude trials of prophylactic intent, such as the polio vaccine experiments. In the latter trials, one was dealing with healthy children, half of whom were to be given a virus vaccine that was supposed to prevent a (clinically) rare disease, but that could (and did, in a few instances) actually *cause* the same disease. Was it ethical to conduct the trial? Was it "fair" to the children who served as controls and might actually have been rendered more at risk than usual because their vaccinated (and protected) playmates might be transmitting live virus to them? Should the latter fact have been discussed in obtaining consent from parents of both the volunteers and the controls?

One experiment with retarded children that superficially seems disturbing turns out to be unobjectionable, in my opinion, on full examination.[8] Newly admitted children to the Willowbrook State School in New York State have actually been infected with hepatitis virus by dosing the children with serum from Willowbrook patients with hepatitis. This seems at first glance abhorrent, but in fact everyone admitted to the school appears to develop hepatitis anyway during the first six to twelve months. In the inoculated children, the dose can be adjusted, and immunity can be acquired by experiencing a disease that is no more severe than the usual (rather mild) illness clinically acquired. Furthermore, the experimental group can be housed separately and exposed to the hepatitis virus without simultaneous infection from other organisms endemic in the institution. In this case, the protocol was reviewed and approved by several agencies, informed consent is always obtained from the parents, and the use of children who are wards of the state is scrupulously avoided.

One final point about pediatric patients. I am completely unclear in my own mind about what and how much should be discussed with the child. If he is an infant, the problem is simple, as it also is if the child is in the late-teens but not yet of legal maturity. But what of the eight- or ten-year-old? How much "consent" should (and can) he give? How much should he be told simply to "inform"?

The use of retardates as subjects should raise no new issues, since the same principles that apply to the normal child, or the psychiatrically incompetent, would seem to apply to the mentally retarded. Surely no one can condone their being treated as subhuman experimental animals. The fact that society may have to pay for their support cannot be construed to allow society free license to use them as subjects cavalierly and without restraint.

The psychiatrically ill may pose some problems in regard to consent. Like the child, the mentally ill person who cannot consent for himself should not, I believe, generally be used as a subject in experiments unrelated to his immediate medical problems. But even in therapeutic trials, there are difficult questions: When is a patient *non compos mentis?* How crazy is crazy? At what point does a neurotic become unable to give informed consent? Can one trust the relatives to be "objective" in giving consent? (This last question applies to all third-party situations, of course, but one has the feeling that relatives of the insane are often almost as disturbed as the patients.)

There is, unfortunately, a tendency for people to moralize about the ethical problems in human research in terms of black-and-white categorical imperatives. I much prefer John Fletcher's statement: "It is far easier to act on the basis of an abstract principle than it is to make a fitting response to new situations on the basis of concrete and immediate responsibility."[9]

Absolutist doctrines seem no more defensible in this area than in others. What sometimes passes for ethical profundity may, in fact, be only shallowness and an irresponsible or arrogant failure to appreciate the richness of the moral alternatives and the subtlety of the ethical issues.

Nothing in my knowledge of the history of medicine, religion, or law supports an ethical approach to medical or experimental practices that is unchanging and dogmatic. Nor would anything in my personal work or reading lead me to believe that there is one "right" answer to such questions as "when does life begin?" or "when does life end?" At the end of the sixteenth century, Pope Sixtus V decided that the previous practice of allowing abortion during the first eighty days of pregnancy was no longer defensible and that abortion at any age of the fetus was sinful. After the death of Sixtus, Pope Gregory XIV decided that abortion was permissible until the time of quickening. In 1869, however, Pius IX returned to the dogma of Sixtus V. During these various periods of history, I suspect, the individuals who were concerned with the problem in question almost certainly believed that they had fastened upon the eternal truth.

The laws of different lands encourage one to believe that "the

272

age of understanding" for a child is a variable and flexible matter. It is said to be twelve or fourteen in the various sections of the British Isles, but is generally placed later in the United States. A knowledge of developmental biology and human variability emphasizes that any rigidly defined age for achieving "majority" is as ridiculous as one inflexible age for retirement of the aged.

Such questions as "who owns a person's body?" may be fascinating as material for discussion and debate, but they are hardly resolvable by logic and reasoning. A Jain sect member believes that to kill a gnat is a sin, and I do not, but neither of us can prove the other wrong (at least in this world).

It would seem preferable to avoid dogma, codes, pontifical stands, and the temptation to talk in capital letters about THE SANCTITY OF LIFE, with the letters written in colored crayons with stars between them, à la Hyman Kaplan. Indeed, at times the greatest regard for human life may be shown by someone who is willing to take a life. We might approach ethical issues in a manner that has been suggested for tackling problems of aesthetic disagreement. One cannot prove that Andrew Wyeth is inferior to Jackson Pollock, or that Mozart is superior to Tchaikovsky, by arguing about one's preferences. But if two people can agree on what they wish a work of art or music to lead them to, on what a piece of artistic creation is supposed to achieve, then they may begin to pick and choose between alternatives and make value judgments relevant to the stated goals. We may agree, for example, that an increase in happiness, serenity, understanding, or creativity is desirable, in which case we can then ask which of the alternatives is most likely to lead us swiftly and predictably to the goal. A piece of music might be said to be better than another if it leads to an appreciation and understanding of other more difficult or complex pieces of music, or if it "wears" better on repeated listening. An individual or a society can and indeed should, I believe, set itself such goals and use them as means of evaluating possible courses of action.[10] I prefer such an ethical stance to one that searches for eternal ethical truths that lie hidden but unchanging in some philosophical vault—a quest for the moral equivalents of the platinum meter rule.[11]

Human experimentation is required in order for medical progress to be made. Such research will of necessity involve risks that can be minimized, but not eliminated. For many reasons, the risks cannot be evenly distributed among the members of society;

the many will continue to benefit from the contributions of a few. As I see it, the basic issue is to keep taking ethical readings on our research approaches so as to be sure that we do not destroy the moral fabric of society in our zeal to improve its physical fabric. Some scientific gains may only be available at a price we are unwilling to pay. We may, for example, be willing to tolerate unpredictable death for hundreds of patient volunteers in return for a cancer cure, whereas we might not be willing to achieve such a discovery if it were only to be made by placating a sadistic god through the public torture and dismemberment of a single child. The problem, then, is to decide when to say "Halt!"

The problem, therefore, boils down to a sober weighing of costs and gains, not a preoccupation with moral clichés and stereotyped mottoes. Much has been written, for example, on the need for "informed consent," but little research has been conducted on what this term actually means. What do we consider a "fair shake" as far as the subject is concerned? How much tailoring of our presentation is required by differences in age, personality, or I.Q. among patients? What minimal information do we want conveyed before we ask whether a subject is willing to participate in an experiment? In one experiment, we have found that lengthy, detailed expositions of risks and purposes may defeat the process of communication, with less comprehension of the problems and dangers than if one uses a brief, straightforward statement.

Have we adequately presented the possible alternative courses of action to the subject? Has society, in its general approach to experimentation, considered what the harm will be of *not* doing research? Have we honestly decided when the rights of the individual must yield to the rights of the group (as they inevitably must on many issues)? There is nothing intrinsically more noble about a concern for the individual than a desire to aid the many; in fact, it might be argued that the opposite underlies the democratic process or the social contract in general. I submit that the less doctrinaire our thinking, the less preoccupied we are with forms, and the more concerned we are with goals and substance, the wiser will be our decisions and the more soundly will we sleep at night.

REFERENCES

1. M. H. Pappworth, *Human Guinea Pigs* (Boston, 1967), p. 61.
2. *Ibid.*, p. 62

3. *Ibid.*, p. 63

4. P. A. Freund, "Ethical Problems in Human Experimentation," *New England Journal of Medicine,* Vol. 273 (1965), pp. 687-92.

5. J. C. McDonald, "Why Prisoners Volunteer to Be Experimental Subjects," *Journal of the American Medical Association,* Vol. 202 (1967), pp. 511-12.

6. R. E. Hodges and W. B. Bean, "The Use of Prisoners for Medical Research," *Journal of the American Medical Association,* Vol. 202 (1967), pp. 513-15.

7. Volunteering can *never* be free of reward, of course, since no one will be able to prevent the inner satisfactions and compensations experienced by the subject.

8. "The Willowbrook Hepatitis Project," *Medical Tribune,* Feb. 20, 1967.

9. J. Fletcher, "Human Experimentation: Ethics in the Consent Situation," *Law and Contemporary Problems,* Vol. 32 (1967), pp. 620-49.

10. This position may be interpreted as moral relativism, but I do not believe that it is. As Alexander Pope has said:

    "Fools! who from hence into the notion fall
    "That vice or virtue there is none at all.
    "If white and black, soften and unite
    "A thousand ways, is there no black or white?"

11. It is interesting that even the platinum-iridium meter bar at the International Bureau of Weights and Measures at Sèvres, France, was replaced as a standard in 1960 by radiation measurements derived from krypton[86] , and the bronze yardstick that was the British imperial standard turned out to lose substance with time.

GEOFFREY EDSALL

A Positive Approach to the Problem of Human Experimentation

THE ORIGINAL subject considered for this paper was "Human Experimentation from the Investigator's Viewpoint." Such a title would be misleading, however, for if this viewpoint could be identified as an isolated entity, it would be too narrow to warrant detailed scrutiny. The majority of investigators known to this writer are part of the mainstream of society; they are concerned over human welfare, staunch defenders of individual rights, and quite disturbed to find themselves put on the defensive for being—as they would see it—in the vanguard of human progress.

Since investigators are, after all, people, generalizations about them are hazardous. But it is safe to say that the great majority of them operate on the assumption that decisions are best reached by the use of reason; they believe that rational thinking is the surest path to right decisions. Being people, however, they may suffer at times from a narrowness of scope in the source material for their reasoning, and they surely must have—to the extent that they are creative—a tendency toward stronger egos than average men are blessed with. Also, being absorbed in the rational process, they may too often be inadequately equipped to perceive the enormous impact of non-rational determinants in the making of individual or social decisions. These and other factors have undoubtedly been largely responsible for the fact that there is an issue here to be resolved.

The striking upsurge of concern over the ethics of human experimentation during the past few years has arisen for a number of well-known reasons set forth elsewhere in this volume. Suffice it to point out that in the tremendous expansion of experimental studies on man that has occurred since World War II, there have been numerous instances in which the ethical approach to the use of human beings for such purposes has appeared to be grossly deficient. There have been other situations in which this deficiency was considered as clear and unequivocal by the average informed layman, even though the scientists concerned may have quite honestly and, indeed, vehemently felt that their actions had been wholly ethical. Be that as it may, documentation of a large number of actual or alleged instances of such violations has been published by H. K. Beecher,[1] by M. H. Pappworth,[2] and by others. Perhaps the most widely publicized example in recent years was the New York episode concerning the injection of cancer cells into elderly and chronically ill individuals who were not specifically informed that malignant cells were being injected into them.[3] At all events, these and other episodes have focused attention upon the actual and potential risks, in our society, that human beings may be used carelessly or callously to accomplish the objectives of investigators whose ultimate goals may have been wholly admirable, but whose judgment as to the means for reaching these goals was unacceptable to the community.

The first reaction has—predictably—been to impose restrictive regulations or laws. Such a reaction tends to be self-accelerating, for a while at least, as a result of the stimulus created by the initial publicity arising from the trigger situations. Questions are raised not only about the events that have led to the issue at hand, but about worse events that may have happened, might happen, or could conceivably happen. Hence the over-all reaction to this type of situation tends to spiral more and more tightly into a set of concepts and terms that give emphasis to only one view of the total situation.

Thus, human experimentation is widely referred to in terms of the *use* of human beings by an investigator. Whenever this *use* appears to have been improper, the investigator is considered to have violated the *rights* of the individual. Major emphasis has been placed on the overriding importance of obtaining *informed consent* from the individual to be utilized in a human experimental study. All of these words, phrases, and concepts—even though they are in themselves totally correct and admirable—tend to narrow the framework of thinking in this field and to force it into a somewhat rigid moralistic-legalistic structure based largely upon the risk of individual "violations" of a code and upon the enforcement of the code by an essentially legalistic system of controls.

Such a structure obviously tends to create and perpetuate a

situation in which the investigator finds himself working in an atmosphere of supervision and suspicion. Once enjoying the exaggerated hero status of an "Arrowsmith," he has suddenly gone a fair distance along the path to the status of a scientific "Elmer Gantry," drawing gullible people into his own sphere for his own interests and plotting to gain power and influence selfishly through exploiting others. (Margaret Mead documents this vividly elsewhere in this issue.) Obviously, both extreme concepts are absurd, but they point up the necessity of finding a reasonable set of concepts and processes that will place human experimentation, and the persons responsible for it, into a harmonious framework in our society. Otherwise progress in medical science and medical practice may be hampered, as progress in the biosciences has been hampered for the last three quarters of a century by the rigid laws against animal experimentation in Great Britain.[4]

What Is Human Experimentation?

At first blush, it would appear easy to define human experimentation: Irving Ladimer describes it as "deliberately inducing or altering body or mental functions, directly or indirectly, in individuals or in groups primarily for the advancement of health, science and human welfare."[5] But the issue is actually not so simple as this. As M. R. Shimkin has pointed out:

Medical experimentation on human beings, in its broadest meaning and for the good of the individual patient, takes place continually in every doctor's office. Hence the general question of human experimentation is one of degree rather than of kind. Deliberate experimentation on a group of cases with adequate controls rather than on individual patients is merely an efficient and convenient means of collecting and interpreting data that would otherwise be dispersed and inaccessible.[6]

Similarly, Sir Geoffrey Jefferson has said: "All medical treatment is also experimental. . . . The prescription of even rest in bed for two or three weeks, or of a bottle of cough mixture, are experiments, the results of which deserve closer observation and quantitative analysis than they get."[7]

Furthermore, as Shimkin has also pointed out: "To do nothing, or to prevent others from doing anything, is itself a type of experiment, for the prevention of experimentation is tantamount to the assumption of responsibility for an experiment different from the one proposed."[8] Nevertheless, the generally accepted concept of what a human experiment is (as distinguished, for example, from medical treatment) is determined by the purpose of the person who initiates the action: If a physician gives a patient a new drug because he believes (even if only on the basis of advertising) that the drug will do the patient good, then he is acting as a physician. On the other hand, if he has doubts about the adequacy of the information furnished to him, wants to resolve these doubts himself, and therefore gives the drug to alternate patients with the disease in question, the others receiving a standard drug, then he is experimenting on his patients. In both cases, his motives may be totally and completely humane, and his desire may well be to do the very best he possibly can for his patients. But in the first instance the physician is seen as acting wholly in the patient's interest, with pure, undiluted humanistic motives, whereas in the second, the interests of the patient are generally assumed to have been subordinated—be it only slightly—to another objective. Somewhat analogous antitheses may be found in situations involving consent for operations. One may take the classic example of the teenage youth who consented—in the absence of his parents—to serve as a skin graft donor for a cousin of his who had been bady burned. The youth became ill and suffered a permanent scar. The physician was sued—successfully—for having used a minor in this fashion without obtaining parental consent. That the donor of the skin had acted idealistically, in the sincere hope of helping his cousin, was apparently considered irrelevant to the decision.[9]

Ten years later arose the landmark case concerning the consent of a minor to donate a kidney for his identical twin brother, who suffered from chronic renal disease that would soon prove fatal.[10] The question at issue was whether or not the operation to remove a kidney from the healthy brother could proceed—even with the consent of the parents and of both twins—without incurring civil or criminal liability. The judge pointed out that testimony by a psychiatrist had indicated that if the sick twin should die without the transplant, the resulting emotional disturbance could well affect the health and physical well-being of the donor twin for the rest of his life. Thus the judge found the operation was necessary "for the continued good health and future well-being of Leonard" (the healthy twin). Here we have clear reaffirmation of the principle implied in the skin graft case: If the action to be taken is at variance with traditionally or legally established procedure, it may be condoned *if it is of self-interest to the person upon whom the operation is to be performed.* On the other hand, the argument that the proposed action has a generous, humanistic, or idealistic basis is apparently inadmissible in court. Thus, in the eyes of the law, the individual is physically inviolable, *his* interests are paramount, and consent for any action that may violate the integrity of his physical being must be based upon the assumption that such action will be for his benefit.

Not everyone agrees with this rank order of values, and some speak out strongly for recognition of the role and the rights of the community. John Dewey, for example, although speaking of animal experimentation at the time, articulated the "community" viewpoint broadly when he said: "The community at large is under definite obligations to see to it that physicians and scientific men are not needlessly hampered in carrying on the inquiries necessary for an adequate performance of their important social office of sustaining human life and vigor."[11] Lord Moulton expressed similar concern over the risk to mankind of erecting barriers to the advancement of knowledge, and the importance of planned experimentation in contrast to passive observation of events: "When we are reduced to observation, Science crawls."[12]

Indeed, in the absence of experimentation, not only science but morality suffers. There are many instances in which the traditional belief that a particular medical procedure was of value has been shattered by carefully controlled experimentation. A widely recognized instance is described by A. B. Hill and his colleagues.[13] Long-term anticoagulant therapy in cerebrovascular disease had given what appeared to be beneficial results in uncontrolled studies; yet by properly controlled studies it was shown that this therapy actually increased the risk of cerebral hemorrhage. Similarly, A. D. Callow and his associates have put to the test an operation that for many years has been taken for granted as being beneficial in extreme cirrhosis of the liver.[14] Only when controlled studies were done was it determined that the operation afforded no significant benefits—a critically important finding for seriously ill patients faced with a major operation that until then was sanctioned by "common knowledge."

The above considerations are cited in order to show as clearly as possible that the ethical issues involved in "human experimentation" are complex and subtle. They overlap into several other areas of medical action, and the whole field is interwoven with traditional ethical and legal concepts that require careful examination and redefinition if they are to be interpreted effectively and constructively in terms of our present-day society, ethics, and communal structure.

The Issue of "Informed Consent"

In keeping with our traditional societal and legal concepts of the sacredness of the individual as noted above, a primary issue that has been raised in conjunction with human experimentation is the establishment of "informed consent." For instance, in the Sloane-Kettering case, the doctors responsible for the study in question did not inform the volunteers that the substance being injected into them consisted of human cancer cells.[15] The doctors maintained that the cells were harmless, that the use of the phrase "cancer cells" would unnecessarily alarm the volunteers, who could not have understood the scientific concept that was being presented to them, and that failure to use such words as "cancer cells" was therefore warranted by the normal criteria of communication, aside from the human value of the study. On the other hand, the Board of Regents of New York State, in considering suspension or revocation of the licenses of the responsible physicians, concluded that they had no right to withhold any of the facts that the volunteer might have regarded as relevant. This is the basic theme of "informed consent." This concept, of course, goes far beyond the specialized situation of human experimentation and applies to medical practice in general. For example: "In a recent malpractice suit in California, the plaintiff received a substantial settlement when convulsions and permanent deterioration followed smallpox vaccination. . . . The basis for settlement was the attorney's argument that the parents of the child were not warned that encephalitis and cerebral damage might result from the vaccination."[16] Thus the underlying thesis here, as in the case of many operative procedures as well as in human experimentation, is that the individual who is to submit to the procedure be given full opportunity to exercise *his own judgment* as to whether or not to go through with it.

Actually, there is essentially no valid argument about the basic principle that informed consent—or whatever may be its legal equivalent in a specialized situation—is a prerequisite for human experimentation. But here again, as in the case of the definition of experimentation, the issue is not so simple. Wolf Wolfensberger has presented an extensive and thoughtful analysis of the complex mechanisms involved in a combination of consent procedures, the responsibilities of the investigator, the value and limitations of legal procedures such as "releases," and the ethical issues that underlie the over-all issue of consent.[17] Yet it is often difficult, if not impossible, to define the limits of the "information" required for such consent. P. J. Burnham has outlined a "consent form" that might represent the extreme requirements for such a simple operation as a hernia[18]; and although his outline is facetious, it nonetheless reminds the reader that even a simple operation may involve mishaps in surgery, accidents while on the hospital floor, or catastrophies resulting from anesthesia that are existing risks, even though they are so rare that they are often disregarded. Thus, the mechanics of informed consent may be made as complicated as the group responsible for defining it chooses to make them.

This may not be the main issue, however, for the implementation of informed consent is in many cases much too easy a hurdle for the investigator to clear. People in general want to trust the doctor and the expert, and they are naturally influenced by his persuasiveness and conviction. Thus, as Edmund Cahn somewhat overstates it:

One of the major malpractices of our era consists in the "engineering of consent." Sometimes this is effected simply by exploiting the condition of necessitous men as in certain Indian States where thousands of consents to sexual sterilization have been purchased by offering a trivial bounty to the members of a destitute caste. Then again, consent may be "engineered" by the kind of psychologist who takes it for granted that his assistants and students will submit to experiments and implies a threat to advancement if they raise objections. Or the total community may "engineer" a consent, as when the President, the Generals and the newspapers call with loud fanfare for a heroic crew of astronautical volunteers to attempt some ultra-hazardous exploit.[19]

On the other side of the coin—as psychiatrists have frequently pointed out—many neurotic patients will give their "informed consent" primarily because of a masochistic desire to be subjected to pain or discomfort, or possibly simply to get attention, to gratify their guilt feelings, or for other reasons that might be suspected of blunting their free-will judgment.

Furthermore, what is the definition of "informed"? Bradford Hill has pointed out: "Surely it is often quite impossible to tell ill-educated and sick persons the pro's and con's of a new and unknown treatment vs. the orthodox and the known.["20] And he goes on to say:

If the patient cannot really grasp the whole situation, or without up-setting his faith in your judgment cannot be made to grasp it, then in my opinion the ethical decision still lies with the doctor, whether or not it is proper to exhibit, or withhold, a treatment. He cannot divest him-self of it simply by means of an illusory or uncomprehending consent.[21]

The problem of consent becomes even more complicated when it deals with special categories of individuals, such as minors, pris-oners, and the insane. Bradford Hill has pointed out the difficulty in reaching rational decisions on this general subject. Take, for example, the item in the code of the World Medical Association that says "Children in institutions and not under the care of rela-tives should not be the subjects of human experiments." Hill com-ments:

Does pasteurized milk contribute less than raw milk to the promotion of health and growth? Does sugar in the diet influence the incidence of caries? Is gamma globulin more or less effective than convalescent serum in the prevention of measles? Was it unethical to find out in the very circumstances in which it was possible (as well as important for the subjects) to do so? The guide says yes.[22]

Yet in Great Britain it is generally not considered permissible to carry out any experiments on minors—even with the consent of the parents—if the experiment is not to be of direct potential benefit to the children and if there is any hazard involved. Largely on the basis of this philosophy, H. K. Beecher and others, such as Senator Thaler, have criticized the Willowbrook studies on infectious hepa-titis in retarded children. Robert Ward and his associates have de-scribed in detail how they thought through this problem:

The decision to feed hepatitis virus to patients at Willowbrook was not undertaken lightly. Consideration was given to many factors before the decision was reached. It was based on the following facts and criteria:

It is well recognized that *infectious* hepatitis is a much milder disease in young children. Hepatitis was especially mild at Willowbrook; it was even benign in adults, and there were no deaths.

Only the local strain or strains of virus already disseminated at Willow-brook would be used.

Since the annual attack rates of jaundice were high—for example, 20 to 25 per 1000—and since in all probability cases of hepatitis without jaundice were occurring with a frequency equal to overt forms, it was apparent that most of the patients at Willowbrook were naturally ex-posed to hepatitis virus.

The advantages were considered of inducing the infection under most favorable circumstances such as special isolation quarters with special medical and nursing personnel to provide close observation and extra care.

The study was planned so as to begin with very small and obviously ineffective doses of virus and to increase the dosage level gradually, in accordance with the results obtained.

The study group would include only patients whose parents gave consent.

A serious uncontrolled endemic situation existed in the institution, and knowledge obtained from a series of suitable studies could well lead to its control.

These factors were instrumental in the decision to proceed with the plan for titrating virus and inducing so-called "passive-active immunity." The plan was sanctioned by the authorities of the New York State Department of Mental Hygiene, and by the Armed Forces Epidemiological Board, Office of the Surgeon General.[23]

The following year, in reviewing the question, they said:

The decision to continue the artificial induction of hepatitis with the Willowbrook strain of virus was made after the following factors had been carefully reconsidered:

It was inevitable that most of the newly admitted susceptible mentally retarded children would acquire the infection in the institution at large. Secondly, infectious hepatitis, a benign disease of children, was especially mild at Willowbrook. Thirdly, facilities were available to provide optimum medical and nursing care in an isolation unit capable of housing 16 patients. And, finally, observations on more than 50 patients who acquired artificially induced hepatitis at Willowbrook revealed that the average experimental disease observed was even milder than the observed natural infection. In fact, many cases would have gone unrecognized if it had not been for careful daily observation aided by serial tests of liver function. In the institution at large these mild transient illnesses would have been missed.

Only newly admitted patients, whose parents gave consent, were accepted for the study. The subjects ranged between three and nine years of age. On entry they were brought directly to the isolation unit and had no contact with other patients in the institution. The nurses and attendants had minimal contact with other patients and personnel. One physician (J.P.G.) made serial clinical observations of all the study patients.[24]

Thus the issue is joined: Is it proper and ethical to carry out experimentation in children in which the experiments would apparently incur no greater risk than the children were likely to run by nature, in which the children received what might well have been better medical care when artificially infected than if they had been naturally infected, and in which the parents as well as the physician felt that a significant contribution to the future well-being of similar children might well result? That some would take the position that even under these circumstances a study such as this was unethical raises another crucial question underlying the philosophy of consent. There does not appear to be any consistent pattern that applies across the board in analogous situations. For example, in this country we permit parents to sign permission for their seventeen-year-old sons to enlist in the military service and thereby run the risk of being killed or permanently maimed. We allow youngsters from the age of sixteen or thereabouts to drive automobiles, take their friends with them, and get killed or maimed individually or collectively. We permit minors to accept many other normal risks—perhaps because they are socially acceptable; they can break their legs, their necks, or their skulls in organized athletics, usually without either the blessing of formal "consent" or the burden of personal liability.

On the other hand, there are many court actions that have, in essence, affirmed the right of society to make decisions concerning minor children—for example, when in the view of prevailing medical opinion the parents were opposing a life-saving procedure recommended by the medical profession. Here the fundamental issue is the right of the individual minor to be protected by "responsible" individuals. Yet the universal recruitment—or conscription—of minors into military service indicates that, under some circumstances, other overriding issues may prevail. There seems to be no clear definition of the delicate balance that exists between the rights of the individual and the rights of society. This balance comes into play over and over again, manifested by the restrictions that are imposed on an individual's right to drive a car, by the vaccinations required of children entering school, and by many other issues where society weighs the rights of the individual against those of the community, and not infrequently imposes its societal will on a specific individual. As Walsh McDermott points out:

As a society we enforce the social good over the individual good across the whole spectrum of non-medical activities every day, and many of these activities ultimately affect the health or the life of an individual. . . . In the decision to impose capital punishment or the selection of only a minority of our young men to become soldiers, the issue is decided by a judgment that is arbitrary as it affects the individual. In short, we play God. When we take away an individual's life or liberty by one of these arbitrary judgments we try to depersonalize the process by spreading responsibility for the decision through a framework of legal institutions. . . . This . . . type of mechanism works only because there is widespread public acceptance that society has rights too and that it is preferable that the power to enforce these rights over the rights of the individual be institutionalized.[25]

René Dubos has gone further in stressing the importance of viewing such problems in terms of the good of the community. He urges that we "redirect our efforts towards those questions of the community as a whole that have a medical basis and that are so grossly neglected at the present time."[26] He illustrates his point with the problem of post-vaccinal encephalitis: "This is a clear case where the individual problem has to be completely dissociated from the total social problem" in deciding on society's right to require vaccination despite this risk.[27]

Thus it is clearly necessary to admit the limitations of the mechanism of "informed consent" and to go beyond it in looking for supplementary or alternative mechanisms for guaranteeing that human experimentation will be ethical.

Additional Criteria Bearing on the Ethics of Human Experimentation

Recognizing the inadequacy of the simple mechanism of "informed consent," a number of attempts to protect potential subjects and to establish workable guidelines, or both, have been made. Outstanding among these have been the codes adopted in connection with the Nuremberg trials by the World Medical Association and other groups. (To this familiar list should be added the highly original and perceptive "Human Studies—Guiding Principles and Procedures" adopted by the Trustees of the Massachusetts General Hospital in 1967.) Since codes, like laws, are relatively unworkable unless they are dynamically interpreted, the general tendency in recent years in this country and perhaps elsewhere has been to establish review groups or "peer committees." Thus, in human investigations as a whole, current attitudes have moved closer to the view expressed by Beecher: "Security rests with the *responsible* investigator who will refer difficult decisions to his peers."[28] The role of such peer groups has been well summarized in an editorial commenting on the directives of the NIH for establishment of minimal standards for human experimentation:

Its central focus is wisely on the establishment of local institutional committees that will act as the proper consultative bodies to safeguard the welfare of patients, approve the procedural aspects of consent (or its lack) and pass on the qualifications and judgment of the investigators as well as the risks and potential benefits of the projects proposed. . . . Just as physicians are reluctant to treat their own families for fear of lack of objectivity, the feeling has grown that the interests of clinical investigation are best met by avoidance of personal bias.[29]

The title of this editorial, "Friendly Adversaries and Human Experimentation," although couched in somewhat legal language, reflects actually the dominant kinetics of modern scientific thinking—that no idea or proposal is valid unless it has been submitted to the most rigorous efforts to refute it. In this spirit, it would seem that scientists and lawyers alike might find a common philosophy around which could be built a mutually workable structure for developing a stable and lasting mechanism for reaching decisions in human experimentation.

Assuming that the investigator has conformed to the best applicable version of the principle of informed consent or its equivalent, and assuming that he has conformed to the best applicable arrangement for review by his peers, then he (and his peers) have additional responsibilities that are in many ways fully as important as the issues of informed consent and individual rights. For example, he has an obligation to get the maximum possible information from the study that he is about to carry out. This requirement is often understated or insufficiently recognized. Bull has pointed out: "Many proposed new treatments are themselves dangerous and it is unjustifiable to use such treatments unless the maximum of information on their possible deleterious effects can also be extracted."[30] Bradford Hill has pointed out the humanistic merits of *controlled* trials in illuminating detail.[31] The human risks incurred by failing to use controls have already been stressed above. Suffice it to state that a clinical trial which fails to yield clearly interpretable, scientifically sound information, and which has thus failed because of inadequate design, inadequate controls, is fully as immoral as a clinical trial that was carried out without the due process of consent.[32] Indeed, as T. C. Chalmers points out, it is ethically important to randomize such studies *at the beginning* of the trial of a new drug.[33] Failure to do this has resulted on innumerable occasions in an incorrect conclusion—for example, that a drug was valuable or dangerously toxic—before conclusive information was actually obtained on the balance between toxicity and usefulness.

There are major dilemmas resulting from the implementation of these principles. I know of one active infectious disease service, for instance, that is faced with the problem of decision when a candidate drug becomes available which might result in a higher cure rate in acute bacterial meningitis. The treatment for bacterial meningitis is on the whole quite successful at present, but still there is a significant number of failures. If one is to test a new candidate drug in such a way as to obtain clearly interpretable information on its relative value, one must administer it to randomly selected patients, another random group getting the currently accepted treatment. Yet in the instance in question, the review committee has hesitated to authorize such studies because they incur the risk that those patients submitted on a random basis to the new treatment *might* do worse than those receiving the standard treatment.

Risk and Progress

This leads to a major philosophical issue that is difficult to discuss within the framework of protecting the rights of human individuals, but is a profoundly fundamental part of human society—namely, the inseparable relationship between risk and progress. The practicing physician has—generally unconsciously—accepted this situation time after time when he has tried out a new drug on a patient because he thought, believed, or hoped that it would be better. Many such drugs have turned out to be disastrously toxic. Even though there are now mechanisms to minimize this hazard, nevertheless progress inevitably brings with it certain risks that must be faced. The development of oral poliomyelitis vaccine appeared, a few years ago, to carry with it a risk of vaccine-associated poliomyelitis—especially Type 3—on the order of one case in a million vaccinated, in adults. The extensive use of the vaccine in children brought about in turn the risk of infecting adults associated with the vaccinated children. This degree of risk—alarming as it was to some people—nevertheless was minor compared to the advantages to be gained by the vaccine. In another country, a cautious decision not to take such a risk has proved to be in error. Because of the apparent risk of vaccine-associated cases of Type 3 poliomyelitis, this type was omitted from their vaccine. Several years later an epidemic of Type 3 poliomyelitis broke out, considerably more serious than the hazard presumably avoided by withholding this type from the immunization program.

Instances parallel to this, of progress linked to risk—in automobile design, airplane development, provision of electricity in homes and elsewhere, and so forth—could be cited to illustrate the inseparability of progress and risk in all human societies. This does not in any way minimize the importance of consent, but it forces us to recognize that risk is an element in human experimentation that cannot be left out of the equation.

Finally, another point often overlooked is the right of the volunteer to volunteer. Perhaps this is most acutely highlighted in the case of the prisoner volunteer. J. C. McDonald has clearly shown the personal value, to prisoners, of the privilege of volunteering for medical studies.[34] This privilege need not be limited to prisoners, however, and should be kept in mind as a part of the social structure of civilized man which—though never to be pushed ahead of the right to refuse to volunteer—must be kept as a part of the total picture when the question of human experimentation is under consideration. Elsewhere in this book, Margaret Mead has focused on the teamwork element in human experimentation, and Jay Katz's happy phrase, the "shared adventure,"[35] re-emphasizes the positive human and community values that are inherent in such experimentation, properly conceived and performed.

Clearly human experimentation is an inescapable fact of our present-day society. It is also clear that the individual rights of the subjects of such experimentation must be observed and protected not merely by obtaining their informed consent, but by establishing reliable procedures for insuring the scientific wisdom of the experiments into which they are drawn. (Here I have used the word "wisdom" rather than "usefulness" of the experiment as a criterion, since emphasis on "usefulness" would be likely to act as a barrier to innovation, which is often the only gateway to genuine progress.)

Human experimentation, like all human adventures, enlists the volunteer into the forward movement of civilization and to this extent enriches him, as does any constructive social act enrich a person. Thus I believe that human experimentation can best be seen in its total place in society as basically not unlike the United Fund; those who can, contribute (theoretically without pressure—but that is another problem); the proposed use of the resources acquired from volunteer donors is evaluated by a mechanism trusted in the community; and all who are able, willing, and invited to contribute may do so according to their own beliefs, capabilities, and limitations. Despite the great differences in detail between the two components of the analogy, there are deep-rooted similarities fundamental to the concept involved. Therefore I propose—as a resolution of the dilemmas that have arisen in the adjustment of human experimentation to our scientific aspirations and our ethical values— that it be seen as a social necessity to the community, inherently dangerous if mishandled, but if wisely handled serving a double role of benefit to the community as a whole and enrichment to the individual who can accept the privilege of participation.

REFERENCES

1. H. K. Beecher, "Ethics and Clinical Research," *New England Journal of Medicine*, Vol. 274 (June 16, 1966), pp. 1354-60.

2. M. H. Pappworth, *Human Guinea Pigs: Experimentation on Man* (Boston, 1968).

3. E. Langer, "Human Experimentation: New York Verdict Affirms Patient's Rights," *Science*, Vol. 151 (February 11, 1966), pp. 663-66.

4. W. J. Dempster, quoted in *Hospital Tribune*, July 15, 1968, p. 2; see also any biography of Lord Lister.

5. I. Ladimer, "Ethical and Legal Aspects of Medical Research on Human Beings, from Law and Medicine, a Symposium," *Journal of Public Law*, Vol. 3 (1955), pp. 467-511.°

6. M. B. Shimkin, "The Problem of Experimentation on Human Beings: The Research Worker's Point of View," *Science*, Vol. 117 (February 27, 1953), pp. 205-207.°

7. G. Jefferson, quoted by Renée C. Fox, "Some Social and Cultural Factors in American Society Conducive to Medical Research on Human Subjects," *Clinical Pharmacology and Therapeutics*, Vol. 1 (July-August, 1960), pp. 423-43.° Jay Katz, elsewhere in this book, has further underlined the difficulty of distinguishing between experimentation and treatment.

8. Shimkin, "The Problem of Experimentation on Human Beings: The Research Worker's Point of View."

9. Ladimer, "Ethical and Legal Aspects of Medical Research on Human Beings, from Law and Medicine, a Symposium."

10. W. J. Curran, "A Problem of Consent: Kidney Transplantation in Minors," *New York University Law Review*, Vol. 34 (May, 1959), pp. 891-98.°

11. J. Dewey, quoted by A. C. Ivy, "The History and Ethics of the Use of Human Subjects in Medical Experiments," *Science*, Vol. 108 (July 2, 1948), pp. 1-5.*

12. Lord Moulton, quoted by D. M. Jackson, *Moral Responsibility in Clinical Research* (London, 1958).*

13. A. B. Hill, "Medical Ethics and Controlled Trials," *British Medical Journal*, Vol. 1 (April 20, 1963), pp. 1043-49.*

14. A. D. Callow, *et al.*, "Interim Experience with a Controlled Study of Prophylactic Portacaval Shunt," *Surgery*, Vol. 57 (January, 1965), pp. 123-30.

15. Langer, "Human Experimentation: New York Verdict Affirms Patient's Rights."

16. E. B. Shaw, "Informed Consent," *American Journal of the Diseases of Children*, Vol. 114 (December, 1967), p. 590.

17. W. Wolfensberger, "Ethical Issues in Research with Human Subjects," *Science*, Vol. 155 (January 6, 1967), pp. 47-51.

18. P. J. Burnham, "Medical Experimentation on Humans," *Science*, Vol. 152 (April 22, 1966), pp. 448-49.

19. E. Cahn, "The Lawyer as Scientist and Scoundrel: Reflections on Francis Bacon's Quadricentennial," *New York University Law Review*, Vol. 36 (January, 1961), pp. 1-12.

20. A. B. Hill, "Medical Ethics and Controlled Trials," *British Medical Journal*, Vol. 1 (April 20, 1963), pp. 1043-49.*

21. *Ibid.*

22. *Ibid.*

23. R. Ward, *et al.*, "Infectious Hepatitis," *New England Journal of Medicine*, Vol. 258 (February 27, 1958), pp. 407-416.

24. S. Krugman, *et al.*, "Infectious Hepatitis," *New England Journal of Medicine*, Vol. 261 (October 8, 1959), pp. 729-34.

25. W. McDermott, Opening comments to Part II of Colloquium on Ethical Dilemmas from Medical Advances, *Annals of Internal Medicine*, Vol. 67, No. 3, Part II Supplement (1967), pp. 39-42.

26. R. Dubos, "Individual Morality and Statistical Morality," *ibid.*, pp. 57-60.

27. *Ibid.*

28. H. K. Beecher, "Consent in Clinical Experimentation: Myth and Reality," *Journal of the American Medical Association*, Vol. 195 (January 3, 1966), pp. 34-35.

29. Editorial, "Friendly Adversaries and Human Experimentation," *New England Journal of Medicine,* Vol. 275 (October 6, 1966), pp. 785-86.

30. Bull, quoted by Jackson, *Moral Responsibility in Clinical Research.**

31. Hill, "Medical Ethics and Controlled Trials."

32. See article by David D. Rutstein elsewhere in this volume.

33. T. C. Chalmers, "When Should Randomisation Begin?" *Lancet,* Vol. 1 (April 20, 1968), p. 858.

34. J. C. McDonald, "Why Prisoners Volunteer to be Experimental Subjects," *Journal of the American Medical Association,* Vol. 202 (November 6, 1967), pp. 511-12.

35. This was a major theme in Dr. Katz's discussion of his paper.

* I am immeasurably indebted to *Clinical Investigation in Medicine: Legal, Ethical and Moral Aspects. An Anthology and Bibliography* (Boston University Law-Medicine Research Institute, 1963) from which these references and quotations came.

JAY KATZ

The Education of the Physician-Investigator

FORTY YEARS ago Francis Peabody opened his famous essay, on "The Care of the Patient," with this challenge:

It is probably fortunate that systems of education are constantly under the fire of general criticism, for if education were left solely in the hands of teachers the chances are good that it would soon deteriorate. Medical education, however, is less likely to suffer from such stagnation, for whenever the lay public stops criticizing the type of modern doctor, the medical profession itself may be counted on to stir up the stagnant pool and cleanse it of its sedimentary deposit.[1]

We are in the midst of another period when the goals and methods of medical education are under intense criticism. The call for reform has questioned the existing rigid temporal distinctions between preclinical and clinical instruction as well as the attempts to teach students all the facts of medicine in four years. Thus proponents of a new curriculum have recommended changes in order to "maintain the motivations of most beginning students to help suffering humanity by introducing them early in their training to patients," to "reduce the amount of factual information and memorizing pressed upon the students and to allow time for students to read, discuss and think in the atmosphere of a graduate school, rather than of a trade school," as well as to "intermingle biological, behavioral and clinical sciences throughout the curriculum."[2] While the need to educate the future physician for the ever broadening scope of service to society has been explicitly recognized, little detailed attention has been given to implementing this aspect of the educational process. Such an inquiry—be it into the allocation of scarce medical resources, experimentation with human beings, or population control—has to be grounded in an exploration of the inherent conflicts between the physicians' responsibilities to their patients, science, and society.

Today, in this age of more deliberate, widespread, and knowledgeable experimentation, the conflicts between the art and the science of medicine, which Peabody tried to reconcile, have come into sharper focus and require a critical analysis of their implications for medical education. In this paper, I intend to comment on the impact of the introduction of the scientific method on current medical practice, to review the major proposals that have been made for the control of human experimentation, and then to discuss the role that education can serve not only for the control of all medical interventions, but also in preparing future physicians for the many obligations which contemporary medicine and society ask them to assume.

Experimentation in the practice of medicine is as old as medicine itself. Hippocrates tells us that while treating a boy whose cortex was exposed, he not only picked out the spicules of bone embedded in the brain, but also "gently scratched the surface of the cortex with his fingernail" and observed convulsions on the opposite side of the body.[3] Physicians throughout history have seized similar opportunities to combine therapy with the quest for knowledge. But only during the last hundred years, since the age of Pasteur, has medicine become more aware of the need for deliberate and well-planned experimentation; at the same time it has realized how difficult it is to separate the practice of medicine from experimentation. The oft-made distinction that the physician is primarily concerned with the patient qua patient and the investigator with the research is not a useful one for the majority of medical situations, for most investigations occur in the context of "clinical research combined with professional care."[4] As A. C. Ivy points out, "the therapy of disease is, and will always be, an experimental aspect of medicine."[5] Moreover, in terms of consequences to the patient and subject, distinctions between therapy and research contribute little. Louis Lasagna has observed, for example, that "the patient is, paradoxically, often better served by the restraint observed in therapeutic approach by the critical experimentalist."[6] What is new in medicine is not experimentation on man, but the realization that experiment and therapy have much in common and that knowledge can only be acquired by experimentation, ultimately only by experiment on man.

Thus the recent increased concern about the ethics of medical experimentation extends to the ethics of therapeutic care. Contributing to the reluctance to examine these issues is the conscious

294

or unconscious realization that any resolution of the problems posed by human experimentation cannot be limited to research settings, but instead has far-reaching consequences for medical practice.[7] The art and the science of medicine are intricately interwoven, but the latter requires a total reassessment of long-cherished convictions about the nature of professional responsibility.

The recognition that experimentation on patients and non-patients alike is both inevitable and necessary raised ethical issues immediately. Thus it is not surprising that Claude Bernard, a contemporary of Pasteur, set forth the first formulation of the scientific rationale and the ethical limits for human therapy-experimentation:

> Physicians make therapeutic experiments daily on their patients and surgeons perform vivisections daily on their subjects. Experiments, then, may be performed on man, but within what limits? It is our duty and our right to perform an experiment on man whenever it can save his life, cure him, or gain him some personal benefit. The principle of medical and surgical morality, therefore, consists in never performing on man an experiment which might be harmful to him to any extent, even though the result might be highly advantageous to science, i.e. to the health of others.[8]

The inadequacy of such general promulgations did not impress itself on the medical community until the disclosures at Nuremberg.[9] The intense soul-searching that followed these disclosures would probably not have led to an uninterrupted scholarly inquiry, for temptation was great to attribute the concentration-camp experiments solely to the "ravaging inroads of Nazi pseudo-science."[10] But other tragedies[11] finally created an atmosphere not only for dramatic indictments, but also for sober and continuing reflection.

The inquiry has led to three recommendations for the control of human experimentation. Taking as a point of departure the ten "basic principles" set forth by the Nuremberg judges, numerous attempts have been made to propose "improved" codes of ethics to guide medical research.[12] The proliferation of such codes testifies to the difficulty of promulgating a set of rules that does not immediately raise more questions than it answers. At this stage of our confusion, it is unlikely that codes will resolve many of the problems, though they may serve a useful function later.[13] Even the much endorsed *Declaration of Helsinki*[14]—praised, perhaps, because it is the newest and therefore the least examined—will create problems for those who wish to implement it. What is meant, for example, by "the subject of [non-therapeutic] clinical research should be in such a *mental, physical,* and *legal* state as to be able to exercise *fully* his *power* of *choice*"? [Emphasis supplied.] Codes, as long as they stand alone and are not surrounded by detailed commentary, are pious exercises in futility. Since they aspire to ideals and are divorced from the realities of human interaction, they invite judicious or injudicious neglect. If codes are to have meaning, they must be tied to procedures that permit constant interpretation of terms like "mental state," "legal state," and "power of choice." The Talmudic version of the Golden Rule states: "What is hateful to yourself, do not to your fellow-man," but then adds "that is the whole of the Torah and the rest is but commentary. Go and learn it." But where can it be learned and how?

The establishment of committees to review the judgment of investigators has been another approach to safeguarding the interests of human subjects. A number of universities and hospitals already had such committees when the U. S. Public Health Service issued a policy statement requiring their establishment for any grants under its jurisdiction. This directive, though, gave a powerful impetus to the creation of such committees for the review of all research proposals carried on in medical institutions. The guiding principles set forth by the Surgeon General were quite broad:

This review should assure an independent determination: (1) of the rights and welfare of the individual . . . , (2) of the appropriateness of the methods used to secure informed consent, and (3) of the risks and potential medical benefits of the investigation.[15]

Thus the directive left to individual committees the determination of what is meant by "rights," "welfare," "appropriateness," "benefits," and so forth. From personal experience, the value of such committees can be considerable. Their weakness, however, rests on the lack of provisions for continuous review of their work both within individual institutions and on a broader national basis. Such opportunities for review must be created in order to accumulate a body of knowledge that would gradually give substantive meaning to the proposed principles and establish, if necessary, additional rules and procedures to safeguard all participants in medical research.

The third approach to controlling medical experimentation led to the strengthening of the regulatory authority of the government over research, as exemplified by the 1962 and 1966 amendments to the Federal Food, Drug and Cosmetic Act.[16] Whatever the assets and liabilities of additional state intervention in the affairs of medicine, physicians were unprepared at the prior congressional hearings either to propose measures that would leave the administration of medical research completely in their hands and yet control the disclosed abuses or to suggest what kind of partnership should be established between the state and medicine. Even without a thalidomide tragedy or a Jewish Chronic Disease Hospital incident, physicians could have predicted that such events might occur and that the general public would react to them. They, therefore, should have begun to reflect on how they might cope with such incidents both before and after their occurrence.[17]

All three of these attempts focus on the control of experimentation without answering whether meaningful distinctions can be drawn between therapy and research. The problems confronting modern medicine are the result not so much of the increase in research activities, but of the awareness that research and therapy, pursuit of knowledge and treatment, are not separate but intertwined. Therefore, the focus on experimentation and the concomitant emphasis on "informed consent" created new difficulties not merely because of the requirement to inform patient-subjects about proposed research, but also because consent raised troublesome questions about what *all* patients should be told about medical interventions.

It is a task of medical education to teach students how to deal with these emerging problems. Yet we have not explored in a systematic fashion whether education can serve medicine well as a method of control. I have often wondered how and by whom the Nazi concentration-camp experiments would have been conducted had the physician's responsibilities toward his patient-subject been exposed to careful scrutiny in the medical education of the nineteenth and early-twentieth centuries.[18] The Nazi studies, despite opinions to the contrary, had their antecedents. There are, for example, reports of French and German experiments in which cancer tissue surgically removed from one diseased breast was transplanted into the apparently healthy other breast or experiments with variola vaccine performed on children in Sweden about which the experimenter commented that "perhaps I should have first experimented upon animals, but calves—most suitable for these purposes—were difficult to obtain because of their cost and their keep."[19]

In my own medical education I have never forgotten Conrad Wesselhoeft's brilliant lecture on "The Care of the Patient." I turned over in my mind again and again one story he told—probably because its "lesson" did not satisfy me, though I was not aware of it then. He related one of his first experiences as a house officer. A patient with appendicitis had come to the emergency room and Dr. Wesselhoeft, once having made the diagnosis, recommended immediate surgery. The patient pleaded an important business engagement and asked that the operation be postponed for a few hours. Dr. Wesselhoeft reluctantly agreed and eventually the operation was successfully performed by him. That evening, at dinner, he related the story and noticed that his father, an eminent physician of his day, looked increasingly disturbed and did not say a word beyond sternly telling him: "Conrad, I want to see you in my study after dinner." There he chided his son severely for having taken too lightly his medical responsibilities by giving his patient leave for a few hours. Young Dr. Wesselhoeft felt that he had learned an important lesson that he wished to communicate to us. But what was the lesson? As I remember, he did not answer this question because it seemed so obvious.

I believe that I now know what troubled me then. Traditionally the concept of medical responsibility has been defined as responsibility for the patient's well-being. While such a definition could encompass, within the context of a medical relationship, concern for the patient's total functioning—physical, psychological, social, economic, spiritual—it is often limited to physical aspects. In order to exercise this more limited responsibility, patients must be carefully diagnosed, given the best treatment for their condition, and not be abandoned. Many students learn well to fulfill these obligations.[20] But there are other aspects to medical responsibility, and the controversy about what to disclose to patient-subjects in investigative settings has put one of them into sharper perspective— namely, the dialogue that should be pursued with the patient about treatment or no treatment or available alternative treatments in light of the risks, benefits, and prognosis as well as the totality of the patient's life situation.[21] Put another way, so long as medical responsibility primarily addressed itself to dispensing physical benefits, it was easier to view the physician as the sole decision-maker. Once physical benefits are placed in the web of the patient's total situation, the patient may have to be given a greater role in the decision-making process.

The Education of the Physician-Investigator

Not only does modern medicine command extensive therapeutic options—each with its known and unknown risks and benefits— but almost daily new therapeutic possibilities are introduced that have not yet met the test of time. Moreover, physicians are much more critical than they used to be about the efficacy of their therapeutic interventions. These considerations raise questions about the extent to which patients should participate in decisions affecting their health. To return briefly to Dr. Wesselhoeft's father, why did he seem so convinced that his son had not behaved with the utmost sense of professional responsibility?[22]

Since medical experimentation is generally conducted with patients, the emphasis on "informed consent" raises questions about the nature of the dialogue between physicians and patients with respect to all interventions. This component of professional responsibility has not received the systematic attention it deserves. In medical commentary on professional responsibility, considerable agreement exists on the extent and limits of permissible physical interventions, but there is less consensus on or little systematic exploration into the dialogue that should take place between physicians and their patients. The Hippocratic Oath is silent on this point; it merely states that "I will follow that system of regimen which according to my ability and judgment, I consider for the benefit of my patients, and abstain from whatever is deleterious and mischievous." Dr. Thomas Percival, whose book *Medical Ethics* influenced profoundly the subsequent codifications of medical ethics in England and the United States, only commented once and in a very restricted fashion on the discourse between physicians and patients:

A physician should not be forward to make gloomy prognostications, because they savor of empiricism, by magnifying the importance of his services in the treatment or care of disease. But he should not fail, on proper occasions, to give to the friends of the patient, timely notice of danger, when it really occurs, and *even* to the patient himself, *if absolutely necessary* [emphasis supplied].[23]

Nowhere in his detailed book, which carries the subtitle "A Code of Institutes and Precepts, Adapted to the Professional Conduct of Physicians and Surgeons," does Percival discuss the obligations of physicians to inform patients about the nature, purposes, and risks of therapeutic interventions. Nor does he comment on when a patient's consent should be obtained prior to a therapeutic intervention. Such omissions suggest that Percival did not consider this issue important. And subsequent codes and commentaries by the American Medical Association[24] have similarly treated this problem, if at all, briefly and without any elaboration.[25]

These considerations put in question statements by commentators that experimental subjects are best safeguarded by the ethical training which investigators have received in their prior education as physicians. If disclosure and consent are posited as important problems for medical research, these commentators forgot to realize that physicians could not draw on systematic prior training. In an article on "Ethics and Clinical Research," Henry Beecher concluded that while "it is absolutely essential to strive" for informed consent, a "more reliable safeguard [in experimentation is] provided by the presence of an intelligent, informed, conscientious, compassionate, responsible investigator."[26] One cannot quarrel with such a prescription, but has medicine trained physicians to analyze the complex and conflicting issues that medical decision-making often entails?

To provide such training requires curricular innovations and, most important, new teaching methods. One goal is to expose students to materials now rarely utilized in medical schools—materials that would facilitate an analysis of the conflicting issues posed by the call for a greater scrutiny of medical responsibility. For example, students must debate whether the traditional distinctions between therapy and experiment are relevant for any decisions vis-à-vis patient-subjects. They must question what values are maximized or minimized in decisions to inform or not inform patient-subjects about the nature of medical interventions. Materials not only from medicine but also from other disciplines will have to be provided for such inquiries.

Another and more significant target for reform is the prevalent, though much lamented, tendency in medical education to teach through lectures and presentation of facts to be learned and memorized. The problems that medical responsibility raises are not amenable to such an approach. Thus, the materials for discussion should be organized to stimulate a continuing dialogue between teacher and students. The quest is not for right or wrong *answers*, but for an appreciation of the conflicting values and purposes at work in all medical decision-making. Medical students must learn to identify right and wrong *questions* in terms of the values and purposes that physicians seek to implement. The Socratic method of teaching, so extensively used in law schools, should be given a more prominent place in the education of physicians. If, as White-head said, physicians are "educated for uncertainty," such a method would teach medical students to confront uncertainty by constantly asking: What do we seek to accomplish, for what ends, by what means, and with what consequences?

I can best illustrate what I have in mind by describing a seminar on "Experimentation with Human Beings" that I teach at the Yale Law School. The materials for discussion are still in preliminary and tentative form and will be shaped further by subsequent class-room experience. They are designed not only for students of law, but for students of medicine and other research-oriented profes-sions. At present, they are ordered in five parts with the over-all heading "Problems for Decision in Experimentation with Human Beings." Part I, which serves as an introduction, presents the case of the Jewish Chronic Disease Hospital. Here we examine the many petitions filed by the participants to the controversy, the opinions of the Court as well as the proceedings before the Medi-cal Grievance Committee of the Department of Education of the State of New York and the report of the Regents Committee on Discipline. In analyzing this case, the students are asked to keep in mind the following preparatory questions:

"(1) What are the characteristics of human experimentation? Do they differ from therapeutic interventions?

"(2) Who are the participants in human experimentation?

"(3) Who should define the rights and duties of the parties in-volved in experimentation and supervise their implemen-tation? More specifically, what role, if any, should be assigned to the state for promulgating and administering rules and procedures with regard to human experimenta-tion?"

Part II explores the possible conflicts between the individual, the investigator, and society—or, put another way, between the goals of advancing science and protecting the rights and welfare of the individual. Commentaries from a variety of disciplines—med-icine, law, sociology, theology, philosophy—and judicial opinions are presented[27] to find answers to such questions as: "Who should decide, how, and under what circumstances to resolve conflicts between science and the individual in favor of either goal? What assumptions about man and society underlie a decision to require or not require his agreement to any intervention by others?" In seeking answers to the latter question, it is suggested that students of human experimentation may first have to pose a series of more specific questions: "Should a decision in favor of advancing science depend on the 'value' of the experiment to science? Should any infringement of individual rights depend on the nature of the physical and psychological 'consequences' of the experiment to the subject? Does it make a difference if there is also an expectation that the experiment may directly 'benefit' the patient-subject?"

In Part III, "Experimentation and Therapy, Distinctions for What Purposes," materials are presented to identify and analyze the variety of settings—"diagnostic," "experimental," "therapeutic," and combinations of all three—in which interventions with human beings take place so that the traditional distinctions between research and treatment can be evaluated in the context of medical decision-making. Three different problems have been selected for intensive study: cardiac catheterization, which has quickly passed from an experimental technique to an important and accepted diagnostic procedure, although it still retains its dual status; the treatment of essential hypertension, which continues to aim for therapeutic goals with and without concomitant experimental investigations; and explorations of man's ability to control behavior, which have led to experimental research with a potential for application to the treatment of society.[28] To illustrate the kinds of materials selected, I will describe in somewhat greater detail the section on cardiac catheterization and angiography. It opens with the Nobel Prize citation to Forssman, Cournand and Richards, and Forssman's Nobel lecture in which he relates the trials and tribulations that he encountered when he began to experiment on himself and others. From the "Judgment at Stockholm," the materials return to writings that questioned the safety and value of catheterization prior to Cournand and Richards' utilization of this technique for the measurement of cardiac output. Papers on the catheterization of the right auricle for "experimental" and "therapeutic" purposes are presented first to examine the relationship between these two purposes. The materials then turn to angiography and explorations of the left heart, techniques that even today are subject to constant modification and carry greater risks than right cardiac catheterization. Among the excerpts included are discussions of the dangers to patients, which initially were thought to be considerable, but were not substantiated by subsequent experience; evaluations of the various techniques by the American Heart Association; and investigations on patients with and without cardiovascular disease as well as on normal volunteers. These materials were selected to give students an opportunity to familiarize themselves with the problems encountered by modern medicine and then to ask: "Are there identifiable criteria which differentiate an experiment from therapy? Even if such criteria can be established, are there reasons for maintaining these differences?"

The inquiry then turns to methods of control, and in Part IV to a detailed examination of the extent to which consent can protect the rights of and resolve the conflicts between patient, subject, physician, investigator, and society. The materials do not distinguish between therapeutic and experimental situations; thus the following question must be kept in mind (if after an analysis of the materials in the last section it still remains pertinent): "What difference does it make if the problem arises in treatment or research and why?" In studying the materials the student is also asked to consider: "What purposes should law and the professions try to achieve by requiring 'informed consent'? To implement these purposes, what must be disclosed and how effective is disclosure to achieve them? In what situations and interactions between which persons or groups is consent either ill-adapted or insufficient to serve these ends? In what circumstances do the purposes of 'informed consent' conflict with other purposes which all the participants, including society, seek to achieve?" The student is reminded that "informed consent" may not be the most significant or adequate method of control to protect the rights of or resolve the conflicts between patient, subject, physician, investigator, and society. The study of these materials should, therefore, begin to raise questions about additional rules and procedures for the control of therapy and experiment as well as about who should be given authority to promulgate and administer them. More specifically, the selections in Part IV are arranged under the following headings: Is consent a basic right? What are the requisites of informed consent? What information about "known" and "unknown" risks will protect physical integrity? What information will minimize threats to self-determination? In what circumstances are physical integrity and self-determination protected or threatened by what kind of information? Next, materials are presented that explore the capacity of the human mind to exercise self-determination and the limits of this capacity in the presence of "health" and "illness," of known and unknown internal and external pressures. Finally, the materials raise questions about the extent to which the right to self-determination should be modified, and the right to consent waived or abolished, in order to protect the physical or psychological well-being of the patient-subject, the interests of science, and the interests of society.

An analysis of the materials in the previous Part may lead to the conclusion that consent is inadequate in certain situations to protect the interests of all participants in the medical decision-making process. Thus, Part V explores other means by which medical interventions might be controlled. Selections are first presented that ask whether physicians within the existing framework of Medical Practice Acts as well as criminal, tort, and contract law should be further restricted in the administration of medical practice and research. If not, should the profession be relied on to supervise and review its practices? Here the functions of codes, review boards, editorial boards as well as the detailed regulations of the National Institutes of Health and the Harvard University Medical School are scrutinized in depth. More specifically, the composition and function[29] of review boards as well as the role of the profession in establishing criteria for the selection of transplant recipients and for the moment of death are explored. The inquiry is concluded with an examination of proposed and enacted federal regulations in order to consider the role of the state in the medical decision-making process. In this context, the recent promulgations by the Food and Drug Administration are examined against the background of controls exercised in other areas by governmental agencies such as the Securities and Exchange Commission.

I do not wish to suggest that the adoption of such a seminar is all that is needed to prepare the future physician for the theoretical and practical challenges of medical practice and research. Indeed, instead of one seminar, a series of seminars integrated in the four-year curriculum are preferable so that, depending on the stage of training, the most meaningful issues can be discussed in depth.[30] The theoretical basis for analyzing professional responsibility could most profitably be presented in the preclinical years. Theory must later be evaluated against practice, and the student will be better able to do so once he has confronted systematically such problems as the limits of professional competence, the value conflicts inherent in his roles of physician, man, and citizen, as well as the assumptions he is making about man in his interactions with patient-subjects. While such seminars will make the student more aware and critical of the approaches to treatment and research during his clinical years, he will continue to learn a great deal about the physician-patient relationship from observing his clinical teachers and identifying with their attitudes. But with a theoretical background, such identifications can become somewhat more reflective and allow for a more active intellectual and emotional agreement with and challenge of what he sees and hears.

Other resources are available for the pursuit of these objectives. It has been suggested that a critical analysis of all papers published during a year in any major medical journal could serve as a useful vehicle for discussions on professional responsibility. Such efforts are of value if they are seen as opportunities to search for the appropriate questions that must be asked before arriving at answers. Through such attempts it may be possible to hammer out theoretical models that can guide the future physician in the analysis of the complex issues posed by modern medicine. One could also draw on the wealth of literature on the care of the patient to deepen the explorations already begun. For example, the challenging papers on this subject by Francis Peabody, Herrman Blumgart, and Walsh McDermott could be employed for a detailed scrutiny of the responsibility of the physician toward his patient. What does Peabody try to convey to us when he writes:

The practice of medicine . . . is an art, based to an increasing extent on the medical sciences, but comprising much that still remains outside the realm of any science. The art of medicine and the science of medicine are not antagonistic but supplementary to each other.[31]

Blumgart offers a variation of the same theme and suggestive insights into how can it be implemented:

Practically all patients should be told the nature of the ailment, the physician bearing in mind that the actual situation must be painted as a painter paints a picture: different colors must be used in terms of the subjective impression to be conveyed, as a snow scene may be painted various shades of gray or white, or, on a bright, sunlit day, as predominantly blue.[32]

Speaking from the vantage point of the investigator, McDermott may or may not be saying something quite different when he states:

When in our cultural evolution it has not yet been possible to develop an institutional framework for a particular kind of arbitrary decision that may affect an individual, there is only one basis on which to proceed and that is on the basis of trust. My position may sound paternalistic as

305

indeed it is. . . . Somehow, somewhere, in this question of human experimentation as in so many other aspects of our society, we will have to learn how to institutionalize "playing God" while still maintaining the key elements of a free society.[33]

I have emphasized the need for theoretical seminars on professional responsibility because such theoretical explorations have been neglected in medical education. The materials for my seminar juxtapose a variety of points of view so that they do not suggest one answer to the problems that confront medicine. At the same time, they are sufficiently structured to permit teachers and students to wrestle with the issues in an orderly fashion and yet to arrive at their own conclusions. To illustrate how they can be used, particularly for the analysis of value preferences, I return to Part IV—"In what circumstances and for what purposes is there a duty to seek consent?" The selections begin with case and commentary that assert: "Every human being of adult years and sound mind has the right to determine what shall be done with his own body."[34] If the value preferences expressed in such opinions are accepted, it could lead to a presumption in favor of disclosure and consent (yet to be defined), for they are prerequisites for the exercise of such a right. And this presumption must rest, in part, on the assumption that man, until declared incompetent by established legal procedures, is competent, intelligent, capable of being informed, capable of making judgments, and responsible for his actions. Juxtaposed are other selections that suggest different assumptions about man—namely, that his decisions and interactions are influenced by unknown and "irrational" determinants that may even lead him to act in ways others might label as uninformed, incompetent, or irresponsible. Class discussion could recognize the difficulty of determining what is rational or irrational for individual man as well as the reality that there is no single best answer for the resolution of man's problems and the danger of other men directing his life. Thus, it could lead to the conclusion that wide latitude should be given to a man to make his own decisions and to deny others the authority to make decisions for him unless he has conferred that right to them. Consent, then, would seek to maximize respect for the individual by providing him with opportunities for self-determination and to minimize assaults on his integrity through undisclosed interventions by others, however "benevolent." On the other hand, physicians have noted, and again materials are provided for analysis, the dire impact of disclosures about poor prognosis or hazardous interventions, the inability of patients to understand medical interventions, and the uncertainty of the effects of any intervention on the individual patient. Such considerations have led physicians to conclude that medical interventions defy explanation and, if attempted, create "unnecessary" anxieties that interfere with hope and recovery. Thus, they suggest that protection of the patients' well-being is in conflict with disclosure. Here the question can be raised as to whether such an attitude rests on a deeply rooted image of man that views experts as being so enlightened with respect to certain objectives (for example, health) and patients as being so resistant to what is best for them because they are ignorant or unaware of their inner wishes that physicians can assume wide discretion in acting on their behalf.[35] Yet to disregard what a person seeks and chooses by assuming that he would choose differently were he "brighter" or more "aware" is a speculative leap and a consequential one for medicine's interaction with patients. If this assumption is posited, physicians must ask what the area is within which a patient should be left to do what he wants to do, and what the circumstances are under which someone else can decide that a patient should do one thing rather than another.

Education is a cornerstone for any meaningful attempt to construct a system of control of medical practice and experimentation. Once its importance is recognized, it has the virtue that something can be done about it. Medical educators must appoint teachers to their faculties who are interested in pursuing the kinds of issues that I have described. The task of a medical faculty is not limited to educating students, but extends to re-examining the entire structure of medical decision-making. New rules and procedures are especially needed, but can only be promulgated after their purposes are clearly articulated. Here lessons from the past and present may serve as a guide to the future.

Throughout the ages, medicine has relied on its codes of ethics as important formal documents for guiding physicians with regard to their professional responsibilities. If codes, like legal statutes, are to endure as living documents, they must be constantly interpreted in the light of new clinical and research experiences, surrounded by a body of medical "common law," and revised from time to time. Medicine has no procedures for such a task, and they need to be created. Publication of articles and medical treatises may be a preparatory step in achieving such a goal. Research that provides data on the impact of disclosure and consent on patient-subjects as well as on participation in investigations is also needed in order to make meaningful recommendations for substantive and procedural reforms. The more difficult problem is to think through who should be given authority, and at what institutional, national, and international levels, to establish guides for decision-making. Thought must also be given to who should be made responsible for appraising, reviewing, and controlling the action of decision-makers.

While. present review committees serve a useful function, the results of their deliberations are generally not available to others; thus there is insufficient opportunity for all to learn from these experiences. During their clinical training, medical students should rotate through these committees and participate in these conferences. The work of the committees should also be presented from time to time to the medical community so that there is a much greater sharing of problems that have implication not only for research, but for the practice of medicine as well.

The National Institutes of Health are in a strategic position to implement the establishment of one or more national review boards, possibly based in universities. Their functions should be both advisory and policy-making, but not decision-making in the narrow sense of either approving or disapproving individual experiments. In their advisory function, they could review the more difficult decisions of local committees as well as invite investigators to submit research studies for consultative opinions. The deliberations of these boards should be published so that everybody can learn from them as well as scrutinize and debate them. In their policy-making function, these boards could address themselves to such questions as the role of the state in the decision-making process and the promulgation of general medical guidelines. If medicine wishes to avoid being regulated more and more by the state, it will have to create its own procedures for medical decision-making.

It has been pointed out that the ethics of human experimentation are best safeguarded "by the presence of an intelligent, informed, conscientious, compassionate, responsible investigator,"[36] and that "the responsibility of the individual physician to an individual patient has been clearly defined, maturely considered, and almost universally accepted; it has been tried and found good."[37] It is the task of medical education to establish, nourish, and reinforce such attributes by identifying and analyzing for and with students their obligations toward patients, subjects, medicine, society, and the advancement of science. Only then will students have the tools—though not necessarily the wisdom or capacity—to become conscientious, compassionate, and responsible physician-investigators. Students will learn that not all that "has been tried and found good" in the past will stand the test of time and that the exercise of medical responsibility is not amenable solely to resolution by conscientious choices. The competing and conflicting values at work in medical decision-making as well as the increased societal concern with the rights of the individual preclude such simple prescriptions.

The practice of medicine has always commanded a remarkable degree of trust. Over the centuries, the physician as a practitioner of the art of medicine fostered this trust. Though he made few therapeutic discoveries, he served his patients well by allaying their pains. Today in his new role as scientist, in an age when the pursuit of knowledge has become a goal in its own right, he could undermine this trust. The responsibilities toward patient-subjects are not different than they used to be, for trust and respect remain, as always, basic goals. What has changed are both the complexity of medicine and our awareness of the complexities. Justice Frankfurter's challenge to law equally applies to medicine:

If [medicine] is to have a strength adequate to the task, the widest learning—constant cultivation of the [medical] mind by exposure to every subject of human investigation—is requisite. Thus only can those through whose decisions [medicine evolves and is practiced] escape shallowness, oversimplification, too quick acceptance of uncritical formulas which, by planting the mind against self-examination, impair its capacity for reasoned judgment.[38]

Education, more than codes and procedures, will teach us not to be led astray, though the latter will then find an important place to nourish conscience otherwise prone to compromise and corruption.

Perhaps there was once a time when medicine could be guided by the ancient maxim—*primum non nocere* (above all, do no harm) —but today it no longer serves us well. The multiple purposes of medical practice—caring for patients, advancing science, improving the health of the community, nations, and future generations —cannot be separated clearly in most decisions that physician-investigators have to make. Instead, more often than not, all these purposes are present in every decision and since the implementation of one purpose may require neglecting and undermining any of the other purposes, conflict is inevitable. Medicine must sort these conflicts, acknowledge the reality of neglect, and even harm and degradation, for only then can it formulate rules and procedures to minimize inevitable risks to individuals and inevitable impediments to the acquisition of knowledge. By addressing itself to this task, medicine could also make an invaluable contribution to other decision-makers—be they in law, science, or politics—for they, too, struggle to resolve the conflicting purposes so pervasive in all affairs conducted by and with man.

REFERENCES

1. F. W. Peabody, "The Care of the Patient," *Journal of the American Medical Association,* Vol. 88 (1927), pp. 877-82.

2. Harvard Medical School: Report of Subcommittee on Curriculum Planning (May, 1966).

3. H. Hoff, "Historical Aspects of Human Experimentation," Report of Fourteenth Conference of Cardiovascular Training Grant Program Directors, National Institutes of Health (1967), pp. 7-17.

4. World Medical Association, *Declaration of Helsinki,* 1964.

5. "Even after the therapy of a disease is discovered, its application to the patient remains, in part, experimental. Because of the physiological variations in the response of different patients to the same therapy, the therapy of disease is, and will always be, an experimental aspect of medicine. [T]he patient is always to some extent an experimental subject of the physician. . . ." A. C. Ivy, "The History and Ethics of the Use of Human Subjects in Medical Experiments," *Science,* Vol. 108 (1948), pp. 1-5.

6. L. Lasagna, "Some Ethical Problems in Clinical Investigation," unpublished manuscript (1967).

7. For example, if consent becomes an important requisite in clinical research combined with therapeutic care, should it be obtained in therapeutic interventions? Does it make any difference whether the same medical procedure is carried out in the context of a research study or not?

8. C. Bernard, *An Introduction to the Study of Experimental Medicine* (New York, 1927).

9. *Trials of War Criminals Before Nuremberg Military Tribunals Under Control Council Law No. 10, The Medical Case* (Washington, D. C., 1947), Vols. 1 and 2.

10. T. Taylor, Opening Statement of the Prosecutor, *United States* v. *Karl Brandt et al., ibid.*

11. For example, the birth defects caused by thalidomide and the experimental injections of foreign cancer cells. On the former, see United States Senate Report of the Committee on Government Operations: Interagency Drug Coordination, 1965; on the latter, *Hyman v. Jewish Chronic Disease Hospital, 251 N.Y.S. 2d 818* (1964).

12. See I. Ladimer and R. W. Newman, *Clinical Investigation in Medicine: Legal, Ethical, and Moral Aspects* (Boston, 1963).

13. See pp. 494-95, *infra.*

14. *Declaration of Helsinki.*

15. Surgeon General, Public Health Service: Clinical Research and Investigation Involving Human Beings (February 8, 1966).

16. W. J. Curran, "Governmental Regulation of the Use of Human Subjects in Medical Research: The Approach of Two Federal Agencies," this book.

17. For an interesting discussion on planning for the future, see H. D. Lasswell, "The Political Science of Science," *American Political Science Review,* Vol. 50 (1956), p. 961.

18. It has frequently been emphasized, and I agree, that no system of control will affect the unscrupulous investigator. Telford Taylor, the prosecutor at Nuremberg, noted that "[t]he 20 physicians in the dock range from leaders of German scientific medicine . . . down to the dregs of the German medical profession." See Taylor, Opening Statement of the Prosecutor. Would *all* of them have participated if the experiences which Prinzmetal described had been scrutinized: "During my training in medical school, as well as during my residency in St. Louis, fellowships at Harvard, New York City, and London, and visits to Vienna, Budapest, and other European medical centers, I was always horrified by the inhumane manner in which charity patients were treated. . . . I distinctly remember the degradation of a poor man with a prolapsed rectum who was asked to defecate in a wastebasket before the class in proctology clinic, which included women medical students." M. Prinzmetal, "On the Humane Treatment of Charity Patients," *Medical Tribune,* September 22, 1965.

19. The American Human Association: Concerning Human Vivisection—A Controversy (1901).

20. Becker and his associates, on the basis of detailed observations of an entire medical school class, have described the development of the "responsibility perspective." They state that "basically the term [responsibility] refers to the archetypal feature of medical practice: the physician who holds his patient's fate in his hands and on whom the patient's life and death may depend." While concern with his "fate" could include the patient's entire functioning, the authors note that "two areas of activity seem most involved with questions of medical responsibility. The first consists . . . of arriving at a correct diagnosis on the basis of a thorough and accurate examination. . . . The second activity consists of performing diag-

nostic and therapeutic procedures containing some element of danger to the patient." The accompanying interview material suggests that in these two activities concern for physical well-being is of primary or exclusive importance and that this aspect of medical responsibility is presented well and in great detail. In contrast, other aspects seem to be neglected. I found only one reference to the problem of disclosure. A student asked what to tell patients "who would die very shortly of an inoperable tumor. . . . The staff member gave a long and complex answer, pointing out that frequently patients figured it out for themselves or, on the other hand, didn't want to know anything about it. In either case the physician had no decision to make about whether to tell or not." See H. S. Becker, B. Geer, E. C. Hughes, and A. L. Strauss, *Boys in White* (Chicago, 1961).

21. As Freidson observed: "[T]he professional expects patients to accept what he recommends on his terms; patients seek services on their own terms. In that each seeks to gain his own terms, there is conflict." E. Freidson, *Patients' Views of Medical Practice* (New York, 1961).

22. What constitutes professional responsibility in such situations? An answer to this question requires a searching analysis of the conflicts of interest and perspective between physician and patient. In pursuing such an inquiry we must ask: Under what circumstances, by what means, and to what extent should these conflicts be resolved in favor of either party?

23. C. D. Leake (ed.), *Percival's Medical Ethics* (Baltimore, 1927).

24. The *Code of Ethics of the American Medical Association,* adopted in 1847, and the *Principles of Medical Ethics of the American Medical Association,* adopted in 1903 and 1912, contain only, and in almost the same words, Percival's statement quoted in the text. The *Principles of Medical Ethics,* adopted in 1957, deleted Percival's wording. Section 2 states instead: "Physicians . . . should make available to their patients . . . the benefits of their professional attainments." The only pertinent sections of the *Opinions of the Judicial Council* interpreting the *Principles* read as follows: (a) "The surgeon's obligation to the patient requires him to perform the surgical operation . . . with complete disclosure of all facts relevant to the need and the performance of the operation" and (b) "Experimentation: New Drugs or Procedures. . . In order to conform to the ethics of the American Medical Association, three requirements must be satisfied: (1) the voluntary consent of the person on whom the experiment is to be performed. . . ."

25. In 1966 the House of Delegates of the American Medical Association endorsed the *Declaration of Helsinki* and at the same time added its own modifications: "[I]n conducting clinical investigation, the investigator should demonstrate the same concern and caution for the welfare, safety and comfort of the person involved as is required of a physician who is furnishing medical care to a patient independent of any clinical investigation." The document then notes that "[i]n clinical investigation primarily for treatment, . . . voluntary consent must be obtained from the patient or from his legally authorized representative if the patient lacks the capacity to consent, following: (a) disclosure that the physician intends to

use an investigational drug or experimental procedure, (b) a reasonable explanation of the nature of the drug or procedure to be used, risks to be expected, and possible therapeutic benefits, (c) an offer to answer any inquiries concerning the drug or procedure and (d) a disclosure of alternative drugs or procedures that may be available." Is the inclusion of (b), (c), and (d) designed to suggest that in "furnishing medical care to a patient independent of any clinical investigation" this information can be omitted? If not, are separate ethical guidelines for "clinical investigators primarily for treatment" needed beyond a statement that in this situation the nature of the intervention must be specifically disclosed to the patient? American Medical Association, *Ethical Guidelines for Clinical Investigation.* Adopted by the House of Delegates (November 30, 1966).

26. H. K. Beecher, "Ethics and Clinical Research," *The New England Journal of Medicine,* Vol. 274 (1966), pp. 1354–60.

27. For example, excerpts are included from law: by Brandeis, Calabresi, Freund, Ruebhausen; from medicine: by Beecher, McDermott, the American Medical Association; from sociology: by Brim, Hollingshead; from philosophy: by Berlin, Mill; from theology: by Pope Pius XII; from judicial opinions: *United States* v. *Karl Brandt et al.*

28. Included, for example, are selections from S. Milgram, "Behavioral Study of Obedience," and J. M. R. Delgado, "Evolution of Physical Control of the Brain." Delgado not only describes animal and human research, but also speculates about their implication for the future of society.

29. For example, should the function of the review board include judgments of the scientific merits of the experiment and the adequacy of the research design; should it be given authority to terminate the investigation if injuries occur that had not been contemplated?

30. Initially it will be necessary to create a series of specific seminars to stimulate interest in such explorations as well as to provide the necessary training for pursuing such inquiries. Eventually most of these seminars should become obsolete since the issues that they are designed to examine are most profitably discussed in the context of the teaching situation in which they arise. Since teaching sessions, including Grand Rounds, can never explore all ramifications of a medical problem because of time limitation, it probably will prove necessary to allocate ethical issues their proper rotation on the agenda.

31. Peabody, "The Care of the Patient."

32. H. L. Blumgart, "Caring for the Patient," *New England Journal of Medicine,* Vol. 270 (1964), pp. 449-56.

33. W. McDermott, "Opening Statement on the Changing Mores of Biomedical Research," *Annals of Internal Medicine,* Vol. 67 (1967), pp. 39-42.

34. *Schloendorf* v. *New York Hospital, 211 N.Y. 127* (1914).

35. See I. Berlin, *Two Concepts of Liberty* (Oxford, 1958), for a detailed exposition, from a different vantage point, of the thoughts expressed in this sentence and the remainder of this paragraph.

36. Beecher, "Ethics and Clinical Research."

37. M. B. Shimkin, "The Problem of Experimentation on Human Beings: The Research Worker's Point of View," *Science*, Vol. 117 (1953), pp. 205-207.

38. F. Frankfurter, "Message of Acceptance on Receiving American Bar Association Medal," *American Bar Association Journal*, Vol. 49 (1963), pp. 876-77.

JUDITH P. SWAZEY AND RENÉE C. FOX

The Clinical Moratorium: A Case Study of Mitral Valve Surgery

THE PURPOSE of this paper is to identify and analyze a particular phenomenon that recurs in the development of new medical and surgical procedures, most commonly during the early phases of their clinical trial. What we shall call "the clinical moratorium" is an event that we consider generic to the process of therapeutic innovation. Its significance lies not only in the frequency with which it occurs, but also in its relationship to some fundamental conceptual, technical, social, and ethical properties of clinical investigation.

Our interest in the clinical moratorium was stimulated by certain observations we made in the context of a socio-historical study of organ transplantation that we are currently conducting.[1] Since the announcement of the world's first human heart transplant, performed by Dr. Christiaan Barnard in December 1967, this procedure has been widely discussed within the medical profession and also by laymen. These debates have been chronicled and to some extent amplified by the lay press, which has covered the one hundred and fifty-one cardiac transplants done through September 25, 1969.[2] Both in professional and lay press contexts, there have been continuing discussions concerning whether or not a moratorium on heart transplants should be called. These exchanges reached a crescendo in Winter, 1969, when the Montreal Heart Institute announced that it was halting cardiac transplants.[3] Hospital spokesmen stated that the Institute would not resume the operation until the high mortality rate accompanying the procedure could be reduced through better control of the immunological processes which cause a recipient's body to reject a transplanted organ.

As we followed the cardiac transplantation debate,[4] it became apparent that there is some confusion over the precise meaning of

315

a clinical moratorium, both semantically and operationally. Partly for this reason, controversy over whether it is justifiable to continue heart transplantation on patients at this stage in its development has repeatedly been accompanied by the question of whether a moratorium on this procedure has already occurred.

The word moratorium is derived from the Latin "moratorius"—"serving to delay"—and is defined in the Oxford English Dictionary as "a legal authorization to a debtor to postpone payment for a certain time." In press accounts of cardiac transplantation, often quoting physicians, the following words and phrases have appeared synonomously with moratorium: *halt, diminish, stop, stop entirely, slow the tide, set aside for the time being, cease, boycott, suspend, defer, slow down, languish, decline, abandon, pause, quit.* As this range of terms suggests, both medical professionals and laymen seem unclear as to whether only the total cessation of trials of a new procedure on human subjects constitutes a moratorium or if a slowdown or temporary halt in its clinical application might also be considered kinds of moratoria. What the press and dictionary definitions have in common is that both turn around the seeking of legitimation for postponing or halting an activity which is felt to be morally binding.[5]

Our interest in cardiac transplantation led us to explore instances of clinical moratoria in recent medical history. This paper will focus upon a case study of the moratorium phenomenon in the development of surgery on the heart's mitral valve over the period 1902 to 1949.[6] We have chosen this case for two principal reasons. First, it represents an earlier innovative period in cardiac surgery. Second, the cessation of mitral valve surgery that extended from 1928 to 1945 is an unusually clearcut as well as prolonged instance of the clinical moratorium.

Based on this study and on our wider acquaintance with medical sociology and history, we will use the word moratorium to mean a *suspension* of the use of a still experimental procedure on patients, a suspension which may last for weeks, months, or years depending upon the particular case.

The first section of our paper will examine critical events in the history of mitral valve surgery. In the light of this analysis, we will then identify numerous of the factors responsible for the halting and resumption of an innovative clinical procedure. Finally, we will attempt to more precisely define the core attributes and patterned variations in the various types of clinical moratoria that can occur.

Mitral Valve Surgery: 1902–1949

On looking at the contracted mitral orifice . . . one is impressed by the hopelessness of ever finding a remedy which will enable the auricle to drive the blood in a sufficient stream through the small mitral orifice, and the wish unconsciously arises that one could divide the constriction as easily during life as one can after death. The risk which such an operation would entail naturally makes one shrink from it, but in some cases it might be well worthwhile for the patients to balance the risk of a shortened life against the certainty of a prolonged period of existence which could hardly be called life.[7]

With this introduction, in 1902, Sir Lauder Brunton, a Fellow of the Royal Society and one of England's leading cardiologists, proposed a surgical technique for correcting stenosis (narrowing) of the heart's mitral valve.[8] At the time of his short note in *Lancet*, Brunton had been working out his procedure on animals, recognizing that "no one would be justified in attempting such a dangerous operation as dividing a mitral stenosis on a fellow creature without having first tested its practicability and perfected its technique by previous trials on animals." As other work was keeping him from further experiments, he continued, he felt he should make his preliminary findings available to the surgeons who might someday perform such an operation on a patient.

Although a growing body of work on mitral stenosis had been conducted in the animal laboratory since the turn of the century, the first operation on a patient suffering from mitral stenosis waited until 1923, twenty-one years after Brunton's proposal. A total of ten operations were carried out between 1923 and 1928; two patients survived (see Table 1). The operation then lay fallow until 1945.

It was not until 1948 that successful surgery for mitral stenosis was accomplished, drew wide attention, and began to be accepted by surgeons and internists despite an initially high mortality rate.

Sir Lauder was "emboldened" to propose intracardiac surgery by the "good results" recently obtained in suturing wounds of the heart. Attempts to treat injured heart muscle, in animals and man, had been the major thrust of cardiovascular surgery in the nine-

317

teeth century, but it was only in 1896 that a patient, operated on by Dr. Ludwig Rehn of Frankfurt, survived suturing of a stab wound.[9] A modern heart surgeon has epitomized Rehn's operation as "a victory of the doers over the doubters,"[10] for the prevalent view since antiquity had been that wounds of the heart were necessarily fatal and that the beating heart could not withstand manipulation. (Aristotle himself had declared that "the heart alone of all the viscera cannot stand serious injury.") The reigning dogma was challenged in 1882 when M. H. Bloch of Danzig successfully sutured heart wounds in animals and demonstrated that the heart rate could be slowed to the stage of cardiac arrest during surgery without necessarily causing death. But Bloch's work was received skeptically at best, and one year later the authoritative German physician Dr. Theodor Billroth declared that "any surgeon who should ever attempt to stitch a wound of the heart can be certain of losing the respect of all his colleagues forever."[11] And in 1896, shortly before Rehn's surgery, the prominent British surgeon, Stephen Paget, affirmed: "Surgery of the heart has probably reached the limit set by Nature to all surgery: no new method, and no new discovery, can overcome the natural difficulties that attend a wound of the heart."[12]

By 1900, despite caveats such as the above, at least seventeen attempts had been made to suture heart wounds with seven survivors—indeed a "good result" considering the general state of thoracic surgery. But when it came to taking the next step, to risk operating within the heart itself, the animus of Billroth and Paget prevailed. A week after Brunton's note appeared, his "sufficiently heroic therapeutic suggestion" was roundly criticized in a leading article in *Lancet*.[13] Brunton's critic (one of the editors of *Lancet*) first faulted him for advising others to try a dangerous operation he himself had not perfected in animals, much less tried clinically. More serious charges concerned "the difficulty of the operation and the doubt as to its efficacy, even if successfully carried out." For example, it seemed possible that the surgically divided valve would quickly heal in its old, narrowed form, or that—a point debated through the 1940's—the stenosis would be converted into a possibly more serious mitral regurgitation (backflow of blood from the ventricle into the auricle).

Criticism of Brunton continued in the next two issues of *Lancet*. This did not preclude the publication of two claims for priority in having suggested mitral valve surgery, presumably in case the operation should be successfully tried. Thus, another leading cardiologist, Dr. Lauriston Shaw, wrote that he had discussed surgery for mitral stenosis at least twelve years ago, but had decided it was not "a justifiable therapeutic procedure." Sir Lauder's "chief task," charged his fellow cardiologist, "is not to show his surgical colleagues that it is possible to enlarge the stenosed mitral orifice, but to persuade his medical colleagues that such a procedure is useful."[14] There appears to have been no further published discussion between Brunton and his colleagues on surgery for mitral stenosis, nor did Sir Lauder ever continue his experiments. He later stated that he developed blood poisoning and had to give up the work,[15] though one may wonder why, given his large subsequent contribution to medical literature, it was this particular endeavor that had to be abandoned.

The twenty-one year hiatus between Brunton's proposal and the first clinical operation for mitral stenosis was marked by a considerable body of experimental work in Europe and the United States, and by two operations on patients with chronic valvular disease.[16] In 1912, Dr. T. Tuffier did a finger dilatation for aortic stenosis, and his patient survived. In 1913, Dr. E. Doyen unsuccessfully operated for pulmonary stenosis. Doyen apparently had also worked out a technique for mitral stenosis, but his death in 1916, during World War I, cut short his career and a possible clinical trial of the procedure.

Experimental study of the anatomy and physiology of mitral stenosis and of its surgical correction was hampered by the inability of investigators to create a stenosis in the laboratory animal. The best that could be done with the various techniques that were developed was to produce defects and a resulting regurgitation or insufficiency. The most successful of these methods was to cut or tear out the valve cusps by the insertion of a valvulotome (knifehook) into the aorta or base of the left auricle. However, a series of significant findings did emerge from the laboratory, and these data helped to resolve many of the issues raised by Brunton's critics. From 1907 to 1909 Dr. W. G. MacCallum and his colleagues at Johns Hopkins showed that the normal animal could withstand experimentally produced mitral regurgitation. In a 1914 summary of their work in experimental heart surgery, Dr. Alexis Carrell and Tuffier pointed out that in pure mitral stenosis the myocardium (heart muscle) is not damaged. They also succinctly reviewed the dangers involved in cardiac surgery, such as injury to the coronary vessels, hemorrhage, air embolism, thrombosis, and so forth. These problems would be encountered by surgeons repeatedly in the next decades. Another important aspect of Carrell and Tuffier's work, as well as that of other researchers, was that it demonstrated how much physical manipulation and trauma the heart would tolerate. In 1922, Allen and Graham using their newly developed cardioscope, with which they could both see the valve and incise its leaflets, found that the cut ends of the mitral valves in experimental dogs did not heal. This suggested that stenosis might not recur in man following surgical division.

On May 20, 1923, after more than two years of laboratory work, the first human case of mitral valve surgery was undertaken by Dr. Elliot C. Cutler, then an Associate in Surgery at Boston's Peter Bent Brigham Hospital, in collaboration with the cardiologist Dr. Samuel A. Levine. Cutler and his research associate, Dr. Claude S. Beck, had learned much of value in their animal work, despite the inability to create a stenosis, but felt they "had reached a point where . . . further knowledge could only be gained by an attempt in an actual case, and much as we feared the difficulties, our experimental work gave us the courage to carry out what must appear as a hazardous trial."[17]

Cutler chose to operate with the valvulotome rather than the cardioscope, feeling that the latter technique was too intricate and time consuming. His account of the operation vividly illustrates the problems of working blindly within the heart, as was generally necessary until the development of open-heart methods in the 1950's.

. . . rolling the heart out and to the right . . . , the valvulotome . . . was plunged into the left ventricle. . . . The knife was pushed upwards about 2½ inches, until it encountered what seemed to us must be the mitral orifice. It was then turned mesially, and a cut made in what we thought was the aortic leaflet, the resistance encountered being very considerable.[18]

Cutler and Levine's patient, a twelve-year-old girl, survived the surgery and four days later was presented to the staff of the Brigham during the hospital's decennial celebration, an index of the importance Cutler attached to the operation. In their first published report of the case, appearing five weeks after the operation, they concluded:

> At this stage of our observations we cannot with accuracy define just what has occurred nor what benefits may have accrued, if any. . . . The experience with this case, however, is of importance in that it does show that surgical intervention in cases of mitral stenosis bears no special risk, and should give us further courage and support in our desire to attempt to alleviate a chronic condition, for which there is now not only no treatment, but one which carries a terrible prognosis.[19]

Cutler and Levine's paper was quickly hailed as a "milestone" in a publication as prestigious as the *British Medical Journal*,[20] and within a year their work had attracted enough attention to have started the priority bandwagon rolling again.[21]

In November 1924, in the best nineteenth-century tradition, Cutler, Levine, and Beck published a paper of over one hundred pages in which they detailed the historical background, experimental work, and protocols of their first four cases of mitral valve surgery. In discussing their "rationale for operative intervention," Cutler and his associates lamented the fact that cardiac surgery had for so long been "practically restricted to wounds of the heart." They acknowledged that the field has many dangers, but affirmed that "since the dangers are chiefly those of technic, they should be surmountable."[22] They went on to emphasize their conviction that there are cases of mitral stenosis in which "mechanical obstruction" of the valve plays the dominant role. Thus, they challenged the prevailing wisdom that weakness of the myocardium, not valvular obstruction, was chiefly responsible for producing the symptoms of cardiac failure seen in mitral stenosis. Despite data such as Carrell and Tuffier's, attention had been focused for many years on the myocardium, chiefly due to the teaching of one of the world's leading cardiologists, Britain's Sir James MacKenzie.[23]

Cutler, like the next generation of surgeons who sought to correct intracardiac defects, was occupied with the critical importance of accurate anatomical diagnosis and the criteria for patient selection. After enumerating the diagnostic criteria he employed, Cutler predicted that "the difficulties of the future will be encountered in the attempt to distinguish the cases of pure mitral stenosis from those in which there is, in addition, tricuspid and aortic valve disease." It would be preferable, he continued, to choose patients who are older than twenty for surgery, for beyond this age repeated infections of rheumatic fever are unlikely to occur. They should also have a "quite marked" valvular obstruction and be individuals in whom "the muscular wall might be expected to be in fair condition."[24]

Though Cutler tried to follow the above precepts, and despite all that had been learned through animal experimentation, only one of his four cases, the young girl on whom he had operated first, survived. The other three patients had survived surgery for ten hours, twenty hours, and six days postoperatively. However, Cutler's faith in his surgical procedures still seemed strong, as he reflected in his comments on these cases.

From such a limited experience no final deduction can be drawn either for or against the proposal or the procedure. We feel, however, that much has been learned that should be of value in the consideration of such cases and in subsequent operations. Certainly, there can be no doubt that the method of exposure used is satisfactory, simple in execution, and that it apparently produced no especially harmful effect on our patients. The fact that there were no operative deaths or any indication that the procedure per se was a factor in the subsequent fatalities is comforting.

A mortality of 75 per cent is alarming, but to those who will analyze the full reports of the separate cases it may not appear so disastrous . . .

Indeed there are so many questions, obviously unanswered, before the first and even after the last operation, that we feel that our mortality rate should be judged, if one wishes to use this as a criterion, only in comparison with figures obtained in the early surgery of other parts of the body, when similar important questions were still unanswered. May we recall the mortality figures in the early surgery of such a relatively simple field as that of the stomach, collected by Dr. W. W. Keen for his Cartwright lectures. Of the first twenty-eight gastrostomies, collected in 1875, all the patients died, and in a series of thirty-five gastroenterostomies in 1885 the operative mortality was 65.7 per cent. Moreover, it took years for these figures to improve. In 1884 the mortality for gastrostomy was still 81.6 per cent.[25]

In 1929, Cutler and Beck reviewed the total of twelve operations reported for chronic valvular disease of the heart through 1928. The subtitle of the paper was significant: "Final Report of all Surgical Cases." For, by then, Cutler had privately, if not publicly, revised his belief in the simplicity and efficacy of mitral valve surgery. As the word "final" suggests, he was calling a personal halt to further trials. A glance at Table One quickly suggests why Cutler, in the words of a colleague, was "just devastated"[26] by the outcome of his pioneering efforts. Of the three valvulotomies and four valvulectomies[27] Cutler and his associates had performed, all patients are listed as "died"—though the first patient had lived a creditable four and a half years after surgery. Out of a total of

TABLE ONE. *Surgery for Chronic Valvular Disease, 1912–1928*[*]

CASE	DATE	SURGEON	DIAGNOSIS	PROCEDURE	OUTCOME
1.	1912	Tuffier	Aortic stenosis	Finger dilatation	Recovery, improved
2.	1913	Doyen	Pulmonary stenosis	Tenotome	Died, few hours postoperatively
3.	5/20/23	Cutler	Mitral stenosis	Tenotome	Died, 4 yrs. 6 mo. postoperatively
4.	8/7/23	Allen & Graham	Mitral stenosis	Cardioscope	Operative death
5.	10/7/23	Cutler	Mitral stenosis	Tenotome	Died, 10 hrs. postoperatively
6.	1/12/24	Cutler	Mitral stenosis	Tenotome	Died, 20 hrs. postoperatively
7.	2/25/24	Cutler	Mitral stenosis	Cardioval-vulotome	Died, 6 days postoperatively
8.	6/11/24	Cutler	Mitral stenosis	Cardioval-vulotome	Died, 3 days postoperatively
9.	5/6/25	Souttar	Mitral stenosis	Finger dilatation	Recovery, improved
10.	11/14/25	Pribram	Mitral stenosis	Cardioval-vulotome	Died, 6 days postoperatively
11.	12/8/26	Cutler	Mitral stenosis	Cardioval-vulotome	Died, 15 hrs. postoperatively
12.	4/15/28	Cutler	Mitral stenosis	Cardioval-vulotome	Died, 3 hrs. postoperatively

[*] Adapted from E. Cutler and C. Beck, "The Present Status of the Surgical Procedures in Chronic Valvular Disease of the Heart," *Archives of Surgery*, Vol. 18 (1929), p. 413

ten operations only one patient was cited as both "living" and "improved." Not only was the mortality rate 90 per cent, but "eight of the ten patients died so soon after operation that the changes brought about in the mechanics of the circulation could not be adequately studied."

The one "successful" case of mitral valve surgery in the 1920's deserves notice. In May 1925, Dr. Henry S. Souttar, Director of Surgery at London Hospital, operated on a nineteen-year-old girl first hospitalized in 1921 for mitral stenosis. After exposing the heart, Souttar reported, he incised the left auricle and began to explore its interior with his left forefinger. He found that he was able to pass his finger into the ventricle through the mitral valve, and "as the stenosis was of such moderate degree . . . it was decided not to carry out the valve section which had been arranged, but to limit intervention to such dilatation as could be carried out by the finger."[28] The patient made an uninterrupted recovery, and all present during surgery were "struck by the facility and safety of the procedure." To the best of his knowledge, Souttar wrote, this was the first time the mitral valve had been reached by the auricular route, or that the interior of the heart had been subjected to digital examination. Comparing his procedure with Cutler's, Souttar commented that although one cannot judge a method on a single case, "it appears to me that the method of digital exploration through the auricular appendage cannot be surpassed for simplicity and directness."

Despite some favorable press from colleagues,[29] Souttar himself never repeated his finger dilatation procedure, and no other surgeon tried to use what then seemed the only successful technique for alleviating mitral stenosis until 1948. We will later explore the reasons for the 1925 to 1948 moratorium. For the present, let us record that Souttar failed to repeat his surgery because, in Meade's words, "he had no more patients referred to him for operation . . . [MacKenzie's] opposition [to surgery for mitral stenosis] prevented Souttar from continuing his work."[30]

Cutler's seventh operation for mitral stenosis, and the last one known to have been performed until 1945, was in April 1928. The conclusion of his "Final Report" reflects the professional outward optimism of the surgeon rather than the inward "devastation" of the innovator who has realized that, for a combination of reasons, his is not a good procedure.

It may seem that the information obtained from the twelve cases of chronic valvular disease in which operation was performed is so meager that further attempts are not justified. However, in view of the preceding discussion, we feel that a few more attempts are necessary in order to answer certain questions already mentioned. Should it be possible to produce experimental stenosis, these questions could be answered in the laboratory. Unfortunately, our own attempts for seven years along this line have been as unsuccessful as the attempts of other and more experienced investigators.

It is our conclusion that the mortality figures alone should not deter further investigation both clinical and experimental, since they are to be expected in the opening up of any new field for surgical endeavor.[31]

The seventeen-year moratorium on the clinical use of mitral valve surgery ended on November 14, 1945, when Dr. Charles P. Bailey, in Philadelphia, attempted a valvulotomy. However, as can be seen in Table Two, this did not precipitate a rapid resurgence of mitral valve surgery. By 1948 only three other surgeons had performed such operations: Dr. Dwight E. Harken in Boston, Dr. Horace G. Smithy in South Carolina, and Dr. Russell Brock in

TABLE TWO. *Mitral Valve Surgery, 1945–1949. Results of the First Series by Bailey, Harken, and Smithy*[*]

Dr. Charles P. Bailey

CASE	DATE	PROCEDURE	OUTCOME
1.	11/14/45	Valvulotomy	Operative death
2.	6/12/46	Finger dilatation	Death, 60 hrs. postoperatively, thrombosis at valve
3.	3/22/48	Commissurotomy	Death, 6 days, "technical difficulty"
4.	6/10/48	Exploratory	Operative death
5.	6/10/48	Commissurotomy	Living, "excellent result"
6.	6/27/48	Commissurotomy	Living, "excellent result"
7.	7/13/48	Commissurotomy	Death, 7 days, cerebral embolus
8.	8/2/48	Valve section (cusp incision)	Death, 3 mo., mitral regurgitation
9.	9/2/48	Valve section	Death, 24 hrs., mitral regurgitation
10.	9/2/48	Commissurotomy	Death, 24 hrs., hemorrhage
11.	9/10/48	Interauricular shunt	Death, 60 hrs., diminished cardiac output
12.	9/16/48	Dilatation	Living, "greatly improved"
13.	2/1/49	Dilatation	Death, 60 hrs., cardiac failure
14.	2/2/49	Commissurotomy	Living, "excellent result"
15.	3/23/48	Commissurotomy	Living, "excellent result"

Dr. Dwight E. Harken

1.	3/22/47	Partial valvulectomy (valvuloplasty)	Death, 24 hrs., pulmonary edema
2.	6/16/48	Valvuloplasty	Living, little improvement
3.	no date	Interatrial septal defect created	Living
4.	no date	Septal defect created	Living
5.	no date	Cardiac denervation	Living
6.	1/6/49	Valvuloplasty	Living, improvement
7.	3/4/49	Valvuloplasty	Operative death
8.	3/18/49	Valvuloplasty	Death, 5 days, pulmonary edema

Dr. Horace G. Smithy

1.	1/30/48	Partial valvulectomy	Death, 10 mo., congestive heart failure
2.	3/1/48	" "	Death, 10 hrs., acute cardiac insufficiency
3.	3/8/48	" "	Death, 48 hrs., pneumonia
4.	4/20/48	" "	Living, "excellent condition"
5.	5/3/48	" "	Living, improved, but persisting auricular fibrillation
6.	6/4/48	" "	Living, improved, limited in activity
7. & 8.	May & June '48	2 operations on 1 patient	Living, improved, but systolic murmur

° Data compiled from: Bailey, *Diseases of the Chest,* Vol. 15 (1949) and *Journal of Thoracic Surgery,* Vol. 19 (1950); D. Harken, *New England Journal of Medicine,* Vol. 239 (1948), and *Journal of Thoracic Surgery* Vol. 19 (1950); H. Smithy, J. Boone, J. Stallworth, "Surgical Treatment of Constrictive Valvular Disease of the Heart," *Surgery, Gynecology and Obstetrics,* Vol. 90 (1950), pp. 175–92 (Dr. Smithy died prior to the publication of this paper). The first eight operations by Brock in England, beginning in September 1948, were not included in Table Two as specific data on them was not available.

England. The revival of mitral valve surgery demonstrates that several kinds of priority are involved and may be claimed in therapeutic innovation.[32] For, whereas Bailey resumed mitral valve surgery sixteen months prior to Harken, his first successful result came only six days before Harken's, and in turn, Harken published on the surgical treatment of mitral stenosis five months before Bailey.

A series of medical and surgical advances facilitated the resumption of mitral valve surgery. A major breakthrough toward resolving the problems that had plagued surgeons in the 1920's came in 1930–32, when methods to create mitral stenosis in the dog were finally worked out. That Elliot Cutler had not lost his interest in the disease and its correction is indicated by the fact that the first man to create stenosis in the dog was one of his residents, Dr. John Powers. Powers went on to study the dog's responses to resection of the mitral valve, the technique Cutler had used in his last four cases, hoping definitively to answer the question of whether an insufficiency could be tolerated. But the dogs, like Cutler's patients, all died after valvulectomy, and on the basis of physiologic studies before and after surgery Powell concluded that the valvulectomy operation was "unphysiologic and should not be used. He suggested that dilatation of the valve . . . might be effective, or that small bits of the stenosed valve might be removed in stages."[33]

Apart from diagnostic and operative problems specific to mitral valve surgery, intrathoracic and intracardiac surgery in general, in the words of Dr. Francis D. Moore, was "still in its infancy" in the 1920's. "Application of [animal work] to the human was still held back by lack of established principles for intrathoracic anaesthesia. There was no good way of following the physiologic progress of the patient."[34] Limitations in diagnostic tools and the dangers of death from hemorrhage during surgery or post-operative death from infection constituted other critical impediments. By the mid-1940's, largely in response to the medical and surgical demands created by World War II, this cluster of problems had been greatly reduced. Major advances included: cardiac catheterization; the improvement of anaesthetic techniques for intrathoracic surgery, particularly the institution of endotracheal anaesthesia; the development of methods permitting rapid blood transfusion; and the discovery and synthesis of antibacterial and antibiotic agents.

Another major technical and psychological stimulus for the relaunching of mitral valve surgery came from the successful initiation of surgery for congenital defects of the heart's great vessels, surgery which also had been proposed but not executed years earlier. In 1907, Dr. John Munro of Boston detailed a method for ligation of patent ductus arteriosus. Ligation was finally attempted, unsuccessfully, by Dr. John Streider of Boston in March 1937, and his presentation of the case at the American Association of Thoracic Surgery meetings two months later drew little notice. Thus, many would date the era of modern heart surgery from 1938, when Dr. Robert Gross of Children's Hospital, Boston, unaware of Streider's earlier attempt, successfully ligated the ductus in a young patient.[35] A second milestone came in 1944 with the implementation of the Blalock-Taussig operation (anastomosing the systemic and pulmonary arteries) to correct the cluster of congenital defects known as the tetralogy of Fallot (which came to be called the "blue baby operation").[36]

If we now look at how Bailey and Harken revived mitral valve surgery, independently, though with awareness of each other's work, we begin to see the confluence of scientific, personal, and historical factors in ending the moratorium.

In 1940 Harken began his residency at Boston City Hospital after a year of work in England with Mr. Tudor Edwards. Studying the heart at autopsies, Harken became absorbed with the challenge of devising a method to enter the heart and remove the vegetations of bacterial endocarditis. For, "endocarditis was one disease of the heart that could be absolutely diagnosed and that we knew absolutely was fatal. And I reasoned that if it was fatal, I had the right to try any operation that might possibly be expected to work."[37] In devising a method to enter the heart through the auricular appendage and remove the vegetations with the visual aid of a cardioscope, Harken made a discovery that we can now appreciate as a fundamental advance for mitral valve surgery. The mitral valve's two leaflets have different functions, and if the major or aortic leaflet is destroyed, the experimental animal soon dies of regurgitation; conversely, regurgitation is not the necessary price of relieving stenosis as long as the aortic leaflet is not destroyed. Bailey was to reach independently the same conclusion, and in their early papers on the subject both surgeons stressed their conviction that it is neither desirable nor necessary to exchange stenosis for regurgitation.

World War II intervened before Harken could try his approach to bacterial endocarditis on a patient, and soon the availability of penicillin removed the fatal threat of the disease. He persuaded Cutler (then in England) and Edwards to use their influence to establish the army's first thoracic surgery specialty unit in England. Subsequently, Harken was named the unit's chief. In that setting he soon had ample opportunity to apply his techniques for intra-cardiac surgery to new problems. In doing the first elective intra-cardiac surgery, Harken and his team removed shell fragments and bullets from the heart and great vessels of one hundred and thirty-four wounded soldiers, in one hundred and thirty-nine oper-ations, without a single fatality. One of the "elementary rules" of cardiac surgery that emerged from this work was that the heart does not readily tolerate dislocation from its position of optimal function in the chest. Such dislocation causes sudden, potentially fatal arhythmias. As Moore has observed, here "was a guiding principle for further work and . . . an explanation for some of Dr. Cutler's difficulties twenty years before . . ."[38]

In a 1945 lecture in London, Harken paid tribute to his prede-cessors who had a made new era in intracardiac surgery possible.

The brilliant work and writing on heart surgery by Doyen, Duval, Tuf-fier, Carrell, Graham, Beck, and Cutler mark the evolution from dreams to experiment and from experiment to bold human adventure. Today it is fair to expect certain simple intracardiac maneuvers to be successful. The door has been opened by modern anaesthesia and the technique of rapid blood replacement.[39]

"Intracardiac maneuvers" for mitral stenosis were in fact attempted that very year, but not successfully. After five years of laboratory study at Philadelphia's Hahnemann Hospital, Bailey felt he under-stood why earlier mitral valve surgery had not succeeded. He at-tributed its failure to using a poor route (ventricular) into the valve and to causing a sudden and large regurgitation by damag-ing the major leaflet. The method which Bailey worked out in-cluded an auricular approach and palpation of the valve with the finger prior to actual valvulotomy.[40]

As previously mentioned, on November 14, 1945 Bailey at-tempted his first clinical case, but before he could enter the heart, the auricle was torn and the patient bled to death. (See Table Two for a resumé of Bailey's and Harken's first operations.) He per-formed a second operation in June 1946: "since [the patient] was deemed hopeless," Bailey reported, "her physicians felt that she might be subjected to valvulotomy."[41] During surgery, as Bailey later wrote to Meade, Souttar's operation was unexpectedly revived when the stenosis was found to be so severe that the knife would not cut the valve.

In desperation, remembering Souttar's report, I inserted my finger through the auricular appendage, palpated the valve and pushed my finger through the diminished slit . . . both commissures split well. . . . For about twenty-four hours post-operatively, the patient's condition improved remarkably and steadily. There was no clinical evidence of regurgitation. However, one day later, she suddenly collapsed and died.[42]

Bailey operated on a third terminal case of mitral stenosis in March 1948; the patient died six days later of hemorrhage from the chest wall.

Bailey's three operations had been performed at three different hospitals in the Philadelphia area, and he was informed that further intracardiac surgery would not be permitted at those institutions. Nevertheless, he scheduled two more cases of mitral surgery for June 10, 1948, at the last two Philadelphia hospitals where he still had operating privileges. Case four died during surgery in the morning, of cardiac arrest judged by Bailey to be unrelated to an attempted finger dilatation. Success finally came that afternoon, at Episcopal Hospital, when a twenty-four-year-old housewife withstood her surgery so well that one week later, "she was transported without incident in a train to a medical convention a thousand miles away for presentation in person."[43]

Six days after Bailey's first success, Harken did a valvuloplasty operation on a twenty-seven-year-old man at Boston City Hospital. The patient survived surgery and five months postoperatively was reported symptomatically improved. Harken's first case, like Bailey's, had ended in failure: the patient died twenty-four hours after his valvuloplasty in March, 1947, in respiratory collapse and pulmonary edema. From his knowledge of Cutler's work and from his own laboratory experiments and clinical experience in the war, Harken ventured into mitral valve surgery with four basic premises:

(1) to approach the mitral valve from above rather than through the ventricle, (2) to operate on the heart without dislocating it from its normal position, (3) to remove only portions of the lesser leaflets . . . thus avoiding regurgitation, and (4) to use the superior pulmonary vein as the port of entry.[44]

By the time he had completed his first five operations for mitral stenosis, Harken had developed a threefold "preliminary classification" of patients and the indicated surgery according to their degree of stenotic incapacitation: (A) low fixed cardiac output: mitral valvuloplasty; (B) normal cardiac output: artificial interatrial shunt; (C) uncontrollable tachycardia or anginal pain: cardiac denervation.[45]

While Harken's only fatality in these cases had been with the first valvuloplasty, it was this procedure, designed to help the most critically ill class of patients, upon which he concentrated. His first paper on mitral valve surgery, for example, is devoted largely to presenting four "basic principles" for valvuloplasty. But like his predecessor, Cutler, and his contemporary, Bailey, Harken soon found that a background of experimental animal surgery, the use of carefully designed instruments, criteria of patient selection, and operative guidelines could not alone ensure the success of mitral valve surgery. In the winter of 1948–49, six out of Harken's first nine patients died, during or shortly after valvulotome surgery.

At this point I went home depressed and said "I quit." Some people suggested I should try my technique on better-risk patients, in order to help me get better results, so I wouldn't "ruin the reputation of cardiac surgery." But I wouldn't do that. After I lost my sixth patient, I had a call from Dr. Laurence Ellis [then President of the New England Cardiovascular Society]. I told him I wouldn't kill any more patients [through mitral valve surgery], and that no respectable referring physician would send me any more patients anyhow. Ellis asked me what I meant: didn't I realize that these patients surely would die if I didn't operate? He said he would still refer patients to me, and didn't I think he was a good cardiologist? This talk with Ellis was a turning point. I went back and operated and my patients suddenly started doing better. But I almost called a moratorium.[46]

Early in 1949, Dr. Harken realized that he "couldn't do an operation successfully with the [valvulotome] and have the patient survive in a substantial number of cases."[47] As he studied postmortem specimens of mitral stenosis, seeking to improve his procedure, he became convinced that the best way to open up the fused bridges of the valve's leaflets, without unduly damaging the valves themselves, was the simple technique Souttar had pioneered: finger dilatation through an auricular entry. After a few cases it "became apparent" that this method, which Harken aptly named finger-fracture valvuloplasty, "had made possible an entirely new evaluation of valvular surgery because it was done with a new order of accuracy."[48]

Apart from some technical refinements, the operation done today for most cases of mitral stenosis differs little from that done by Souttar in 1925. By the early 1950's, with the reports of successful mitral valve surgery by Bailey, Harken, Smithy, Brock, and others, surgical intervention for mitral stenosis became generally accepted by surgeons and cardiologists. Overall mortality rates began to decline as experience was gained and as patients not in the last stages of the disease were referred and accepted for surgery. For critically ill patients (Harken's Class IV), the mortality rate took longer to decline. In Harken's first eighty cases there were twenty-nine deaths (twenty-five of them surgical), a 35 per cent mortality rate. "Why do we keep operating in that situation, with such an overwhelming mortality rate?" Harken asked rhetorically in a talk at the Brigham. "Because if we don't, we think these people would die in the normal course of their disease. And if we do, people look like some of the patients you see here . . ."[49]

The Clinical Moratorium: Contributory Factors

Study of the development of surgery for mitral stenosis has served as a starting point for defining the parameters of what we believe to be a common occurrence in the process of therapeutic innovation, the calling of a moratorium on the use of a new medical or surgical procedure. From the history of mitral valve surgery, and that of cardiac transplantation, we have been able to identify a number of factors that contribute to a clinical moratorium. Depending upon specifiable circumstances, the interplay of these factors may either help to induce, deter, or terminate a moratorium. They include: the stage of medical knowledge and practice (state of the art factors); the experiment-therapy dilemma inherent in clinical research; facets of the dual role of physician-investigator; certain social structural characteristics of relations between the physician, his colleagues, and the hospital in which he carries out his investigative work; the impact of media of mass communication and lay opinion on the medical profession; the influence of cultural conceptions and beliefs, such as attitudes toward the human heart.

The Clinical Moratorium

Virtually every medical and surgical procedure, even the most established, carries with it a certain modicum of uncertainty as to its efficacy and safety. Gaps in knowledge, technical inadequacies, and the problems of uncertainty that stem from them are inherent to medical research and practice. These problems occur in a dramatic form during a period of therapeutic innovation, creating intensive strains for research physicians and their patients alike. This is one reason why a moratorium is likely to occur during the early phases of clinical trial, error, and evaluation. The investigator continually weighs the known and probable risks and the benefits of a new procedure for the patients on whom he is conducting clinical trials. On the basis of this dynamic calculus, decisions are made and remade concerning the circumstances under which a new treatment may justifiably be used, and on what categories of patients.

The most immediate and manifest reason for suspending a therapeutic procedure is that the mortality rate associated with it is judged to be "too high." However, as we will see in the next section, there is no simple definition of therapeutic "success" and "failure," and no ready answer to the question of what constitutes an "acceptable" mortality rate at different points along the experiment-to-therapy spectrum, and with various kinds of patients.

We have seen in the development of mitral valve surgery that numerous state of the art factors may influence the decision to initiate, suspend, or resume use of a given procedure on patients. The levels of development of the following elements play determining roles: relevant basic science knowledge; an animal model (an animal in which one can reproduce or simulate a human disease state and test therapies); knowledge about the specific applicability of the procedure to given disease states and individual patients; the degree of relevant technical proficiency (in surgery, for example, anaesthesia, transfusion, and other areas of operative management, and in medicine, the control of a drug's unanticipated side effects).

Our case study of mitral stenosis provides numerous examples of the role that state of the art factors can play in the "stops" and "starts" associated with moratoria. A major reason why American surgeons did not adopt Souttar's finger dilatation method, despite the success of his one case, was expressed by Dr. Evarts Graham. As he wrote to Meade, Graham was "much interested" in Souttar's operation, "but felt that his procedure would never amount to very much because it lacked precision and was a blind one."[50] When next we look at the resumption of mitral valve surgery in 1945–1948, we find that Smithy revived the valvulectomy operation used by Cutler, knowing that six of Cutler's seven patients and all of Power's experimental dogs had died. In Smithy's case, with the major strides in intrathoracic surgery and anaesthesia since the 1920's and his own work on a partial valvulectomy technique in dogs, beginning with aortic valve surgery, five of his first seven patients survived surgery and the immediate postoperative period. (Of those five, one died ten months later; three showed slight improvement, and one great improvement in the course of the first year.)[51] The importance of instrumentation and technique in the mitral valve surgery done by Bailey and Harken, in turn, has been well summarized by Meade.[52]

It is generally agreed that for a satisfactory result the commissures must be opened all the way to the myocardium. Souttar had planned to use a tenotome, as Cutler had used in his first and only successful case. Until Bailey demonstrated the correctness of Souttar's ideas, everyone working on the valves of the heart had devised and used instruments with which segments of the valve leaflets could be excised. Indeed it was with such an instrument that Bailey had planned to attack the valve which he was forced to treat by finger dilatation. Bailey's first successful case was treated by finger fracture. Harken, six days later, used an instrument with which he cut through the commissures. He and Bailey then devised knives with which the commissures could be cut without resecting segments of the valves. Since then a great variety of knives have been made. It is interesting that Harken, who first used a knife, became one of the chief advocates of the finger fracture method, and Bailey came to feel that more of the valves needed to be enlarged by the use of knives.

Partly as a consequence of these and other technical advances, by the mid-1940's the medically prevalent view of the heart as an organ too vital and fragile to withstand manipulation or surgical trauma changed. Gradually, the heart came to be seen as a strong, resilient, and fairly simple muscular pump. In turn, this conceptual shift facilitated the work that opened the modern era of intracardiac surgery.

THE EXPERIMENT-THERAPY DILEMMA[53]

One of the most fundamental problems shared by all physicians trying out new treatments on sick patients is that of determining how experimental and/or therapeutic that treatment is. Such an evaluation depends heavily on the state of the art factors discussed above, and as earlier mentioned is a primary criterion for deciding on whom and under what circumstances the new procedure may justifiably be used. The usual discussions of this calculus, under the rubric of the "ethics of human experimentation," are too often couched in dichotomous terms of "experiment" or "therapy."[54] In practice, however, one sees a *process* of therapeutic innovation which generally progresses from animal experiments to clinical trials with terminally ill patients beyond conventional therapeutic help, to the use of the treatment on less and less critically ill patients.

In the evolution of surgery for mitral stenosis, as in all clinical research and innovation, there were no clear guideposts telling physician-investigators that the time had arrived to move from one stage to another. Rather, physicians had continually to assess the state of the art, their own capabilities, the probable risks and benefits to their patients, the possible yield in knowledge that might help other patients,[55] and the proper allocation of scarce resources (manpower, equipment, facilities, funds).

As illustrated by the responses to Brunton's proposal in 1902 and by the short-lived course of valve surgery in the 1920's, the transition from animal experimentation to clinical use, for any procedure, is one "which is inherently 'premature' [particularly in the absence of an animal model], and for that reason is often judged to be controversial, and, sometimes, 'immoral.' It typically involves a stressful and discouraging period. . . . For, as a combined consequence of the many unknown and uncontrolled factors in this stage of experimentation, and of the drastic, complicated illness of the patients who undergo the clinical trials, successful outcomes are rare and ephemeral. Failure and death rates are high."[56]

In order to evaluate what constitutes the justifiable use of a new procedure and to appraise "success" and "failure," physicians characteristically make what Joseph Fletcher has termed "mathematicated decisions" based upon a "statistical morality."[57] They estimate and express in terms of probabilities and percentages the differential diagnosis of a disease, and its course under different circumstances, especially its prognosis in response to alternative treatments. This way of reasoning is not peculiar to the clinical investigator; rather, it is inherent in all medical practice.

We have noted that after his first four valvulectomies Cutler acknowledged that a 75 percent mortality rate is "alarming," but maintained that in terms of each case it is not "disastrous," and affirmed that his results must be judged in comparison with other pioneering surgical efforts—mortality rates of 65 to 81 per cent were long common in surgery "of such a relatively simple field as that of the stomach." Similarly, in his "Final Report" of 1929, Cutler insisted that "the mortality figures [90 per cent] alone should not deter further investigation . . . since they are to be expected in the opening up of any new field for surgical endeavor." Another form that "statistical morality" reasoning may take is that the critically ill patient, beyond the help of conventional therapy, will most probably die if the new therapy is not tried. For example, Brunton argued that "the risk of a shortened life" with heart surgery should be balanced against "the certainty of a prolonged period of existence which could hardly be called life" without surgery. Harken explained that this is why he kept operating on class IV mitral stenotics despite an "overwhelming" mortality rate of 35 percent. Similarly, Moore in 1950 emphasized that Harken's decision to operate initially only on severely ill patients was "realistic", for "of sixteen patients selected for operation but who were not operated upon, fourteen are now dead, eleven within six months of the time when surgery was advised."[58]

Cutler's argument, that surgery for mitral stenosis must go on despite high mortality, expressed the research physician's moral commitment to the continuing perfection of new clinical methods. Beyond this, Cutler was the kind of "first pioneer" who, as Moore has put it, is likely to have "a certain amount of inspirational vision. . . . He is driven by this to do something that his own insight tells him can be accomplished. This may be done, and either he or others may be lost in the process. But he points the way."[59]

Despite this kind of drive and commitment, the stresses Cutler experienced in losing his valvulectomy patients seem to have impelled him to call a personal halt to this operation. It is significant

336

to note that it is only through the ambiguous subtitle of his 1929 paper—"Final Report of All Surgical Cases"—that Cutler publicly signaled his moratorium, and that in his paper he desisted from urging other surgeons to do likewise. Nevertheless, as we have seen, no mitral valve surgery was performed for the next seventeen years. This moratorium is associated with a classical phase in trailblazing scientific advances. "There is . . . a gap or pause or moratorium before others—ordinary mortals—can undertake it. They usually have to wait for collateral and technological developments to occur so that the visionary adventure becomes a pathway taken by other people."[60]

The criteria for the kind of surgical failure that Cutler experienced seem easier to define than those for success. Using failure as synonomous with death, Moore has pointed out that failures in surgery of mitral stenosis, like all surgical failures, fall into at least three categories: the disease was too far advanced to stand the stress of surgery; postoperative complications occurred; or technical methods were not adequate to the problems encountered.[61] One might also include in the category "failure" cases in which no improvement is effected, and those in which the procedure results in another serious problem, such as mitral regurgitation. On the other hand, as was true for Souttar's patient, Cutler's first case, and for mitral valve surgery patients in the 1940's, merely to survive a radical new surgical procedure and the postoperative hospitalization may be rated as a success. Thus, the meaning of a surgical success, depending on the nature of the operation and its stage of development, may range from survival to palliation through correction of a condition. Another criterion for success is the decision that a therapy can be employed on other than terminally ill patients. When this occurs, a new treatment moves into a less experimental phase of its development. For example, in 1950, Moore judged that:

The surgery of mitral stenosis has now been through its "dark days," days when the surgeon, his medical colleagues and those with whom he sought counsel were tried as to whether or not the effort should be maintained through such difficulties. It is through those dark days and into a phase where its scope should be broadened. Recently a group of six patients who were *not* in the last stages of the disease have been operated upon. All of them have done well and showed a gratifying return to normal heart function.[62]

JUDITH P. SWAZEY AND RENÉE C. FOX

THE DUAL ROLE OF THE PHYSICIAN-INVESTIGATOR

In any historical era, a significant number of the patients for whom a research physician cares are ill with diseases that are not well understood and can only be imperfectly treated. The institutionalized role of such a clinical investigator is dualistic. On the one hand, like all physicians, he is responsible for the diagnosis, treatment, and mitigation of his patient's suffering. On the other hand, he is obligated to conduct research that bears directly or indirectly upon the maladies of his patients, using some of them as his subjects.

For all of its intellectual, professional, and humanitarian gratifications, the role of research physician is accompanied by characteristic problems and stresses. We have already discussed some of the problems of uncertainty such a physician encounters, resulting from limitations in medical knowledge and practice at a given time. To these may be added those uncertainties that are artifacts of the inability of any physician personally to command all available medical knowledge and skill. Furthermore, the research physician deliberately works in the realm of the uncertain, focusing on those questions which medicine still has not answered, seeking to make some headway with their solution.

Given the fundamental nature of his orientation and activities, the clinical investigator is confronted with more numerous and grave problems of therapeutic limitation than are other types of physicians. He seldom can help to effect the total recovery of his patients; more often, he can only ameliorate or palliate their conditions; and frequently, he can do nothing more than postpone their imminent death.

Under optimal conditions, the research and clinical responsibilities of such a physician are complementary. His investigative work bears directly on the diagnosis and treatment of his patients' conditions, which in some sense it benefits, and conversely, his clinical activities on behalf of his patients also advance his research. However, the clinical and investigative responsibilities of the research physician are not always perfectly reconcilable, and they may openly conflict. Some of the procedures he conducts on research patients may help future generations of persons ill with similar disorders or contribute to general medical knowledge rather than to his subjects' own immediate welfare. What the research physician does to aid or protect his patients may undermine an experi-

338

ment he ideally would have liked to bring to its logical conclusion. And the research in which he asks patients to participate often exposes them to discomfort or risk.

These attributes of their double-edged role cause stress for most physician-investigators. The strains that they experience are intensified by their typically close and continuous relations with the patients who are also their subjects; by colleagues' scientific and ethical judgments of their work; and by a certain vested interest not only in protecting their professional reputations, but also, in advancing them through recognition for being eminently successful with breakthroughs in knowledge or technique.

When the role strains associated with clinical experimentation become acute and especially burdensome, one of the options open to research physicians is that of calling a moratorium. Physician-investigators also have other patterned ways of coming to terms with their professional stresses, which may either push them toward a moratorium or pull them away from it. From a certain point of view, their research constitutes one of their primary intellectual and moral mechanisms for coping with the problems of uncertainty and the unknown. For research activities provide investigators with a way of trying to do something about the hiatuses in knowledge and therapeutic limitations that currently exist. Through this medium they can express their hope and belief that medical advances eventually will come through their efforts. Partly for this reason, unless other factors intervene, a medical investigator tends to continue a particular line of research in what from the outside may seem a self-propelling way.

A good deal of contemporaneous medical research is organized and carried out in a group. Membership in such a team may provide investigators with a way of sharing responsibility, and with the kind of day-by-day collegial counsel, support, and tension release that helps them continue their research despite its concomitant strains and frustrations. However, the fact that by and large the solo investigator pattern has given way to a team model also means that research physicians are more immediately subject to being criticized, contradicted, or overruled by their collaborators. Thus, the sense of the group may be a powerful factor in compelling an investigator to call a moratorium on clinical trials which his colleagues believe ought to be discontinued.

The nature of the relationship between a team of research physicians and their patient-subjects is one of the cardinal factors that may lead them to feel they cannot go on with certain of their experimental procedures. Such physicians and patients are typically drawn closer together by the inexorability of the patients' illnesses, the tragic outcome that awaits many of them, the prolonged contact of patients with physicians over the course of their repeated hospitalizations and periodic follow-ups, and by the collegial relations between patients and physicians that develop as a consequence of their mutual participation in clinical research.[63] Thus, when it seems to research physicians that their clinical trials are exposing patient-subjects to too much discomfort or risk, are not benefitting them in any ostensible way, or are accompanied by an excessive mortality rate, they may decide to call a halt to the trials. Under these circumstances, the pressure to invoke a moratorium comes as much from physicians' subjective reactions to the fate of their patients as from their responsiveness to more impersonal ethical constraints.

Several of these "push-pull" factors, emanating from the stresses of the physician-investigator's dual role and the ways he may respond to them, were encountered in our case study of mitral valve surgery. For example, we can infer that the strong criticism which Brunton's 1902 proposal met was largely responsible for his not undertaking clinical trials of his technique for mitral valve surgery. When such trials were attempted two decades later, Cutler was "pushed" into calling a moratorium because he could not personally tolerate the high mortality rate encountered with valvulectomy and related procedures such as anaesthesia and postoperative management. We do not know the role that the opinion of his colleagues played in Cutler's decision. But we do know that when mitral valve surgery was next attempted, in the 1940's, Harken was deterred from calling a halt in the face of repeated failures by the strong personal and professional encouragement he received from Ellis, an eminent colleague.

THE RESEARCH PHYSICIAN, HIS COLLEAGUES, AND THE HOSPITAL

As the case of Harken and Ellis suggests, relations with colleagues that are more occasional and distant than those with members of his own research team may also be key elements in determining whether or not an investigator pursues a line of experimentation on which he has embarked. If such "outside" or remote colleagues enjoy high professional status and prestige, their influence on a research physician's course of action may be all the greater. For the opinion that a high-ranking physician may have of his work can affect an investigator's own professional reputation and, as a consequence, both the facilities put at his disposal and his state of morale. The impact that Ellis's opinion had on Harken, for example, was enhanced by the fact that Ellis was a respected cardiologist and president of the New England Cardiovascular Society.

An authority figure can also exert a deterring influence on clinical trials. This is exemplified by the role played by Sir James Mac-Kenzie in mitral valve surgery during the 1920's. MacKenzie, one of England's, and the world's, leading cardiologists, believed that a diseased heart muscle was the major feature of mitral stenosis, and thus he opposed valvular surgery as an essentially useless measure. In the face of MacKenzie's influence on other cardiologists in England, Souttar had no more patients referred to him for mitral valve surgery. This was in spite of the fact that he was one of England's leading surgeons (Director of Surgery at London Hospital) and that his first patient to undergo valvular surgery survived and seemed to show improvement. The impact of Mac-Kenzie's opinions was also felt in America. This impact, however, was less strong in the United States than in England, partly due to the geographical distance and professional insulation that working in another society provided. Thus, as Meade records, in Boston, Dr. Samuel Levine, a leading American cardiologist, "stood out in opposition to Sir James and was responsible for Cutler being able to operate."[64]

The particular "social circles"[65] within the medical profession to which a research physician belongs may also act as a stimulus for his undertaking and continuing certain forms of clinical investigation or may lead him to abandon them. There is good circumstantial evidence for assuming that Cutler's decision in 1928 to call a personal moratorium on mitral valve surgery was instrumental in its nonresumption by the profession at large for almost two decades. In this respect, he may be said to be an authority figure who, like MacKenzie, exercised a profession-wide deterring effect on valvular surgery, albeit for different reasons and in a more latent and general fashion. However, despite his moratorium, Cutler continued to exert a positive influence, in his social circle, on surgery for mitral stenosis. Younger physicians of the Peter Bent

Brigham Hospital who had contact with him conducted relevant animal experiments. And it seems more than coincidental that Harken, one of the two surgeons who ended the moratorium in the 1940's, had significant contact with Cutler both in Boston and England during the period when Harken was working out his valvuloplasty procedure. Although Harken, Bailey, Smithy, and Brock were not close friends, they all knew each other and followed the course of each other's laboratory and clinical work.[66]

Since the turn of the century, most clinical medical research has been conducted in a hospital setting. A significant proportion of such investigative work now takes place in university-connected hospitals committed to the advancement of medical knowledge as well as to the care of patients, the training of medical professionals, and, in recent years, more generalized community-oriented health functions. Affiliation with a hospital that can provide a research physician with a site for his investigations, the complex facilities, highly trained personnel, and kinds of patients necessary for his work is indispensable to him.

The hospital as an institution can not only do a great deal to foster a physician's research, it can also impede or terminate it by refusing to grant him affiliation, or by withdrawing certain rights and privileges from him once association has been accorded. In the 1940's, three hospitals in the Philadelphia area used the second kind of social control over Bailey by forbidding him to do any more operations after he had lost a mitral commissurotomy patient in each institution. This could easily have brought his early attempts to perform a successful commissurotomy to an involuntary close. Were it not for the boldly manipulative ways in which he utilized the surgical amphitheaters of the two Philadelphia hospitals still open to him, Bailey might have gone down in medical history as a surgeon on whom a moratorium was imposed.[67]

MASS MEDIA AND LAY OPINION

Advances in medicine are of great interest and concern to the lay public in many contemporary societies. News of the latest basic and applied biomedical developments is continually conveyed to the public through the various media of mass communication. The media not only accord a good deal of space and time to such reporting, but frequently they also assign it the prominent status of "front-page news." As we have suggested elsewhere, the great

342

amount of popular attention accorded to medical science is "indicative of a high cultural value attached to health, longevity, relief of suffering, and the 'conquest of disease.' "[68] It is also associated with the role that medical research and those who conduct it or collaborate in it are presumed to play in the achievement of these goals. To an ever increasing extent, the media have the power to reflect and shape lay attitudes toward medical research and innovation, in ways that may help to facilitate or impede it.

We have not made a systematic study of the role that the mass media played throughout the history of mitral valve surgery. But, as far as we know, this surgery was not extensively covered until the early 1950's. At this time, the operation had developed to the point where it was technically successful and had begun to benefit numerous patients in a still restricted number of hospitals. The content of all the news articles that we have examined from this period is highly positive and even triumphant in tone. Valvular surgery is presented as a harbinger of a new era of open heart surgery, and emphasis is placed on the "new life" that such operations can make possible for former cardiac invalids.

The treatment of organ transplantation, especially human heart transplants, by the press and other media has been much more copious and extensive than the coverage of mitral valve surgery. Dr. Irvine H. Page has characterized it as "instant reporting," and contended that "there has never been anything like it in medical annals."[69] The same kinds of positive themes run through the press treatments of heart transplantation as those of surgery for mitral stenosis. The surgeons who have performed this trail-blazing procedure have been presented as heroes, along with the heart recipients, donors, and their respective families. Those who have survived surgery and shown improvement have been depicted as undertaking activities that not only surpass what they were able to do preoperatively, but that also demonstrate unusual "physical prowess or endurance."[70] It may be assumed that these aspects of reporting have helped to encourage many of the sixty surgeons who have thus far conducted heart transplants to perform them. Such presentations have given them public support, recognition, and, in some cases, fame. Publicity about heart transplants has also facilitated their work by emphasizing the need for donors as well as the promise this operation holds for desperately ill recipients.

However, certain themes that the mass media have emphasized

may have undermined rather than reinforced the continuance of heart transplantation. Medical spokesmen have stated their feeling that a "too optimistic" impression of the present state of cardiac transplantation has been given and that this has had some boomerang effects on the lay public. This has been made all the more likely by the fact that newspapers have kept a "box score" on all heart transplants done and their outcome, demonstrating the typically high mortality rate for a therapeutic innovation in this very early stage of development. Furthermore, as some physicians have pointed out, the "transplanter" has often been presented as a taker of organs, rather than as a healer and the patient's guardian. Debates about the pros and cons of cardiac transplantation have taken place as much on the pages of daily newspapers as within the confines of the medical profession. And, to some extent, the spectacular, "circus trappings and glitter"[71] way in which some of the heart transplant surgeons have been presented to the public has subjected them to collegial criticism rather than increasing their professional standing, because such publicity violates professional norms of privacy, modesty, and disinterestedness.

CULTURAL CONCEPTIONS AND BELIEFS

Both the evolution of mitral valve surgery and cardiac transplantation demonstrate that concepts, ideas, and beliefs deriving from the cultural tradition of a society may latently affect the occurrence or nonoccurrence of a moratorium. The fact that in Western society the heart was considered to be a delicate, vital organ by physicians as well as laymen was long an impediment to cardiac surgery. The Judeo-Christian conception of the heart as a mystical organ, where the soul and the most noble motives and sentiments of man reside, has also forestalled and slowed down attempts to manipulate it.

These underlying ways of thinking about the human heart surfaced during the period of early clinical trials of mitral valve surgery and receded once the operative technique had been sufficiently perfected to demonstrate its viability and therapeutic benefit. In the more recent era of cardiac transplantation, these same conceptions have again manifested themselves, indicating that they have not been dispelled. These notions about the heart have been especially visible in the attempt by some members of the medical profession to redefine death as cessation of brain activity rather than of cardiorespiratory function and to have their new criteria accepted by physicians and laymen alike.[72]

Attributes of the Clinical Moratorium

Clinical moratoria rarely occur in as total and clearcut a form as the moratorium on mitral valve surgery that began in 1928 with Cutler's last operation and ended in 1945 with Bailey's first. Slowdowns or suspensions in the experimental use of new therapeutic measures on patients are more commonly of shorter duration. The moratorium period is usually one of reflection, re-evaluation, and study for the research physicians formerly conducting clinical trials. During this time, they often return to laboratory experiments in an attempt to solve certain of the problems that led them temporarily to cease human trials.

As the foregoing implies, a moratorium does not mean a permanent abandonment of a therapeutic innovation, either because it has proved to be unfruitful or noxious, or because, in the natural flow of medical scientific advance, it has been superseded by a better one. Nor, according to our definition of the phenomenon, does the failure to move from the level of animal to human trials constitute a clinical moratorium. Thus, for example, we do not define as a moratorium the period 1902 through 1922 when no one tried Brunton's technique "for dividing a mitral stenosis on a fellow creature."

The two major subtypes of clinical moratoria that we have identified, then, are total cessations and slowdowns of the use of a new clinical procedure on human subjects.

Slowdowns may occur for a number of reasons, singly or in combination: After a certain number of clinical trials, some physicians may cease to use an experimental procedure; other physicians may try it once or twice and then stop; physicians working in a particular institution may collectively withdraw from further clinical trials; all or most of a group of pioneer physicians may continue with their trials, but at a decelerated pace.

We have not studied a sufficient number of moratoria to generalize about their average duration. And we do not have enough data to determine whether it is more common for a short-lived moratorium (lasting weeks or months) to take the form of total cessation or of a slowdown.

In the previous section of this paper, we discussed various factors that bear upon a moratorium. When these factors converge to push toward a moratorium, they do so either by virtue of "internal" or "external" pressures. By internal pressures toward a moratorium, we mean those that originate primarily with the research physician who feels that he ought to discontinue clinical trials. A classical example is Cutler's conviction that he should terminate mitral valve surgery in the face of a mortality rate that was "devastating" to him. External pressures conducive to a moratorium are generated by the opinions of colleagues or lay persons that trials should not proceed, and by the actions they may take to implement their judgment. This type of pressure is illustrated by the fact that after Souttar had attempted one mitral valve operation, patients with mitral stenosis no longer consulted him, partly because colleagues did not refer such patients to him. Another example is seen in cardiac transplantation. Dr. Denton Cooley, the surgeon who has performed the greatest number of these operations, attributed the decline in heart transplants from December, 1968 through February, 1969 to the fact that "the stream of heart donors . . . dried up" because critics among the lay public and in the medical profession had become "faint hearted . . . in the face of a few initial defeats."[73]

Moratorium pressures may also be "formal" or "informal" in nature. When three Philadelphia hospitals withdrew operating privileges from Bailey, they exercised a formal constraint over his ability to conduct more mitral valve surgery. In contrast, when Harken's colleagues suggested that he would damage the reputation of cardiac surgery if he continued to operate with such a high mortality rate, they exerted informal pressures upon him. A research physician may or may not consent to arrest trials in response to external pressures. If he does not agree, as the case of Bailey shows, those generating the pressures may decide to use formal sanctions to ensure his compliance.

The actual moratorium may be formally or informally declared. For example, when Dr. Pierre Grondin of the Montreal Heart Institute decided to halt cardiac transplants in Winter 1969, his decision was formally made public through press announcements issued by the Institute. A moratorium may be formally proclaimed not only through the mass media, but also in a professional publication or in a presentation at a medical meeting. Cutler's halt occurred in a more informal way. Although he published a final report on his valvular surgery attempts, he "signed off" in this article without explicitly declaring that he was doing so. The more usual informal manner of declaring a moratorium is through face-to-face exchanges with colleagues.

To summarize, the pressures toward calling a moratorium can logically and empirically take the following three forms: internal, external-formal, and external-informal. The actual declaration of a moratorium, in turn, can be made through formal or informal channels.[74] Our view of the process through which a moratorium comes to be called can be schematized as follows.

INITIATION OF A CLINICAL MORATORIUM

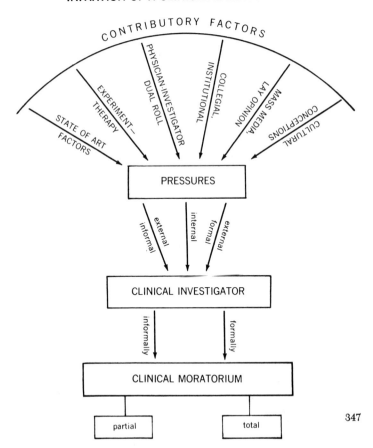

Clinical moratoria only take place when the pressures on the research physician to desist from certain trials on patients are stronger than those counterpressures generated by what would ordinarily be his scientific and therapeutic obligations to continue. Here, we return to an essential attribute of the clinical moratorium referred to earlier in this paper. The physician who commits himself to the career of clinical investigator incurs the obligation to conduct research with patients. His goal is to advance medical science and practice in ways that he hopes will benefit his subjects and other patients with similar or related medical problems. Within the limits of what the ethics of human experimentation permit him to do, the research physician has an obligation to contribute to an ongoing investigative process. In and through these research activities, he is bound to bring the latest developments in knowledge and technique to bear upon diseases that cannot otherwise be adequately prevented or treated. If for some reason an investigator wishes to interrupt or roll back this process, as is the case when a physician would call a clinical moratorium on his own or colleagues' work, there is a sense in which the burden of proof falls on him.[75] In some form, he must explain to colleagues and patients why he feels this step ought to be taken. For, when he invokes a moratorium, he challenges institutionalized values that work to keep the process of clinical research ongoing: "We have made a beginning; now it is time to proceed. . . . Why do we continue? Because if we don't, these people will die, and if we do, some will improve." A call for a clinical moratorium, then, entails the seeking of legitimation from significant others temporarily to bring a halt to an otherwise obligatory research activity, on the grounds that this suspension will ultimately serve the values of clinical investigation better than continuing the trials in question.

APPENDIX

As pointed out at the beginning of this paper, our analysis of the clinical moratorium grew out of our study of cardiac transplantation. We feel that we have established the moratorium as a normal, recurring phenomenon in clinical investigation, and have identified the key factors contributing to its occurrence, and its essential attributes. Methodologically, working with both an historical medical development (mitral valve surgery) and a contemporary one (heart transplantation) has taught us what kinds of data are needed to ascertain whether or not a moratorium has occurred. For example, the following graph, in and of itself, does not tell us whether cardiac transplantation through September, 1969, has undergone suspensions or slowdowns that meet the criteria of moratoria. The facts that no transplants were done in March, 1968, or that there was a dramatic drop in the number carried out from November to December, 1968, might both constitute moratoria. But it might also be true that during these months there were no facilities or personnel free to care for new heart recipients or that the surgeons who have performed the majority of transplants were meeting other professional responsibilities, such as attending medical congresses.

Ideally, one needs personal interviews with the relevant clinical investigators and their close colleagues, study of what they and other physicians are writing and saying about cardiac transplantation in both professional and lay contexts, and a survey of mass media coverage of transplantations during this period. The absence of such systematic data accounts for the fact that physicians as well as laymen are not sure whether moratoria on cardiac transplantation have taken place.

NUMBER OF HUMAN HEART TRANSPLANTS PER MONTH

January 23, 1964 to September 30, 1969

Data supplied by the National Heart Institute. The total of 151 transplants reported through September 30, 1969 included two patients who received a second transplant, and the use of 2 calf, 1 sheep, 1 chimpanzee, and 1 artificial heart.

number of patients

30

25

20

15

10

5

1

REFERENCES

1. Our study, being done under the auspices of the Harvard University Program on Technology and Society, will be published as a book in 1971. For some of the study's major themes, see R. C. Fox, "A Sociological Perspective on Organ Transplantation and Hemodialysis," New York Academy of Sciences Conference on New Dimensions in Legal and Ethical Concepts for Human Research, May, 1969. To be published in the *Annals* of the New York Academy of Sciences.

2. Data supplied by the National Heart Institute. It is interesting that the "box score" reporting on cardiac transplantation has virtually ignored the chimpanzee-to-human heart transplantation performed by Dr. James Hardy at the University of Mississippi Medical Center on January 23, 1964. The recipient, a sixty-eight-year-old male, died some two hours after surgery, because the implanted heart was too small to pump an adequate supply of blood.

3. We would have predicted that the death of Dr. Philip Blaiberg on August 17, 1969, the first patient to survive a heart transplantation for almost two years, would cause an increase in calls for a moratorium on this procedure. However, our survey of major professional and lay press publications indicates that this did not occur. Although Blaiberg's death was prominently and extensively covered by the press, for example, most statements about its implications for cardiac transplantation went no further than to advocate "moving ahead . . . with a renewed sense of caution." The only article we found that asked for an *in memoriam* stoppage of heart transplants appeared in the London *Times*, and was written by its medical correspondent (August 18, 1969):
   What is certain . . . is that Dr. Blaiberg must not be allowed to have died in vain. The heart surgeons of the world must show their respect for this gallant soul by vowing to carry out no more heart transplantations until the full lessons of those already done have been absorbed.

4. In addition to covering professional publications, we have been following national and local American press coverage of organ transplantations via articles provided by a national press clipping service.

5. It is interesting that the word moratorium, which originally had a very specific legally defined debtor-credit referent, is now applied to a number of different kinds of situations, in which the delay or stoppage involved is normatively, rather than juridically, invoked and authorized. In clinical investigation, a research physician or group calling for a moratorium implicitly or explicitly appeals to colleagues for the right, at least temporarily, to withdraw from participation in the ongoing stream of medical research. The moral commitment involved is that of contributing to the

351

general process of clinical research, rather than to a particular procedure, such as cardiac transplantation. We will discuss this point at greater length in the final section of the paper.

6. Three other instances of clinical moratoria, which we would like to study in more detail, have occurred in the development of brain surgery and of kidney and liver transplantation. In the latter case, for example, we find that when human whole liver transplantation was first attempted in 1963, four out of five patients survived surgery, but died of various complications within six to twenty-three days. In the face of these results there occurred what Dr. Francis Moore has termed a "spontaneous moratorium" in liver transplantation until Spring, 1967. A few isolated operations were attempted, but "most authorities were in agreement by this time that major improvements [in immunosuppression, organ preservation, and tissue typing] would be necessary before further clinical trials were justified." (F. D. Moore, quoted in the *Boston Globe,* February 8, 1969, p. 1; *Status of Transplantation, 1968.* A Report by the Surgery Training Committee of the National Institute of General Medical Sciences, National Institutes of Health, p. 36.)

7. L. Brunton, "Preliminary Note on the Possibility of Treating Mitral Stenosis by Surgical Methods," *Lancet,* (February 8, 1902), p. 352.

8. Oxygenated blood flows from the left auricle into the left ventricle through the mitral valve. Mitral stenosis is a narrowing of the valve, caused by an inflammation following a severe attack of rheumatic fever. As the valve progressively constricts, a reservoir of blood builds up in the auricle, putting an extra strain on the heart and causing an increasing back pressure which may eventually clog the lungs and leak through the lung tissue to cause dangerous, perhaps fatal congestion.

9. For detailed histories of cardiac surgery see L. A. Hochberg, *Thoracic Surgery Before the Twentieth Century* (New York, 1960), and R. A. Meade, *A History of Thoracic Surgery* (Springfield, Ill., 1961).

10. Dr. Dwight E. Harken, personal communication.

11. Quoted in T. Simon, *The Heart Explorers* (New York, 1966), p. 3.

12. S. Paget, *The Surgery of the Chest* (Bristol, 1896), p. 121.

13. "Surgical Operation for Mitral Stenosis," *Lancet* (February 15, 1902), pp. 461–62.

14. Letter to the editor, *Lancet* (March 1, 1902), p. 619. See also *Lancet* (February 22, 1902) for letters by Brunton, Lane, Fisher, and Samways.

15. Meade, *Thoracic Surgery,* p. 433.

16. For a review of clinical and laboratory work up to 1923, see E. C. Cutler, S. A. Levine, and C. S. Beck, "The Surgical Treatment of Mitral Stenosis: Experimental and Clinical Studies," *Archives of Surgery,* Vol. 9 (1924), pp. 690–821.

17. E. C. Cutler and S. A. Levine, "Cardiotomy and Valvulotomy for Mitral Stenosis. Experimental Observations and Clinical Notes Concerning an Operated Case with Recovery," *Boston Medical and Surgical Journal*, Vol. 138 (1923), pp. 1023–27.

18. *Ibid.*, p. 1025.

19. *Ibid.*, p. 1027.

20. "Operative Treatment of Mitral Stenosis," *British Medical Journal* (September 22, 1923), pp. 530–31. The article notes that "Sir Lauder Brunton's suggestion appears to have inspired too much apprehension to be followed except by Doyen, whose patient did not survive the operation."

21. For example, see J. S. Goodall and L. Rogers, "Some Surgical Problems of Cardiology. Technic of Mitralotomy," *American Journal of Surgery*, Vol. 38 (1924), pp. 108–12. Commenting on Cutler's operation, and describing the technique for mitral surgery that they have designed (but not tried clinically), Goodall and Rogers stated: "It was about [1913] that one of the writers [at Middlesex Hospital, England] was working at the possibility of introducing surgery for relief of mitral obstruction."

22. Cutler, *Archives of Surgery*, Vol. 9, p. 691.

23. J. MacKenzie, *Diseases of the Heart*, 3rd ed. (London, 1918). It is interesting to note that one of Brunton's critics in 1902 had suggested that the prognosis in mitral stenosis probably depends as much on the condition of the myocardium as on the degree of stenosis.

24. Cutler, *Archives of Surgery*, Vol. 9, pp. 696, 698.

25. *Ibid.*, p. 812.

26. D. Harken, Personal communication.

27. The various kinds of surgical techniques used to open a stenotic heart valve have included: (1) a simple incision of a valve cusp, also called valve section or valvulotomy, (2) excision of the valvular ring, or valvulectomy, (3) finger dilatation, (4) commissurotomy: Dr. Charles Bailey's term for a combination of finger dilatation and use of a knife to partially excise the valve, and (5) valvuloplasty: the term used by Dr. Dwight Harken to indicate his goal of restoration of valvular function. Harken first used a partial valvulectomy technique, and then employed a method of finger dilatation he called "finger-fracture valvuloplasty." As one reads the literature on mitral valve surgery, one has the impression that innovators in the field have been anxious to gain credit for coining a new term as well as perfecting a new technique.

28. H. S. Souttar, "The Surgical Treatment of Mitral Stenosis," *British Medical Journal* (October 3, 1925), pp. 603–06.

29. For example, four letters, generally favorable in tone toward the Souttar operation, appeared in the *British Medical Journal* (October 17, 1925),

p. 722; (October 31, 1925), p. 818. Although there is no indication that they tried finger dilatation, Cutler and Beck felt that "The method may be worthy of trial." E. Cutler and C. Beck, "The Present Status of the Surgical Procedures in Chronic Valvular Disease of the Heart," *Archives of Surgery*, Vol. 18 (1929), p. 415.

30. Meade, *Thoracic Surgery*, p. 447.

31. Cutler and Beck, *Archives of Surgery*, Vol. 18, p. 416.

32. The basic study of priority disputes in science is by Robert K. Merton, "Priorities in Scientific Discovery: A Chapter in the Sociology of Science," *American Sociological Review*, Vol. 22 (1957), pp. 635–659. As Merton did not deal with clinical medicine, however, his analysis of priority disputes does not cover cases such as credit for performing a certain operation for the first time versus credit for performing that operation successfully for the first time.

33. Meade, *Thoracic Surgery*, p. 440.

34. F. D. Moore, "Report of the Surgeon-in-Chief," Peter Bent Brigham Hospital, Boston, *Thirty-seventh Annual Report*, for the year 1950, p. 55.

35. The nonpursuit of ideas proposed or techniques tried is a common occurrence in the history of science, medicine, and technology. We have several examples of these kinds of discontinuity in the development of cardiac surgery which provide insight into some of the bases of this phenomenon. These include: the unresponsiveness of Streider's colleagues to his technique for ligation of a patent ductus; Gross's unawareness of Streider's previous attempt at ligation; the deterring effect of collegial criticism on Brunton's proposal to move from the animal to the human level in surgery for mitral stenosis.

36. For a fuller discussion and references to these developments see Meade, *Thoracic Surgery*, chapters XVII, XIX.

37. D. Harken, personal communication. The account of Harken's work is also drawn from: D. Harken, "Foreign Bodies in, and in Relation to, the Thoracic Blood Vessels and Heart, I. Techniques for Approaching and Removing Foreign Bodies from the Chambers of the Heart," *Surgery, Gynecology and Obstetrics*, Vol. 83 (1946), pp. 117–25; D. Harken and P. M. Zoll, "Foreign Bodies . . . III. Indications for the Removal of Intracardiac Foreign Bodies and the Behavior of the Heart During Manipulation," *American Heart Journal*, Vol. 32 (1946), pp. 1–19; D. Harken, L. Ellis, *et al.*, "The Surgical Treatment of Mitral Stenosis, I. Valvuloplasty," *New England Journal of Medicine*, Vol. 239 (November 25, 1948), pp. 801–09; D. Harken, L. Ellis, and L. Norman, "The Surgical Treatment of Mitral Stenosis, II. Progress in Developing a Controlled Valvuloplastic Technique," *Journal of Thoracic Surgery*, Vol. 19 (1950), pp. 1–15; D. Harken, L. Dexter, *et. al.*, "The Surgical Treatment of Mitral Stenosis, III. Finger-fracture Valvuloplasty," *Annals of Surgery*, Vol. 134 (1951), pp. 722–42; D. Harken, L. Ellis, *et al.*, "The Responsibility of

the Physician in the Selection of Patients with Mitral Stenosis for Surgical Treatment," *Circulation*, Vol. 5 (1952), pp. 349–62; Moore, *Annual Report*, 1950, pp. 54–61; Meade, *Thoracic Surgery*, chapter XXVII.

38. Moore, *Annual Report*, 1950, p. 56.

39. Harken, *American Heart Journal*, Vol. 32.

40. The account of Bailey's work is drawn from: C. Bailey, "The Surgical Treatment of Mitral Stenosis (Mitral Commissurotomy)," *Diseases of the Chest*, Vol. 15 (1949), pp. 377–93; C. Bailey, R. Glover, and T. O'Neill, "The Surgery of Mitral Stenosis," *Journal of Thoracic Surgery*, Vol. 19 (1950), pp. 16–45; T. Simon, *The Heart Explorers;* Meade, *Thoracic Surgery*, chapter XXVII; L. Engel, "Heart Surgery: A New Attack on our Number 1 Killer," *Harper's Magazine*, 1957; "Surgery's New Frontier," *Time*, March 25, 1957, pp. 66–77.

41. Bailey, *Diseases of the Chest*, Vol. 15, p. 85.

42. Meade, *Thoracic Surgery*, pp. 440–41.

43. Bailey, *Diseases of the Chest*, Vol. 15, p. 390.

44. Moore, *Annual Report, 1950*, pp. 356–57.

45. Harken, *New England Journal of Medicine*, Vol. 239, p. 802. Harken next evolved a fourfold classification: benign, handicapped, hazardous, terminal.

46. Harken, personal communication.

47. From a speech by Harken at the Peter Bent Brigham Hospital, quoted in R. C. Fox, *Experiment Perilous* (Glencoe, Ill., 1959), p. 24.

48. Moore, *Annual Reports, 1950*, p. 58. Harken's first finger-fracture valvuloplasty was covered widely and, historically, somewhat innaccurately, by the lay press. Accompanied by a photo of the patient as she prepared to leave the hospital, stories on March 2, 1950 had headlines such as "First Restoration of Heart Valve by Surgery Reported," and "Radical Operation Inside the Heart Hailed as a 'Startling Success.'"

49. Harken, quoted in Fox, *Experiment Perilous*, p. 58.

50. Meade, *Thoracic Surgery*, p. 448.

51. H. G. Smithy, J. Boone, and J. Stallworth, "Surgical Treatment of Constrictive Valvular Disease of the Heart," *Surgery, Gynecology and Obstetrics*, Vol. 90 (1950), pp. 175–92.

52. Meade, *Thoracic Surgery*, pp. 445–46.

53. Material in this and the following section is partly drawn from R. Fox, *Annals* of the New York Academy of Sciences (in press), and *Experiment Perilous*, chapters 2 and 3.

54. The difficulties of either-or decisions emerge clearly if one tries to categorize a procedure such as kidney transplantation. Although twenty-five years have passed since the first human trial, the operation is neither manifestly experimental, nor conventional therapy, and those involved in the field have trouble articulating its status.

55. A statement attributed to the pioneer neurosurgeon, Victor Horsley, epitomizes this element of benefit to other patients. When his colleague Dr. Charles Beevor, said, "But Victor, if you operate on this man for a brain tumor, he will surely die." Horsley responded "Of course he will die, but if I don't operate on him, those who follow me won't know how to perform these operations." E. Thomson, *Harvey Cushing. Surgeon, Author, Artist* (New York, 1950), p. 134.

56. R. Fox, *Annals* of the New York Academy of Sciences (in press).

57. J. Fletcher, "Our Shameful Waste of Human Tissue," in *The Religious Situation: 1969* (Boston, 1969), pp. 223–52.

58. Moore, *Annual Report, 1950,* p. 58.

59. Moore, personal communication.

60. *Ibid.*

61. Moore, *Annual Report, 1950,* p. 59.

62. *Ibid.,* p. 58.

63. For further discussion of the properties of the relationship between research physicians and their patient-subjects, see: R. C. Fox, *Experiment Perilous,* especially pp. 85–109, and "Some Social and Cultural Factors in American Society Conducive to Medical Research on Human Subjects," *Clinical Pharmacology and Therapeutics,* Vol. 1 (1960), pp. 423–43; and the papers by M. Mead and T. Parsons in this volume.

64. Meade, *Thoracic Surgery,* p. 447. The history of mitral valve surgery suggests that it might be fruitful to explore more generally the relative impact that different kinds of medical specialists have on the occurrence or nonoccurrence of a moratorium. For example, MacKenzie, the cardiologist, blocked Souttar, the surgeon; and conversely, it was two cardiologists, Levine and Ellis, who encouraged Cutler and Harken to perform mitral valve surgery. Historically, surgeons and physicians have more frequently than not represented different, sometimes complementary and more often conflicting, points of view. We hypothesize that the encouragement that Cutler and Harken received from Levine and Ellis was all the more forceful and effective precisely because it came from colleagues belonging to a medical specialty from which they, as surgeons, would not ordinarily have expected such firm support.

65. The best recent statement by a sociologist of the concept of social circles and appropriate methods for studying their influence is: C. Kadushin, "Power, Influence, and Social Circles. A New Methodology for Studying

Opinion Makers," *American Sociological Review,* Vol. 33 (1968), pp. 685–99.

66. The influence of social circles in the development of cardiac transplantation seems to have been much greater than in mitral valve surgery. As Diana Crane has documented, ten out of twenty-three surgeons in the United States and Canada (no information on five other surgeons) who had performed heart transplants by May, 1969, had been associated as teacher or student with two universities, Johns Hopkins or Minnesota (D. Crane and D. Matthews, "Heart Transplant Operations: Diffusion of a Medical Innovation," presented at the 64th Annual Meeting of the American Sociological Association, San Francisco, Cal., September 4, 1969).

67. By 1957, Bailey's own professional status and that of cardiac surgery had changed radically, as witnessed by the following passage from a story in *Harper's Magazine:* "In 1957 the Prince of the operating room, the man the big league hospital can't afford to be without, is the heart surgeon. . . . In the Philadelphia area, there are several hospitals where Bailey is now a power and, within limits, can do very nearly anything he wants." L. Engel, *Harper's* (1957), pp. 38, 41.

68. Fox, *Annals* of the New York Academy of Sciences (in press).

69. I. Page, "The Ethics of Heart Transplantation," *Journal of the American Medical Association,* Vol. 207 (1969), pp. 109–13. We realize that this increase in coverage is partly a consequence of the general growth of the mass media in the past two decades, and of their increasing reportage of developments in the life sciences.

70. *Ibid.*

71. *Ibid.*

72. See, for example, "A Definition of Irreversible Coma. Report of the *Ad Hoc* Committee of the Harvard Medical School to Examine the Definition of Brain Death," *Journal of the American Medical Association,* Vol. 205 (1968), pp. 337–340.

73. Cooley's statement, delivered during an interview at the annual meeting of the American College of Cardiology in New York City, was carried in newspapers across the country on February 28, 1969.

74. Thus, we would redefine the slowdown in liver transplantation termed by Moore a "spontaneous moratorium" (see note 6 above) as an informally declared moratorium generated by internal pressures.

75. A similar burden of proof falls on the non-physician (for example, clergyman, lawyer, journalist) who advocates the calling of a clinical moratorium.

FRANCIS D. MOORE

Therapeutic Innovation: Ethical Boundaries in the Initial Clinical Trials of New Drugs and Surgical Procedures

THIS VOLUME of essays and the conferences from which it sprang seem to have been initiated by widespread concern over the precise details and clinical practices of human experimentation in biomedical research. By "human experimentation" was meant either the intentional employment of normal human subjects as volunteers for physiologic experiments, or the study of patients (in a way that would not directly benefit them) to gather information on a disease or its treatment. While both of these ethical problems are worthy of consideration, they do not appear to me to present any severe ongoing ethical or technical difficulty in American medicine today. There are far more severe ethical problems in the Armed Forces, where chemical and biological warfare systems are studied on normal human volunteers who suffer the coercion intrinsic in military activity, or in the Space Program with its high lethality-potential in failed missions.

Nonetheless, public discussion of the purely medical problems, such as they are, has led to efforts at regulation and standardization; public attention to the climate of clinical investigation has helped to rectify ethical irregularities.

A far more important biomedical-ethical problem arises daily in thousands of hospitals concerning the initial use of drugs, treatments, or operations and the initial employment of untrained personnel in the care of patients. Here, the subject-patient stands to benefit from the "experiment" if it is properly done; the line between experiment and therapy is never clearly drawn. Every new operation, for example, is an experiment; indeed every operation of any type contains certain aspects of experimental work. Likewise the employment of a familiar drug on a new patient for the first time constitutes an experiment in the precise determination of the proper dose, and there is an inevitable period of uncertainty about unusual reactions that the patient may exhibit.

Medical education in America aims to inspire in every physician a sense of inquiry, an intuition for biological variables, and an innate desire to evaluate evidence realistically. Each doctor should employ some of the essential features of the scientific and experimental method in the daily treatment of every patient. Without such an approach, the patient would suffer through the application of blind dogma and arbitrary rule-of-thumb; without the experimental method, medicine would become traditional, since it could not move ahead on the basis of established observations and experience.

Despite these clear advantages of the scientific and experimental approach, severe and pressing problems remain when new treatments are applied to man and when new personnel carry out standard operations for the first time. This latter problem—that of educating and gradually transferring responsibility to young men without, at the same time, jeopardizing the patient's safety—is the central focus of clinical education. It is most especially pressing and obvious in surgery. The young surgeon passes from the status of a "greenhorn" intern at the age of twenty-six to a phase of technical perfection at about the age of thirty-two, when, frequently, his sheer operative skill is unequaled by an older generation. But he has yet to acquire judgment, wisdom, forbearance, and human insight—qualities that require the passage of time in any physician's education. Nevertheless, during those seven or eight years the young man has operated on many patients, and in many instances has carried out an operation for the first time on some patient. The clear recognition of the joint responsibility of the professor and the intern in such a setting is one of the most fascinating ethical problems in all of American education, but this is not our concern here.

Instead, we are concerned with a few of the ethical questions of therapeutic innovation raised by the application of new treatment to sick people. These are initial trials, carried out in human patients, of drugs or operations that may benefit the subject. This is the largest single category of medical experimentation—if that is a suitable term for therapeutic innovation—currently practiced at the clinical level.

The problems posed in such innovations are legion, and public reactions to their accomplishment range from malpractice suits to

359

the Nobel Prize. Our problem here is to distinguish the various degrees of acceptability within this spectrum. Why do some of these activities most ennoble the biomedical sciences, while others elicit more adverse comment among scientists than any other category of clinical experiment?

A Historic Example of Mass Human Experimentation

A familiar though remarkable historic example of therapeutic innovation which took place in Brookline, Massachusetts, about 250 years ago raises questions as appropriate for review in 1969 as they originally were in 1721.

An epidemic of smallpox had carried away many of the colonists in Boston and eastern New England in 1702. Accounts vary as to what brought word of smallpox inoculation to the keen ear of the Reverend Cotton Mather. But to this enterprising clergyman belongs the full credit for stimulating physicians to activity. Whether he saw accounts of the Turkish experiments or learned from talks with his own Negro slave that the practice of inoculation had been tried among primitive African populations (the latter being the more dramatic version which he himself preferred), the fact remains that he stimulated others to action with such promptness that the inoculation in Britain carried out by Lady Montagu took place only a few weeks prior to his, and the much larger New England experience became the prototype for widespread application both in this country and abroad.

The practice of inoculation against smallpox in the early-eighteenth century consisted in the intentional infection of a normal person with virulent unattenuated smallpox virus obtained from a patient who himself might later die of the disease. This inoculation was done with the hope that the recipient would be afflicted with a mild case of smallpox—a "distinct case" as it was then called—and that the resultant "non-susceptibility" would last the rest of his life. By contrast, the practice of vaccination introduced seventy-five years later by Jenner in England and, following his lead, by Waterhouse in the United States consisted in inoculating the recipient with the virus of the cowpox. This mild and rarely lethal disease confers immunity to smallpox by virtue of an antigen shared by the two viruses.

Cotton Mather could find none of his Boston medical cronies interested in such a heterodox undertaking. So he turned to the nearby town of Brookline where he discussed the matter with Zabdiel Boylston, then thirty-seven years of age. Boylston was the son of a doctor who had studied at Oxford, yet he himself had no medical degree. He was still a young man who had not emerged as a medical figure in a society that was already teeming with strong medical characters. Among these were the men who, a few years later, were to found the Harvard Medical School and the Massachusetts Medical Society. This large conservative wing of practitioners would have no part of the Reverend Mather's suggestion. But Zabdiel Boylston saw it for what it was—a chance to reduce the mortality from smallpox epidemics.

Accordingly, Zabdiel fetched some pus from a pock and proceeded to inoculate his thirteen-year-old son by rubbing this material on a scarification on the boy's arm. This epic experiment occurred on June 26 or 27, 1721. It is generally conceded that Boylston did not select himself for this experiment because he had already suffered the disease and was immune. In any event, the deed was successfully accomplished—at least the son did not die of the disease—and Boylston inoculated 247 persons in the next few months. Of these, six died. There was a clamorous and riotous opposition to the procedure both among fellow practitioners and among the laity who were aroused by their friends the doctors. Not long thereafter, out of a group of 5,759 cases of the naturally occurring disease, 844 died, according to Boylston's own account. Other figures from contemporary literature state that Boylston inoculated 242 persons of whom six died, and that there were 5,889 cases in the epidemic of whom 844 died. Whichever figures are correct, it was evident that the mortality was lower in the inoculated form of the disease, and that those who had been successfully inoculated rarely, if ever, contracted the naturally occurring epidemic form of smallpox.

After a time of persecution, Boylston won out. He was acclaimed and honored here and in England. The practice spread to the other colonies. Benjamin Franklin, who had been a severe critic, later became a strong proponent. It is alleged that this stimulated an interest in medical science which resulted in his founding of the School of Medicine at Philadelphia in 1765. Although never really systematized, inoculation against smallpox was carried out for the next eighty years in the colonies, often in hospitals built expressly for that purpose—such as that built at Salem for Dr. Holyoke in 1773. This practice of inoculation unquestionably led to the understanding and rapid widespread acceptance of vaccination, once it became available following Jenner's lead in 1796.

This was a lethal experiment. It carried a mortality of over 2 per cent. It was undertaken to protect the individual, and through him the larger group, from the ravages of an epidemic disease. It was undertaken by people who had little idea of the nature either of the disease or the infectious agent, although Mather wrote of the "animalculi" that were involved. The basis for any confidence that this experiment would be successful was in large part hearsay from the Middle and Far East. There was no animal trial or laboratory work. A cloud of fantasy and petty controversy surrounded the actual details of inoculation techniques. Little effort was made to isolate those who had been inoculated with the disease, and they could become carriers of a virulent virus. Curiously enough, opponents of the procedure based their claims on the assertion that inoculation would not protect against the epidemic disease; they were not so interested in its public hazards or mortality, although this hazard to society was quite evident at the time. (Princess Caroline, for example, following the lead of Lady Montagu, inoculated convicted criminals and pauper children before she did her own family. She evidently hesitated to inflict an experiment that she considered hazardous on people whom she considered to be of great importance.) Finally, and most remarkably, the entire mass experiment carried out in Boston and Brookline was proposed and urged by a man of the church and was opposed almost to a man by the medical profession.

Could this experiment be conducted today? Certainly not. The mortality was prohibitive. There was no scientific basis or preliminary laboratory work. It is quite evident that both Cotton Mather and Zabdiel Boylston perceived a potential social benefit that was greater in their minds than the immediate sacrifice of six lives. From this experiment was born the initial awareness of active immunization as a means of protecting society against the scourge of epidemic disease. The first mass trials of the Salk polio vaccine and all the other inoculations from Pasteur to Enders went through moments when they shared precisely the same ethical problems faced by Mather and Boylston.

Although Dr. Boylston (and the many others who have worked with preventive inoculations) were dealing with the prevention of disease rather than with its treatment, the subjects of the experiment stood to benefit. For this reason, the ethical problem raised here falls into that general family of ethical issues involved in therapeutic innovation.

Other Examples of Initial Therapeutic Trial

The first use of ether anesthesia, the first injection of insulin, the first use of liver extract, and the first application to a patient of any one of a host of new drugs are all part of the same ethical family. At the present time, we are engaged in one of the largest mass human experiments of this type ever considered: the widespread use of oral contraceptives. It has been estimated that more than twenty-five million women have taken these tablets and that at any one time fifteen million women are taking them. Their effects after prolonged administration are entirely unknown. There is virtually no animal work reporting the continuous administration of these drugs for more than three years, and their impact—either on the psyche, ovaries, endometrium, or breast—on women after twenty years of continuous administration remains entirely unknown. Although their administration seems to be a matter of great social and human urgency, urged by many national and international groups, the ethical problem is real and the unknowns are serious. Oral contraception has certain features that set it apart from ordinary therapeutic innovation because it is a medicinal treatment given to a healthy person to prevent a normal occurrence, rather than an inoculation given to prevent fatal epidemic disease or a drug (or operation) employed to treat human illness. Oral contraception must, therefore, be even more free of taint than innovations involved with the treatment of disease.

New surgical operations pose problems similar to those raised by other therapeutic innovations. At the present time, they are assuming a new order of magnitude in ethical implication. There was a time when new surgical operations depended for their success only on the drainage of pus, the removal of some gangrenous or diseased part known to be dispensable, or the rearrangement of musculo-skeletal anatomy. So long as the surgeon could rely on the unfailing tendency of wounds to heal, of blood to clot, and of bacteria to be overcome by immune defenses, his success was virtually assured. Fortunately, the natural process of evolution had already provided these solutions. The body perceives no essential difference between injury incurred accidentally in the traumatic life of a higher vertebrate and an injury inflicted by the surgeon.

363

Wound-healing, blood-clotting, and immunology are the first line of defense that enables the survival of the fittest; these Darwinian mechanisms are used every day by the surgeon—or, strictly speaking, by his patient.

This simple state of affairs no longer obtains in surgical innovation. For the last twenty-five years and with increasing frequency, new operations are being employed that depend for their success on complicated physiologic or pharmacologic interactions. At the simplest, these may involve such a thing as the removal of an entire lung—a procedure that depends for its success on the fact that, in man, cardiac output and normal respiration can both be accomplished in a single lung. Other recent examples of this type of physiologic readjustment involve operations on the autonomic nervous system, interference with tracts in the brain, or the rearrangement of the anatomy of the bowel or of the heart. In all of these, the surgeon must depend upon a physiologic readjustment to assure recovery. These physiologic adaptations are complex, often specific to man, and the initial period of human trial of such new operations is much more difficult and demanding. Furthermore, unlike the basic recovery-drive after simple surgical injury, these complex physiologic adjustments are often paradoxical or unpredictable. Although the surgeon may be removing cancer, curing pain, or helping high blood pressure, he is silently depending upon an adaptation that was unheard of in the evolutionary process. Vagotomy does not occur in nature.

In the past ten years, surgery has invaded an entirely different area of fundamental biology—one in which it must rely for success not on an evolutionary response or a physiologic adjustment, but on the outright abolition of a normal response established in the species during epochs of evolution. A specific example of this is to be found in transplantation, where success depends upon the abolition of normal immunologic defenses. In fact, in transplantation we have for the first time a surgical procedure that was "tried out" on patients (after a long laboratory trial) and depends for its success on a state of immunologic nonreactivity produced by drug treatment which, if applied generally, would result in illness and death. The transplant procedure involves the simultaneous application of dangerous drugs and a new operation; the success of both depends upon the interaction of each.

To complicate the ethics of transplantation further, there is always another individual involved. Either he is quite healthy and undergoes a major surgical injury to help another, or he is so recently deceased that bystanders sometimes wonder if he indeed is dead since so many organs and tissues of his body are still obviously alive.

As the constellation of biological variables around new surgical operations becomes more complicated, as in transplantation, so also does the ethical problem become more pressing. Many of us concerned in the development of tissue transplantation have felt that the questions which it has raised have been responsible in great measure for the renewed interest in the ethical standards of biological research.

The Need for Guidelines

These problems are urgent and press for solution; if a teaching hospital or a university medical school is doing its job and carrying out its responsibility to the public, it must be involved with initial trials and therapeutic innovations that raise ethical problems.

Is it possible to design a set of principles that protect the patient under conditions of therapeutic innovation and yet maintain some atmosphere of permissiveness? We must always insist that these guidelines protect society by enabling a continuous advance of biomedical science in the clinical areas. By establishing arbitrary ethical standards, one might be surprised to find that while he is protecting the individual patient, he is exposing society to the hazard of a static rather than a dynamic medicine. The power to restrict becomes the power to stifle the enthusiasm that has brought forth the advance of modern medicine and public health.

Can Consent Be Informed?

In this context, the principle of informed consent has two special limitations. The first unique feature of informed consent in therapeutic innovation is that the patient actively seeks the untried therapy with an earnest plea to become the willing subject. To those who have never dealt with such desperate patients, it may come as a surprise to witness the enthusiasm with which the patient with late cancer or the family of children with severe heart disease approach an entirely new and untried procedure. This willingness is especially notable if the family knows or suspects, with or without suggestions by the doctor, that the new procedure is the only source of hope for survival. The cancer patient himself

365

seeks out the new drug or the new treatment; people of education and considerable scientific sophistication become blinded and will transgress the boundaries of the simplest common sense not only in accepting new drugs, but in seeking quackery in the hope of a cure. The posture of "informed consent" in therapeutic innovation is, therefore, not a matter of trying safely and sanely to explain to a volunteer what is going to be done, but rather the much more difficult task of explaining alternatives to a worried patient who wishes, above all else, to have the experiment carried out on him.

The second aspect of "informed consent" that is so limiting in its application to therapeutic innovation (as indeed it is also in experimental investigation of any sort) is the obvious fact that there is no means of becoming informed other than by the experiment itself, even if there is a desire to give consent. The very fact that the procedure has not previously been carried out in man indicates that the scientist himself lacks the critical information required for informed consent. If the doctor knew the most likely outcome of the procedure, such information could only have come from previous experience, and in that event the patient would hardly be at risk.

An intrinsic feature of consent lies in the presentation of sound alternatives to the patient. If I were to identify any one feature of the doctor-patient relationship that is most frequently colored by unconscious subjective factors on the part of the doctor, it is this question of clinical alternatives. One or two examples will illustrate. A colostomy or ileostomy is a form of diversion of the gastrointestinal tract made so that the fecal contents are emptied onto the abdominal skin. Here the discharge is received in some sort of a bag or receptacle that the patient empties from time to time. While unpleasant and unhygienic, most intelligent persons accept this as the price that they pay for the treatment of severe disease—usually malignancy. The more intelligent the patient and the more fastidious his care of his own physical person, the less difficulty he has with colostomy or ileostomy, since he takes special time each day to care for himself in a way that is acceptable to his own high standards. On many occasions I have borne witness to conversations between physicians and patients in which the picture painted of this colostomy or ileostomy was entirely the product of a physician's imagination, based on the fear that he himself might one day have to have such a procedure. A patient suffering from ulcerative colitis or cancer of the rectum who is given an offensive or frightening verbal description of colostomy or ileostomy would be so biased in his approach to the operation that he may actually refuse a procedure that offers him the greatest likelihood of survival. By contrast, the over-enthusiastic description of the state of well-being which may result from the surgical treatment of ruptured intervertebral disc, bursitis of the elbow, or hypertrophy of the prostate (considering only three of many examples) will sometimes result in a patient entering into an operation for benign disease, not life-threatening, with an optimism born of the surgeon's tone of voice rather than a realistic estimate of his own response to the projected treatment.

When we move from these rather familiar examples in the explanation of alternatives to such desperate measures as kidney or liver transplantation for fatal disease, it is evident that the hopes of the surgeon, the fears of the patient, and the inborn optimism of youthful science combine to push the patient onward. Ethics in clinical care bring a sense of balance between these two extremes.

Preliminary Laboratory Trial

There is no way of trying out a surgical operation in small doses, and, as with oral contraception, there is no quick way to reproduce in the laboratory the passage of years. In addition, many surgical operations remove structures or rearrange anatomy in an irreversible or irreparable manner; there is no turning back. Even in the case of therapeutic innovation with drugs, hormones, or vaccines, the human experiment always carries a few surprises when contrasted with preliminary laboratory work.

Despite these limitations, preliminary laboratory trial occupies a position of unique importance. In the opinion of most scientists, physicians, and surgeons, laboratory study puts the stamp of human and ethical acceptability on therapeutic innovation more than does any other characteristic. Preliminary laboratory trial is the only way to provide information, however incomplete or inadequate, that might lead to an acceptable informed consent. Preliminary trial in animals is not always easy and is frequently expensive. For example, it is almost impossible to produce in a dog the type of chronic renal failure that has been the setting for most kidney transplantations carried out in man. It is entirely impossible to reproduce in the dog either the type of chronic valvular disease of the heart that has been the basis for open-heart surgery, or congenital heart disease that will provide an important indication for transplantation. Despite these limitations, preliminary laboratory work must be carried out with the greatest care and in an effort to reproduce as many features of the situation as possible. New drugs or operations should be employed in the dog or in some other large animal, as well as in the small laboratory rodent. The larger mammals are truer models for human application, and they permit repeated clinical observation and blood chemical sampling, together with physiologic monitoring, in a way that is not possible in the rat, mouse, or hamster.

But before leaving this matter, we should mention the present crisis in laboratory finance in the biomedical sphere. While the 1968 cutback is considered by the Congress in terms of budget savings, and by the scientific public as one of the highly undesirable consequences of our military involvement in Southeast Asia, the sudden withdrawal of large amounts of federal support for biomedical research is going to have an inevitable ethical consequence: The necessary preliminary laboratory work is going to be severely curtailed in the instance of many forthcoming therapeutic innovations.

During the past ten years, the expense of conducting laboratory experimental work has doubled as a result of inflationary spirals in all the goods and services concerned. Prior to 1967, the National Institutes of Health budget increases had barely kept pace with laboratory inflation, but these had been sufficiently large so that other sources of laboratory support (such as certain philanthropic foundations and industry) had tended to withdraw from the field. With the withdrawal of laboratory financial support due to the congressional policy of pursuing military action in Southeast Asia, we are greeted with an almost unsupportable situation in biological research. An ironic example will illustrate. A certain young man of excellent medical background had just completed two years of service as a military surgeon in Vietnam. Here he had been handsomely supported in one of the largest and most wasteful of military encounters, and had worked himself without stint and without surcease to assist in the care of the wounded. Returning to civilian life, he was to become a Research Fellow in our laboratories to study the transplantation of the liver (liver transplant being a potential help to babies born with bile duct anomalies, to individuals with liver tumors, and to soldiers with severe bullet wounds of the liver). On returning to civilian life, he was told by the government that although his name had been accorded one of the highest places in the priority list for Senior Research Fellowships, funds were not available to support him. In the Sunday Supplements that week, there was an account of new research being done to make a lunar module perform in a high vacuum simulating the surface of the moon, a research expending more money each month than has ever been spent on any aspect of tissue transplantation. It is clear, then, that ethical considerations in preliminary laboratory trial go to the roots of our society and to the question of what we regard as suitable priorities for human effort at this time.

The Ethical Nature of Clinical Science: An Historic Example of Its Violation

The subtitle to this section might easily have been "The Ethical Nature of Clinical Investigation," and as such it would have been a perfectly proper heading. The term "clinical investigation" has unfortunately become almost a term of opprobrium, and many people regard the term as meaning exclusively research that is carried out on normal subjects or on patients who do not stand to benefit thereby. Actually, the terms "clinical research" and "clinical investigation" are synonymous and apply to any sort of research or investigation that is carried on in relation to patients. The term "clinical" is an ancient word which means "reclining in bed"; as an adjective applied to investigation, it merely refers to the human patient. Modern medical care cannot be pursued without an element of clinical research or clinical investigation. Careful study of the patient, careful recording of the results, and careful consideration of variables with statistical accuracy are essential to any sort of clinical research or investigation, just as they are essential to the ethical climate in the initial trial of new drugs or operations. In this way, the normal hospital environment of a high-grade university hospital becomes a cloak of protection that surrounds the patient. The history and physical examination, the complete workup, the inquiring though sometimes bothersome medical students, the interns and residents, the full view of the event by the rest of the staff—all protect the patient from premature, willful, ill-advised, or secret therapeutic innovations. The ethical content of science itself lies in careful observations, honest reporting, and an unbiased review of the results.

This essentially ethical nature of the scientific process provides

369

protection when the scientific process is applied to the medical act. By the same token, when a new operation is attended by the most perfect pre- and post-operative management, skillful anesthesia, and expert surgical technique, these hospital surroundings enable the surgeon to carry out a new procedure with a minimum of hazard to the patient. Such safeguards cannot rescue a poorly conceived operation from failure, but they can surround a well-conceived procedure with the greatest likelihood of success and the least chance of accidental ill effects. The same is true in the therapeutic innovation of drugs, hormones, vaccines, and antibiotics.

The borderline between acceptable clinical science and unacceptable human experimentation is most frequently violated through breach of scientific method. Outright quackery posing as therapeutic innovation includes such nostrums as goat-gland grafts for virility, or electronic devices that tune sinusitis to the wave-length of the planets. Such absurd examples, though surprisingly common, do not illuminate our problem because they are patently ridiculous, and those persons who seek such release from the realities of illness, infections, and aging might almost be considered as fair game.

Much closer to home are those recent examples of breach of scientific method that have brought down the reputations of outstanding scientists and have led to the fraudulent marketing of cancer cures with the apparent support of renowned institutions. In such examples, some sort of psychiatric insight is required to understand the scientist as he slowly swings from the dignity of recorded public knowledge to a frantic search for notoriety as the great discoverer of a cancer cure. A recent example of this process involves a substance called "Krebiozen," a name coming from the Greek and meaning "that which regulates growth." The Krebiozen episode illustrates how a highly sophisticated scientist, in mid-twentieth century, can go astray despite the protective surroundings of modern science and a self-conscious approach to ethics. (In my account, I am drawing heavily on the Boylston Society Essay of Dr. William D. Morain, entitled "Krebiozen: Nineteen Years of Controversy," which gathers together many loose ends of this still controversial case.)

The story began in 1947 when Dr. Andrew C. Ivy of Chicago published an article in *Science* entitled "The Biology of Cancer." In this piece he advanced the concept that a unified method would be found to deal with all cancer. In 1949, two brothers named Durovic came to Chicago, bringing with them a drug called

"Kositerin," allegedly extracted from cattle and alleged to cure 98 per cent of the people with high blood pressure. The Durovics refused to disclose the nature of this drug. They were referred to Dr. Ivy, who was at that time at the peak of his authority and brilliance, the author of many scientific publications, a representative of American medicine at the Nuremberg trials, and Executive Director of the National Advisory Council of the United States Public Health Service. Evidently the Durovics then told Dr. Ivy of another substance called Krebiozen which was extracted in milligram quantities from blood pooled from hundreds of horses. Again, the Durovics refused to state what the material was or how it was actually produced. It is probably only a coincidence that Dr. Ivy had advanced in his article in *Science* the thought that the normal body contains tiny traces of an anti-cancer substance.

Dr. Ivy administered the drug to a dog, then to himself (as per the *Nuremberg Code*), and within three weeks to a patient. Even at this time, one can perceive the seeds of disaster. Dr. Ivy claimed that Durovic was a widely known former Professor of Medicine at the University of Belgrade who had gone to Argentina after being expatriated during the war and had published extensively in the scientific literature. No such publication could be found. An investigation of his activities in Buenos Aires revealed that most of them centered around a private office where he injected hypertensive patients with Kositerin at the price of 5,000 pesos per treatment. Fifteen bulls, but no horses, were found to have been bought by his sponsoring company. It is stated that South American officials of the company involved with Kositerin were quite astonished when public press reports began to arrive of Durovic's success with a second drug unknown to them and made from horses.

Dr. Ivy then held a press conference to which he invited many persons, including prominent politicians and philanthropists. He issued an attractive booklet on Krebiozen with an optimistic report on a very small group of cancer patients, of whom ten had already died. A press release appeared shortly thereafter, and there was an immense public pressure to obtain Krebiozen, which was made available at a price.

Many friends and associates tried to dissuade Dr. Ivy from involvement in the study of a material the nature of which was held secret; but nothing could move his resolve. Seven months after the press conference, the *Journal of the American Medical Association* published a "Status Report on Krebiozen" which stated that the commission appointed to study it ordinarily "would not attempt to evaluate the clinical benefits, if any, of a substance whose character and method of manufacture were not known." It was stated that 98 of the 100 patients reviewed had not shown any improvement and 44 of them had expired.

Battle had thus been joined between an eminent scientist and an established organization of the medical profession, one regarded by many as reactionary to all advance or change. Dr. George D. Stoddard, then President of the University of Illinois, was given the role of referee. He appointed a committee of eminent clinicians and scientists. Within a year, a report was published indicating that the material had no curative value in the treatment of cancer, and again indicating total dissatisfaction with research on a material of unknown origin or composition. The door was left slightly open in that the committee could not state categorically that the material was entirely free of biological effect.

There is not space here to detail the rest of this unhappy story save to point out the subterfuge of the Durovics in stating, as increasing pressure arose to identify the material, that all the existing Krebiozen powder had been dissolved in the 200,000 ampules of mineral oil. A chemist had evidently been unable to find anything in the mineral oil. Countercharges of conspiracy were leveled against Dr. Ivy and the Durovics; a legislative committee was appointed; certain officials of the University ultimately sided with the harassed Durovics and Ivy; and Dr. Stoddard was forced to resign. Dr. Stoddard's book, due to be published in Boston in the middle-1950's, was banned by injunction prior to publication; when it was finally published, it was met by a libel suit by Dr. Ivy. As recently as 1963, Krebiozen was still being distributed for "clinical testing." The Food and Drug Administration entered the controversy in 1963, the Thalidomide scandal having forced it to take a much closer look at all new drugs. Discussion in the United States Senate and a picket line in front of the White House both became features of the controversy.

Finally on August 14, 1963, the riddle of almost fifteen years' duration as to the exact chemical nature of the substance was solved. A chemistry student at the University of Pennsylvania had found an infrared tracing in an atlas of 20,000 tracings of known chemical compounds which exactly corresponded to a substance found in tiny quantities in Krebiozen. This powder was creatine monohydrate. It was administered to the cancer patients in tiny quantities, a miniscule fraction of the amount of this normal chemical constituent that the human body normally metabolizes each day. To make it soluble in mineral oil, it had been heated with other compounds, yet even this was difficult; evidently the ampules dispensed after 1963 contained absolutely nothing other than mineral oil.

The trial that followed is of historical importance in indicating the way in which popular lines are drawn between anything that smacks of the Scientific Establishment, on the one hand, and intuitive public sympathy with the Underdog Innovator, on the other. The defendants were not found guilty of fraud or conspiracy. Dr. Durovic left the country, and the conflict still rages.

"The main question left standing in the Krebiozen controversy," wrote Elinor Langer in an article in *Science* in 1966, "is how so many people could spend so much time on a problem so limited and come up with so little."

The breach in scientific method was clear in one important regard—that the actual nature of the material was unknown, not disclosed, and kept secret. But more important than this was the consistent breach in the search for scientific evidence; the evidence had to be sought in the clinical results of the administration of the drug to cancer patients. Here was the flaw. Clinical investigation (as opposed to laboratory work) had not been a part of Dr. Ivy's long and brilliant career. Dr. Ivy became entrapped by the difficulties of clinical investigation in cancer patients, well-known to all clinical scientists, but new to him as a laboratory man.

The cancer patient has a tremendous investment in anything done to help him; he wants to see helpful results to give him new hope and relieve his pain. The most junior surgical intern daily sees cancer patients arousing from operations with hope and confidence, even though nothing whatsoever could be done; it takes many days or weeks for this reality to become evident. To gather scientific evidence under such circumstances requires special techniques and special disciplines. Although clinical research is seemingly simple when compared with some of the more rigorous or expensive laboratory techniques, clinical research places the investigator in a position of self-discipline that is almost unknown to the laboratory investigator who is surrounded by the conventional safeguards of the laboratory and shielded from the uncertainty of frail human patients who wish to bear witness to a favorable result.

373

To the outside world, and particularly to that segment of our society that is anti-rational, anti-intellectual, and anti-scientific, the conventional trappings of science appear to be but an expression of the establishment. Individuals—often unknown to science—who are fighting against the establishment become heroes to those same persons who would restrict the activity of the universities, do away with professors and a free press. The public espousal of the cause of the lonely warrior fighting the great and powerful medical establishment provides strong popular support for the claim of either the quack or the misled scientist that he has "never received a fair trial." In the case of Krebiozen, this claim would have aroused greater sympathy had the protagonist sought the active collaboration of other scientists who might have borne witness to the chemical nature of the secret drug and the validity of the clinical trials.

Checks and Balances: The Collaborative Enterprise

A new policy was recently formulated by the National Institutes of Health requiring a review of projected new drugs or procedures in man by a local panel of peers. To our view, this formality confers little security on the patient and is far less important than the active collaboration of scientists from a variety of disciplines and backgrounds. Such workers provide a balance for one another's ideas; they act as a damper on ill-advised enthusiasm; and they become a check on personal ambition.

There can be little question that personal ambition, usually for career advancement or public acclaim, underlies much intense motivation in research work and in the trial of new ideas, drugs, operations, or treatment. Such personal ambition is usually well hidden under the sophisticated affect of the dedicated clinical scientist and, far from being remiss, is the sign of a healthy society. While social convention requires its disguise in the masquerade of scientific intercourse, this ambition is not a thing to be ashamed of. Personal ambition for advance and recognition is a far better motive for the work of difficult or protracted clinical investigation than is the seeking of political advancement or financial reward. No matter how deep the urge for pure knowledge, few scientists have not derived some excitement from a general acceptance of their ideas or procedures, particularly if these were of potential social benefit. The possibility of such acceptance provides a more stimulating environment for scientific work than the even temper of an apathetic society where, because of the heavy system of penalties placed upon failure, there is neither a channel for innovation nor an interest in departure from tradition.

But ambition, no matter how praiseworthy, can certainly lead individuals astray. A common example is found in the premature publication of scientific results. Personal ambition for recognition has clearly outstripped the cooler judgment of awaiting more definitive data. The active collaboration of scientists provides the best way of harnessing these fine qualities of excitement and ambition so as to maintain their force for forward motion and yet prevent them from running wild. For this reason, a collaborative group with open discussion, avoidance of secrecy, and frequent review of plans and policies seems far more important than the short-term arbitrary review of some one drug or operation by a formal panel with a strictly *ad hoc* mission. Such formal panels are usually composed of individuals who know little of the work contemplated, and they may even come to include individuals who for reasons of jealousy or ignorance would rather not see the old order challenged anyway. The ethical acceptability of therapeutic innovation documented in a research application, for example, is far better attested by the nature of the scientific consultants working on the project than it is by the nature of the hospital panel that is to review each case.

Ethical Climate of the Institution

Nearly all these remarks can be included under the general heading of "the intellectual and ethical climate of the institution." Such a climate is difficult to regulate or standardize, difficult at times even to recognize or describe. Yet it is more important than any other single consideration in protecting the willing patient from unwise, inexpert, or ill-advised therapeutic innovation. As one reads Zabdiel Boylston's own account of his inoculation experiments, one is impressed by his misgivings, the care with which he nursed each patient through the illness, the careful records he kept, and his plea to others to avoid secrecy and proceed with these innovations freely and openly. In these qualities, one senses his intellectual and ethical approach, and feels that although none of the other more familiar modern safeguards were present, all was right in Brookline in 1721.

In terms of the modern hospital, this ethical climate must be appreciated by direct personal participation. It has been said that no one knows whether a football game is rough unless he plays in it; the sideline spectator cannot really tell whether the kick in the ribs is necessary, accidental, or intentional. The same applies to a hospital. One cannot really see the inner workings of men's minds by reading the article or even visiting for a day. One must join the hospital staff for weeks or months as observer, visitor, research fellow, physician, or surgeon before he can decide that the ethical climate is suitable for the site of therapeutic innovation.

Only by visiting a hospital does one gain an impression as to whether or not the choice of subjects for therapeutic innovation indicates a fundamental unease on the part of the investigators. We have already alluded to the practice of selecting poor people, criminals, native populations, under-educated or backward people, or even the feeble-minded for certain types of hazardous innovation. When one discovers that doctors are selecting patients in this way, then one has identified a major flaw in the ethical climate and a severe chink in the scientific armor. It means that those carrying out the therapeutic innovation are ill at ease with it, would not wish to have it carried out on their own person or families, and are looking for some "easy game" to get over the first few barrier cases. If, by contrast, the therapeutic innovation has been researched and studied with such care that it is regarded by those carrying it out as a blessing to a properly selected patient, one then finds that these initial patients represent a true cross section of the hospital population rather than a hand-picked selection of underdogs. In this area, the Golden Rule finds its expression. The mere statement that somebody would like to have it "done on himself if needed" is meager comfort. What is significant is the demonstration that those selected for therapeutic innovation represent the full spectrum of the hospital population and not just a group for whom recourse would be scanty. When a new vaccine is first given trial in a primitive African tribe, one needs to go no further; the investigator feels insecure and unsafe with the material and wants to get his quick answer from a group in whom consent is impossible, information is totally lacking, and the backlash is insignificant.

Protection of Science and the Scientist

Finally, restrictions and guidelines can become so rigid that society risks a static science in which the scientist (biologist, clinician, physician, surgeon) is constantly bombarded by criticisms, suits, and penalties.

This problem, more than any other feature of our topic, is a matter of public relations, the public image, and the willingness of those in the scientific establishment to stand up and be counted on the side of intelligent therapeutic innovation carried out in an ethically acceptable setting. A large segment of the public, possibly lacking educational opportunity, may always be biased by bitter experiences with biomedical science, and perhaps biased without such experiences. These people will cry "guinea pig" when they hear of anything new being tried by doctors. It is but a step from this anti-rationalism to congressional unease with "what's going on in our hospitals and laboratories," restrictive legislation, inspection of laboratories and hospitals, the establishment of external review boards, and finally stifling of effort.

To offset this danger, we need repeated public statement of the meaning of and the need for therapeutic innovation, the teaching of scientific history in a realistic way to emphasize the hazards and sacrifices as well as the rewards involved, defense in congressional hearings of the "open scientific society," and publications to define those elements that can make therapeutic innovation an ennobling and absolutely essential feature of modern scientific and medical growth, one more essential to our society than the man on the moon and far less expensive.

REFERENCES

O. T. Beall and R. H. Shryock, *Cotton Mather: First Significant Figure in American Medicine* (Baltimore, 1954).

Zabdiel Boylston, *An Historical Account of the Small-Pox Inoculated in New England* (Boston, 1730).

W. L. Burrage, *A History of the Massachusetts Medical Society with Brief Biographies of the Founders and Chief Officers, 1781-1922* (Privately printed; Boston, 1923).

T. H. Harrington, *The Harvard Medical School, 1782-1905*, Vol. 1 (New York, 1905).

A. C. Ivy, "Biology of Cancer," *Science*, Vol. 106 (1947), pp. 445ff.

E. Langer, "The Krebiozen Case: What Happened in Chicago," *Science*, Vol. 151 (1966), pp. 1061ff.

Memoirs of E. A. Holyoke, M.B., LL.D. (Prepared in compliance with the vote of the Essex South District Medical Society; Boston, 1829).

F. D. Moore, "Symposium on the Study of Drugs in Man. Part II. Biologic and Medical Studies in Human Volunteer Subjects; Ethics and Safeguards," *Clinical Pharmacology and Therapeutics,* Vol. 1 (1960), pp. 149ff.

F. D. Moore, *Give and Take. The Biology of Transplantation* (Philadelphia, 1963).

F. D. Moore, "Ethics in New Medicine. Tissue Transplants," *The Nation,* Vol. 200 (1965), pp. 358ff.

W. D. Morain, "Krebiozen: Nineteen Years of Controversy." Unpublished essay, Boylston Medical Society, Harvard Medical School (March 18, 1968).

J. G. Mumford, *A Narrative of Medicine in America* (Philadelphia, 1903).

"Status Report on Krebiozen: Committee on Research," *Journal of the American Medical Association,* Vol. 147 (1951), pp. 864ff.

G. D. Stoddard, *"Krebiozen": The Great Cancer Mystery* (Boston, 1955).

DONALD FLEMING

Comment on "Therapeutic Innovation: Ethical
Boundaries in the Initial Clinical Trials of
New Drugs and Surgical Procedures"

DR. MOORE's account of the famous inoculation controversy in
Boston in 1721 is misleading in various respects. The sources of
Cotton Mather's original knowledge of the procedure are not seriously in question. He did hear reports of inoculation for smallpox
in Africa from his Negro servant Onesimus; and he did read a
letter in the *Philosophical Transactions* of the Royal Society of
London from Dr. Emanuel Timonius, a graduate of Oxford and a
medical graduate of Padua, who described and commended inoculation out of his own experience as a practitioner in Constantinople
and his observation of other practitioners. To describe Timonius's
role in alerting Mather to the value of inoculation as dependent
"in large part" upon "hearsay from the Middle and Far East" is
grossly unfair to both men. Timonius was not dealing in hearsay,
but recounting his own observations—so for that matter was Onesimus—and Cotton Mather for his part was responding to the nearest
equivalent of "clinical evidence" in his time.

Dr. Moore, who seems in general to be identifying with Cotton
Mather or at any rate with Zabdiel Boylston, is here conceding
too much to their contemporary critics. The most vigorous of these,
William Douglass, was the only M.D. (from Edinburgh) among
the physicians of Boston. Moreover, Douglass had a voracious
appetite for natural history and aspired as passionately as Cotton
Mather himself to make a lasting contribution to empirical science.
Once the importance of Douglass's role in the whole controversy
is grasped, one is forced to pose more incisively the question as to
why Mather's and Boylston's activities aroused such vehement
opposition at the time, and opposition led by one of the best-
informed men of a scientific bent in Boston.

One answer leaps to the eye—jealousy; Douglass's jealousy
of Mather, compounded with the other physicians' jealousy of

379

Boylston. Yet this was a motive, not an argument, and the medical opponents of inoculation could not have struck an echo from the community at large unless they had had reasons that would bear public inspection.

Dr. Moore observes that "opponents of the procedure based their claims on the assertion that inoculation would not protect against the epidemic disease." Doubts on this score were certainly expressed on both sides of the Atlantic, but after all that was what the trials in Boston were about, and some skepticism was in order. This skepticism was inflamed by dogmatic assertions by Mather and Boylston, after the first ten (successful) inoculations, that the procedure properly administered could *never* fail. Happily, this did not induce them to conceal the deaths of inoculated persons; for they were prepared to attribute all such fatalities to smallpox contracted in the ordinary way before the inoculation. This argument had the merit of keeping their statistics honest. Yet one can imagine the baffled indignation of Douglass and other skeptics on being confronted with an unprovable, but unanswerable, excuse for every apparent failure of inoculation. Douglass had never heard of a "self-sealing argument," but he instinctively knew one when he saw it.

Apart from this, Douglass fully appreciated and dwelt upon a major objection to inoculation that Dr. Moore implies was unimportant in contemporary debates. Douglass held that Mather and Boylston were making a reckless trial, not only upon the inoculated but upon the uninoculated as well. Boylston with Mather's complacent approval let his patients have friends in for a social glass in the sickroom, and got them back into circulation as soon as possible. For Douglass and many others, this amounted to willful scattering of contagion among those who declined to be inoculated at Mather's bidding. Douglass's point was irrefutable. The trial of inoculation could have been made with more care to prevent the inoculated from infecting other people; and Mather and Boylston would not have sacrificed any conceivable scientific gain by delimiting the experiment to this end.

Dr. Moore's account of Mather's and Boylston's experiment omits any reference to the overriding theological issues that pervaded the entire debate. William Douglass and others regarded inoculation as irreligious in forestalling God's providence. Nobody questioned the propriety of using "means" to cope with sickness once it took hold. God sent the "means" as well as the scourge.

Comment on "Therapeutic Innovation"

The novelty that many professed to detect in inoculation was to bring sickness upon one's self in anticipation of God's providence or, worse still, to avert it definitively. Thus, one of the principal channels by which God communicated His anger might be stopped up and His people in Boston might neglect to make the saving motions toward reform by which, alone, His wrath could be diminished. If undiminished by contrition in the face of an epidemic, it would have to find some other and conceivably more appalling vent.

The parallel is evident between the scientific and the theological objections to inoculation. Douglass and others were concerned about the spread of infection from the inoculated to the uninoculated. By an identical process of involving others involuntarily in the consequences of their own decisions, the inoculated by eluding God's visitation of smallpox might bring something worse upon the whole community. The irony was that Cotton Mather and many other Congregational clergymen in Boston rejected this argument out of hand. It was not the last time that progressive clergymen were ahead of their congregations.

The inoculation controversy in Boston did not turn primarily upon the specific details or scientific validity of the trials, but upon a much larger issue that was troubling the entire Western world in the eighteenth century: How far could men disown their old legacy of fear and trembling before God without bringing retribution upon themselves? The identical scruples were canvassed in the wake of the earthquakes in Boston and Lisbon and of the introduction of lightning rods. These free-floating anxieties about men's relation to God were periodically focused by a particular controversy, but we miss the whole point if we confine ourselves to the specifics of that occasion.

The inoculation debates of 1721 are now a remote chapter in medical history. It would not be worth criticizing Dr. Moore's account of these if his discussion of current developments in medicine did not betray the same limitations. Speaking from his own wealth of experience in this generation, he makes valuable discriminations among the ethical issues posed by contemporary surgery, as in differentiating traditional forms of surgical intervention from the newer operations requiring unprecedented physiological adjustments. Organ transplants are an even more obvious example of drastically new procedures in surgery. To grasp the appropriate ethical distinctions for coping with such innovations is clearly of the first importance. But as a strictly *historical* judgment, is it correct to imply, as Dr. Moore does, that the ethical ferment in contemporary medicine is solely a function of these new developments in therapy and surgery?

The alternative is to look for essentially extraneous factors at work in the world at large and impinging upon medicine—the equivalent of the theological issues that got mixed up with the fate of inoculation. For better or worse, one such factor is increasingly evident. Many intellectuals, and some non-intellectuals as well, have the sense of being confronted with the phenomenon of runaway science—science out of control, a body of technical possibilities racing uncontrollably ahead of any ethical restraints upon their application. In this general context, there has been an almost convulsive embrace of the only overtly ethical tradition associated with any branch of experimental science—the Hippocratic restraints upon the practice of medicine. After Hiroshima, Aldous Huxley proposed an appropriately modified Hippocratic oath for physicists. Even Albert Einstein ruefully mocked at this as quixotic, but one can judge from Huxley's proposal the magnitude of the investment by people concerned about runaway science in protecting the ethical tradition of medicine itself from erosion. If the wraps were taken off scientific medicine, the last restraint upon science for its own sake would be gone. This is the extra ingredient in every agonized scrutiny of a medical innovation, and it has very little to do with the details of the procedure in question.

DAVID D. RUTSTEIN

The Ethical Design of Human Experiments

THIS ANALYSIS of the ethical considerations governing human experiments is based on the assumption that it is ethical under carefully controlled conditions to study on human beings mechanisms of health and disease and to test new drugs, biological products, procedures, methods, and instruments that give promise of improving the health of human beings, of preventing or treating their diseases, or postponing their untimely deaths. Without such an assumption, there can be no systematic method of medical advance. Progress would have to depend on the surreptitious, illegal, or unsupervised research and testing of new modes of prevention and treatment of disease. The ethical standards of such irregular activities would certainly be at a far lower level than can be guaranteed when the testing of new methods of treatment is openly practiced.

Proceeding on that assumption, how can one design experiments upon human beings that will yield the desired scientific information and yet avoid or keep ethical contraindications to a minimum? This question is asked in the belief that in the design of the experiment itself many ethical dilemmas may be resolved. Attention must be given to the ways an experiment can be designed to maintain its scientific validity, meet ethical requirements, and yet yield the necessary new knowledge.

Let us concentrate on laying out new guidelines that might lead to the solution of ethical problems rather than on focusing our attention on the difficulties that these problems present. The ethical requirements that have created the most difficulty are obtaining informed consent from the potential subject; the need for the subject to derive a health benefit from the experiment; and keeping the risk to the subject as small as possible. Such questions are important and relevant because ethical considerations are paramount when experiments are to be performed on human subjects. It is the thesis

383

of this essay that in the design of a human experiment it is mandatory to select those experimental conditions, subjects, and methods of measurement that impose the fewest ethical constraints. Such an approach will not cause the ethical problems of human experiments to disappear. If a definitive attempt is made, during the planning stages of an experiment on human beings, to keep the ethical as well as scientific criteria in mind, it is possible often to perform the necessary research to yield the desired information.

Scientifically Unsound Studies Are Unethical

It may be accepted as a maxim that a poorly or improperly designed study involving human subjects—one that could not possibly yield scientific facts (that is, reproducible observations) relevant to the question under study—is by definition unethical. Moreover, when a study is in itself scientifically invalid, all other ethical considerations become irrelevant. There is no point in obtaining "informed consent" to perform a useless study. A worthless study cannot possibly benefit anyone, least of all the experimental subject himself. Any risk to the patient, however small, cannot be justified. In essence, the scientific validity of a study on human beings is in itself an ethical principle.

How, then, can the experimental human subject be protected from incompetent investigators so that he will not become a victim in feckless studies? There are two lines of defense. The research committee of a medical school, institution, or hospital must be concerned with the ethical principles as well as the scientific validity of the proposals placed before them. To perform this task effectively, every committee must have among its membership a biostatistician to insure scientific validity and an expert (for whom there is as yet no name) who is concerned with the ethical aspects of human experimentation. The biostatistician can assist the committee in evaluating the scientific quality of the proposed investigation and make recommendations for improvement of the scientific aspects of the study design. Experiments on human beings must not be performed without a carefully drawn protocol, which in turn can best be prepared in consultation with experts in study design. In the same way, experts in the ethical aspects of human experimentation should assist the committee in passing on the ethical issues of proposed studies and in recommending modifications that might make the studies ethically acceptable.

The Ethical Design of Human Experiments

The second line of defense can be provided by editors and editorial boards of journals that publish scientific reports of human experiments. If higher scientific standards of publication were established and adhered to, it would soon become clear to investigators that there would be small likelihood that improperly designed studies would be published. Automatically, many human subjects would be protected against participation in unsound and unethical medical research. When there has been a clear-cut violation of ethical principles, scientific reports of human studies should be refused publication. The reason for such refusal should be clearly stated.

For appropriate evaluation of manuscripts, therefore, the membership of editorial boards should include biostatisticians and experts in the ethical aspects of human experimentation to provide advice to the board and to the editor in their respective fields.

Anticipating Ethical Problems

Whenever possible, it is necessary to anticipate serious ethical problems in human experimentation in order to explore ways in which they can be avoided or kept to a minimum in the design of the experiment. The experiments in human heart transplantation are a case in point, particularly in the selection of the heart donor.

Death is not a simultaneous, instantaneous event for all of the organs of the body. Some organs die earlier than others—the brain being the most vulnerable. It is evident that the heart must be "alive" and free of disease at the time of transplantation if it is to be useful to the recipient. The selection of the heart donor, therefore, cannot be based on his "total death" in the usual sense—that is, a lack of any spontaneous activity and the complete absence of cerebral, cardiac, and pulmonary activity and of spinal reflex function.

As experience with this operation is accumulating, everyone concerned is becoming increasingly aware that to comply with both the scientific and ethical constraints, donor selection must be the responsibility of a specially constituted committee in hospitals where transplantation is performed and must not have among its members any member of the transplantation team. Within such a protective structure, the eligibility of the donor will in effect depend primarily on his having complete and irreversible cessation of cerebral function while the heart remains as normal as possible.

Indeed, there may be clinical or electrocardiographic evidence at the time of donor selection that the heart continues to beat.

These criteria of eligibility represent a revolution in our cultural concept of death—and it has occurred by default. The dramatic nature of the heart transplant operation has obscured the underlying change in our ethical concept of deciding when an individual is dead—that is, when a physician may act as if there is no longer any need for treating the patient "to save his life." Until recently, if the heart were still beating, treatment would continue. It is remarkable that this major ethical change has occurred right before our eyes, and that this change is more and more widely accepted with little public discussion of its significance.

This new definition of heart donor eligibility that substitutes "irreversible brain damage" for "total death" raises more questions than it answers. Does acceptance of this concept mean that it is no longer necessary to treat, for example, the senile patient who would meet such criteria? How do eligible donors differ in principle from totally feeble-minded individuals? What are the implications for the inheritance of property if the heart of an intestate donor is kept beating with a pacemaker while the search for a recipient goes on and the donor's wife dies during the interval? Does this new definition of death for the heart donor open up new channels of criminal activity that will lead to the burking of patients to increase the supply of eligible donors?

Let us examine the nature of this revolutionary change in our ethics and pursue its implications to their logical conclusion. Substituting "irreversible brain damage" for "complete absence of any living manifestations in any organ" as essential in the diagnosis of "death" forces us to examine the meaning of the phrase "irreversible brain damage." The presently recommended definition of "irreversible brain damage" demands a complete absence of all manifestations of brain function, all the way from the higher levels of cortical activity down through the centers governing the emotions, sensations, automatic functions, and muscular control and including the spinal reflexes with, however, two special exceptions— the centers controlling respiration and circulation. These centers are excluded for practical and not for ethical reasons. In severely ill patients, the function of these centers can be taken over by machines that may not be stopped until the diagnosis of death is made on other counts. Moreover, for successful heart transplantation, the heart must be "alive" if it is to benefit the recipient.

Why do we insist on the absence of all activity of all of the other subcortical centers if we are willing in our diagnosis of irreversible brain damage to disregard these two centers of essentially automatic function? Again the reason is a practical one. We do not yet know how to make a firm diagnosis of irreversible brain damage limited to the higher cortical centers. We therefore turn in our ignorance to the requirement that all nervous activity be absent (with the exceptions noted) as the basis for the new diagnosis of "death." Again we are confronted with a practical and not a conceptual or ethical reason.

It is clear that in accepting the new definition of "irreversible brain damage" as equivalent to death in man, we are really concerned only with irreversible damage of higher cortical centers. We are saying that in man "life" exists only when he is aware of and can respond to his environment or, if he cannot, that he may recover to a point where he will react consciously within his environment. It remains then for intensive research to be conducted so that physicians will be able to identify specifically the irreversible loss of activity of higher cortical centers and distinguish it from lower reflex function. If, as a result, a reliable diagnosis of irreversible damage of higher cortical centers could be made and this concept generally accepted, the new diagnosis of death would be concerned only with the permanent loss of those functions that distinguish man from other animals. Eventually, many of the great problems imposed on society with its growing senile population might be overcome. In the meantime, however, it should be clear to all of us that such a concept has already been accepted in principle by those who would replace "irreversible brain damage" for "total absence of the functions of all organs" as satisfactory for the diagnosis of death in man.

It would have been better if some of these questions had been explored before the first heart transplantation was performed. Heart donor eligibility is becoming so complex that in the present stage of diagnosis the ethical problem of donor eligibility might best be avoided by the development of a suitable mechanical heart.

Asking the Right Question

The design of an experiment depends at first on the question asked by the investigator. Some questions are in themselves unethical. One cannot ask whether plague bacilli are more virulent in human beings when injected into the bloodstream than when they are sprayed into the throat. One may obtain hints as to the answer to such a question by epidemiologic comparison of the spread of pneumonic plague (spread from the lungs into the air) and bubonic plague (spread by insect bite). Anecdotal information on the spread of plague can also be obtained through the study of laboratory accidents. But a deliberate experiment to answer this question cannot be performed.

The human experiments performed by the Nazis during World War II horrified the world because they were designed to answer unethical questions. "How long can a human being survive in ice cold water?" will, it is to be hoped, never again be a question to be answered by a scientific experiment. Thus, as a first step in the design of any human experiment, we must first be sure that the question itself is an ethical one.

Moreover, an unethical experiment can sometimes be converted into an ethical one by rephrasing the question. In drug testing, for example, it is not ethical to design an experiment to answer the question: "Is treatment of the disease with the new drug more effective than no treatment at all?" In answering such a question, the patients in the control group would literally have to receive "no treatment" and that is completely unacceptable. Instead, if the patients in the control group are given the best possible current treatment of the disease, we may now ask an ethical question: "Is treatment with the new drug more effective than the generally accepted treatment for this particular disease?"

We faced this problem in the design of the United States-United Kingdom Cooperative Rheumatic Fever Study, which was concerned with measuring the relative effectiveness of cortisone and ACTH in the treatment of that disease.[1] We could not give rheumatic fever patients in the control group "no treatment." We would have had to go so far as to prohibit bed rest, which in itself may be helpful to rheumatic fever patients, because patients in bed have a slower heart rate. Instead, we asked the question: "Is treatment with ACTH or cortisone better, worse, or the same as the best generally accepted drug treatment for this disease?"

Our control group, in addition to all the other non-specific treatments which the treated groups also received, were given large doses of aspirin—the generally accepted drug treatment of the time. A question that compares the new treatment with the most effective treatment of the time is not only ethical, but it is also the most practical question. If the new treatment is to replace the generally accepted treatment, it must be demonstrated clearly to be better.

With a question framed in that way, one may obtain consent from the patient by explaining that he will receive either the best treatment of the time or the new drug. It is made clear that, although promising in animal and other experiments, the new drug has not yet been shown in human experiments to be better, worse, or the same as the generally accepted treatment. Most patients will accept these alternatives. The investigator himself would be reassured that he has done the best for his patient's health and safety, while evaluating a more promising remedy for his disease.

When designing a human experiment, the question under study must not be so trivial as not to justify any risk to the human subject. One may not ask whether large doses of a cortico-steroid agent would remove freckles. Nor may there be an excessive risk when compared with the possible benefit of a successful experiment. One may not test in humans a "sure cure" for the common cold which causes paralysis in experimental animals. Thus, in selecting a question for human experimentation, the expectation of benefit to the subject and to mankind must clearly far exceed the risk to the human subject.

Ethical considerations that prohibit certain human experiments are similar in their effects as are scientific constraints on the design of experiments. At the moment, much research on infectious hepatitis, a serious human disease, is impossible because there is no method for isolating infectious hepatitis virus. No laboratory animal has been found which is susceptible to it and no other procedure for its isolation has been developed. This scientific constraint is serious because without isolation of the virus a vaccine cannot be made for the protection of susceptible human beings. Human beings are susceptible and theoretically could be used for the growth of large quantities of virus needed for vaccine manufacture, but now we face the ethical constraint. It is not ethical to use human subjects for the growth of a virus for any purpose. Here, then, we have an example of a scientific constraint that in turn creates an ethical constraint, both of which interfere with the conduct of experiments important to life and health. When asking a question that might be answered by human experimentation, both the scientific and ethical demands must carefully be taken into account. Unless both are satisfied, the experiment cannot be performed.

The Ethics of Controlled Human Experimentation

Controls are essential in such human experiments as the testing of a drug or a surgical procedure. In order to evaluate new therapy, it is necessary to identify those additional benefits of the new remedy which exceed the improvement that might be expected in the course of the natural history of the disease. To be sure, in a disease such as human rabies, which is practically 100 per cent fatal, controlled observations are not needed because any recovery of treated patients is an obvious benefit. Acute leukemia and virulent tumors such as reticulum-cell sarcoma are other examples of diseases whose natural history is one of immutable progression to death and where benefit can be identified without a controlled experiment.

Most diseases do not fall into such a clear-cut category. Even diseases such as cancer of the breast have such a variable course that one is not certain to this moment if surgery prolongs the life of the patient suffering from this disease. The variability of the disease from patient to patient makes it difficult, if not impossible, to evaluate the additional effectiveness of the surgical remedy without a controlled study.

Controlled studies also keep the investigator from leaving the world of reality. The enthusiastic research worker often concentrates on whether the new treatment seems to work. Psychologically, he is apt to pay less attention to possible harmful effects of the new treatment. The result of this attitude is documented repeatedly by the myriad of treatments that make the headlines and promise miraculous cures on the front pages of our best newspapers, only to be completely discarded a few years later. This phenomenon is not without its harmful effects. The definite, albeit limited, benefits of established treatments are often cast aside in favor of the dramatic new, but as yet unproven method of treatment for a human disease. For example, before the advent of the sulfa drugs and antibiotics, there were fairly effective procedures that alleviated and at times cured urinary-tract infection. When these new therapeutic agents became available, some physicians concentrated on intensive therapy with one of the new agents and often felt that it was no longer necessary to practice many of the important details of treatment that had been given in the past. Now, after several decades, there is a gradual return to a more balanced regimen of treatment that places each of the antibiotics in proper perspective in the total treatment of urinary-tract infection. In such situations, a controlled study that is properly performed permits a clean comparison of the helpful and harmful effects of the new treatment and of the older established method of therapy. If, in addition, circumstances permit the ethical use of a placebo control, information can also be obtained about the natural history of the disease.

One might ask whether it is unethical not to perform a controlled human experiment. The Pasteur experiment with rabies vaccine is classic. Controlled human experimentation was completely unknown when Pasteur first tested his new vaccine on those Russian *muzhiks* who were bitten by rabid wolves. All were given the vaccine and all recovered. The result was so dramatic and so electrifying that further experimentation seemed unnecessary. When it was later learned, however, that the chances were relatively low of developing this uniformly fatal disease—human rabies—even after a bite from a known rabid animal, and that the vaccine itself causes paralysis which is not infrequently fatal, it became important to determine whether the vaccine really does more good than harm.

But it became impossible to do a controlled experiment on rabies vaccine. After the general acceptance of the treatment, if a controlled experiment were to be performed, and if a subject in the control group developed rabies, the experimenter might not only be sued for malpractice, but might even be deemed criminally culpable for not having given the patient the "accepted treatment of the time." This same situation is now developing in the estimation of the benefits of heart transplantation and in measuring the value of intensive-care units in the treatment of heart attacks from coronary disease.

In hospitals where heart transplantation is performed, there are many more eligible recipients than donors. It would be relatively easy to randomize the procedure and measure the effectiveness of this new operation. Whenever a heart from a human donor became available, a random selection could be made among all of the eligible recipients. Those not selected would then comprise a control group whose course and outcome could be compared with those of the recipients of a transplanted heart.

The same situation obtains in the treatment of heart attacks from coronary disease in intensive-care units. There is as yet no published control study demonstrating the effectiveness of intensive care in the treatment of acute myocardial infarction. Once again, a control study is possible because in any one center the numbers eligible for care may far exceed the available facilities. A randomly allocated control study would provide the precise information that is needed to estimate the value of this procedure.[2] Instead, we are already beginning to hear ex-cathedra statements of the effectiveness of intensive-care units that are unsupported by the required scientific evidence.

Even up to the present moment, many patients suffer severe discomfort or are permanently harmed from treatments whose validity has been based on uncontrolled observations. Thousands of hypertensive patients in the 1930's and '40's were subjected to extensive surgery for the removal of their thoracolumbar sympathetic nervous system in the belief that the progress of the disease would be arrested. The treatment is no longer used.

Would this problem have been resolved had controlled studies been performed by means of random allocation in which half of the patients would have had sham operations? In an analogous situation when uncontrolled evidence suggested that the internal mammary artery operation might be helpful in the treatment of angina pectoris, Dr. Henry Beecher recommended a study in which the patients in the control groups would be given a sham operation.[3] He indicated that a far smaller total number of human subjects would have been needed and a definitive answer could be obtained by such a procedure. Although scientifically sound, I do not believe that it is ethical to perform sham operations on human subjects because of the operative risk and the lack of potential benefit to the patient. Instead, controlled studies could have been performed with the randomly allocated control patients being given the best medical treatment of the time together with a period of bed rest similar to that of the surgical convalescent.

The history of diseases of unknown etiology is replete with serially accepted and discarded fads of treatment. Peptic ulcer is an example. The Sippy rigid alkali and milk diet became the Meulengracht meat diet and in time became a bland diet with enough alkali to relieve the patient's symptoms. The short-circuiting surgical operation of gastro-enterostomy changed to one for removal of a large portion of the acid-secreting part of the stomach—partial gastrectomy—and then to the less traumatic procedure of removing the nerve supply to the stomach and upper intestine—vagotomy. Along the way, a procedure for freezing the stomach was introduced, then discarded, not because the fad had worn itself out, but because it was obviously harmful. All these treatments might or might not have been accompanied with psychiatric therapy. To this day, the treatment of peptic ulcer, as is the case of many diseases of unknown etiology, is an art with little solid scientific support.

In essence, a new treatment of a disease may be better, worse, or the same as the generally accepted one. The controlled clinical trial has not only been effective in rejecting useless treatments, but perhaps even more helpful in recognizing a harmful therapy, such as the anticoagulant treatment of cerebral thrombosis. That treatment was earning growing acceptance until, in a controlled clinical trial, it was recognized that cerebral hemorrhage was a more frequent complication in the group treated with anticoagulants than among the patients in the control group.[4] The trial was terminated.

One may conclude that if the question under study is an ethical one, and if the design of the study is sound, taking both the scientific and the ethical constraints into consideration, controlled studies when indicated impose fewer ethical problems than uncontrolled human experiments.

"Benefiting" the Subject

Years ago, after I had administered the first dose of streptomycin to a human patient, there was a need to obtain "normal" values for the absorption and excretion of this new antibiotic.[5] Because of the toxicity (subsequently eliminated) of early lots of the antibiotics, it did not seem ethical to test normal subjects who could not conceivably benefit from the procedure.

A satisfactory compromise was reached. Streptomycin in early laboratory experiments gave promise of being effective in the treatment of infections due to gram-negative enteric bacilli—one of which is the typhoid bacillus. A typhoid carrier—that is, an individual who has recovered from typhoid fever, but continues to carry this pathogenic bacillus in his gall bladder, intestine, or genito-urinary tract—is relatively "normal" so far as the aims of our experiment were concerned. Moreover, he could have conceivably benefited from the experiment by elimination of his carrier state.

As a result of strict public health controls, the typhoid carrier is the pariah or leper of modern society. Everyone who knows him avoids him. Invited guests will not enter his home, and he will not be invited elsewhere. Indeed, the entire family suffers. Because of the great desire to be relieved of this burden, many typhoid carriers willingly volunteered, and the experiment on the absorption and excretion of streptomycin was performed on them. Unfortunately, the eradication of their carrier state was temporary, and it returned after drug therapy was stopped. But there was a possible benefit to the subject that could only be ascertained by experiment. The necessary human data on the absorption and excretion of streptomycin were collected.

A Proposed Design for Testing New Drugs

We will explore the hypothesis that a system of drug testing can be developed that will satisfy scientific requirements, meet a higher standard of ethical principles than now obtains, and yet release a new drug for general use more rapidly than is now feasible.

Now that the Federal Food and Drug Administration has imposed and implemented rigorous scientific standards for drug testing, there are frequent complaints that the procedure itself may be unethical in that it is so costly, time-consuming, and demanding of highly qualified investigators that the benefit to the public of the new therapeutic agent is unnecessarily delayed. And, yet, the critics are properly loath to recommend a return to a system that might permit a toxic drug, such as Thalidomide, to be sold in the open market. The horns of the dilemma are clearly visible—potential benefit, on the one hand, and potential harm, on the other.

In outlining a plan to resolve this dilemma, let us first explore the existing process of rigorous testing through which a new drug becomes available for widespread use. From time to time, evidence is presented that a new medicament may be useful in the prevention or treatment of a particular disease. At that point, it is tested in animals for toxicity and for therapeutic efficacy in an appropriate model (for example, an animal disease or a laboratory test for inhibiting the growth of or eradicating a pathogenic micro-organism). If such efforts are successful—that is, if the drug continues to demonstrate therapeutic usefulness without serious toxicity—a decision finally is made to explore the use of the new drug in a few carefully selected patients.

Ideally, this next stage is carried out by a few investigators who have had great experience with the disease under study and who are most likely to detect in relatively few patients variations produced by the drug from fluctuations in the natural history of the illness. Let us assume that this hurdle has been surmounted and that the drug is deemed apparently effective, relatively safe, and ready for a large controlled clinical test. Assume also that an estimate has been made of the number of patients needed for a precise evaluation of the drug were its effectiveness to continue to be the same.

A controlled clinical trial is then instituted. An appropriate question is asked and a protocol of experiment is developed to satisfy scientific and ethical requirements. Patients are randomly admitted to treatment and control groups. Measurements of effectiveness and toxicity are made, recorded, and analyzed sequentially. If the results are satisfactory, a final decision is reached concerning the widespread availability of the new therapeutic agent. The drug may then be released and then monitored for continued effectiveness and for rare manifestations of severe toxicity.

At the present time, this process—performed in accordance with an ethical and scientifically precise plan—postpones the widespread use of an effective drug, involves too many competent investigators for too long a period of time, and through repetition in many countries throughout the world imposes the hazards of testing the same drug on an unnecessarily large number of human subjects. The process raises ethical questions because it is unethical to expose to unnecessary risk more human subjects than are needed to ascertain the scientific fact. Fortunately, when the situation is carefully analyzed, many of these difficulties may be overcome without sacrificing scientific standards or ethical principles.

The time required for testing can be reduced, and there can be an earlier release of the drug, if the trial is performed collaboratively, instead of haphazardly, by a group of investigators in different hospitals using a common protocol of experiment. In a coordinating center, the data are analyzed sequentially to be sure that the dose is maximal, the method of administration effective, and toxicity minimal. When satisfactory results are obtained, the drug could be released immediately for general use.

The collaborative clinical trial avoids one of the great ethical problems of drug testing. In any one hospital, when evidence that a new drug may be effective begins to become manifest, there are increasing pressures on the investigator to release it for general use before a statistically significant sample of patients has been studied. At that point, in a collaborative study, the number of cases in all of the centers in the study is usually large enough to provide a solid estimate of the efficacy of the agent as well as of the nature and the degree of its toxicity.

A collaborative program by itself in any one country will not necessarily reduce the number of human subjects who are exposed to the risk of testing a particular drug. The number of human subjects can be reduced, however, by international agreements among developed countries that adhere to drug testing standards similar to our own.[6] A well-designed international collaborative and cooperative study in which the new drug could be tested on a specified but much smaller number of human subjects could suffice for all. At present, in many advanced countries a valid sample of treated and control patients is collected, and with relatively little exchange of information, the same experiments are repeated in many countries. The present process wastes professional skills and medical resources, unnecessarily exposes too many human subjects to the risk of drug testing, and is thereby unethical.

Experience in the United States-United Kingdom Cooperative Rheumatic Fever Study has demonstrated that international cooperation in drug testing can be successful.[7] From that experience, it is urged that an international agency, such as the World Health Organization, or an international pharmaceutical manufacturers' association explore the possibility of rapid, efficient international drug testing.

There are, of course, political and economic objections, including conflicts in patent policy, protection of trade secrets, and disturbance of international drug marketing agreements. These should be faced squarely to see whether or not a solution can be found so that the benefits of international testing might be reaped. One obvious benefit is much earlier marketability of the drug.

Another benefit for pharmaceutical companies adhering to the agreement is protection against damage suits resulting from relatively uncommon toxicity of the drug. For example, if it is determined by the international agency that to assure effectiveness and lack of serious toxicity a drug should be tested on a specified number of cases and the requirement is met by the manufacturer, it should be *prima facie* evidence that he cannot be responsible for severe drug reactions that occur less frequently than the number of cases treated. Thus, if it is estimated from preliminary testing that five hundred cases should be included in the clinical trial, and this requirement is satisfied and the drug released, a manufacturer could not reasonably be expected to be responsible for a rare, severe reaction that might occur in only one of two thousand patients.

In summary, then, an international drug testing program, including a monitoring system for following the continued effectiveness and the rare manifestations of toxicity of the drug, would decrease the number of human subjects at risk and bring the benefits of the new agent to the world in a shorter period of time.

Modern Design of Human Experiments

The advent of the electronic computer has increased the efficiency of biomedical research and, in turn, has had its ethical implications. In the days of collecting laboratory measurements on the smoked drum, it was easier to collect data than to analyze them. Indeed, final interpretation of experiments was often delayed for months as data were collated and analyzed by hand tabulations, often made by the investigator himself in odd moments between the pressing needs of laboratory duties and teaching. Rarely was the analysis of data given priority over his other activities. At the top of the list was the next experiment, the gross results of which were eagerly anticipated while the detailed analysis was again postponed.

As a result of these traditional limitations on data handling and processing, and with the increasing complexity of our understanding of biological systems, there has been a growing tendency to design experiments in simplified systems where at any one time a few variables can be measured with great precision. This method of research has yielded a great deal of generally applicable biological knowledge. But because the systems of the human body are so complex and the new simplified approach to research so remote from them, the research results have become less and less applicable to the solution of problems of human health and disease. Indeed, the clinical problem that may have originally inspired the research program may often be forgotten as the scientist concentrates on further and further detailed study of his simplified system. As a corollary, when such clinical investigation became more remote from human subjects, fewer ethical problems were created.

With the advent of the electronic computer, the underlying situation was completely reversed. The revolution in data handling and processing has now made it much easier to analyze and interpret than to collect scientific data. The analysis of scientific data, if the experiment's design is sound, should now take relatively little time and effort. Indeed, the immediate availability of an analysis of the data of an experiment should permit the scientist to concentrate on the significance of the experimental results. The scientist now has the time to take into consideration the results of this last experiment so as to plan better the next one.

More importantly, clinical experimentation no longer need be limited to the study of a few variables at any one time in simplified systems. Experiments can presently be designed to study the complex interrelationships of many variables at the same time. For example, instead of studying the salt and water metabolism of the kidney as if it were completely independent of all the other functions of this organ, it is now possible to study total organ function. Indeed, computer handling of data makes it feasible to study total body functions. Furthermore, with on-line data collection and analysis in real time, it is feasible, for example, to build into a physiologic experiment many contingent measurements depending upon what happens in the earlier stages of the experiment. With such study design, medical research can deal more directly with complex systems in the human subject. Moreover, because the research system is closer to that of the human being, the experimental results should be more easily applicable to the improvement of health and the prevention and treatment of human disease.

This modern method of research—with its more complicated design and more intensive and thorough study of each human subject—is uncovering new ethical questions: How long can one safely run a particular experiment on a patient with a certain disease? How much blood may be collected for research purposes over a specified period of time and how frequently may the experiment be repeated? Will a particularly long continued intensive experiment interfere with the best treatment of the patient? It is clear that more comprehensive clinical experiments requiring more intensive scientific planning will also demand more careful attention to the protection of the human subject. Moreover, now that more complete experiments can be performed, human subjects must not be "wasted" in trivial experiments. This is not to say that simple but complete and penetrating experiments should not be performed. It is a plea for more meticulous planning based on modern technology, computer facilities, and biostatistical consultation to yield more applicable experimental results without increasing the risk to the human subject. It will force us to ask the question: "Is it ethical to perform *limited experiments* if, with more careful planning and with no increased risk to the patient, much more valuable information could be collected of more immediate applicability to patients, including the subject himself?"

The design of medical experiments may also under certain circumstances help to surmount existing ethical problems. It is often difficult to justify ethically a human experiment concerned with the study of normal metabolism or physiology or with the changes produced by a particular illness, because benefits to the subject are likely to be limited. To be sure, the more profound study of the patient's condition implicit in the research measurements may yield information that permits better treatment of his disease. But we can do better than that. A properly designed experiment with on-line computer analysis of properly programmed data makes feasible the study of a physiologic, metabolic, or pathologic mechanism and simultaneously the evaluation of a therapeutic agent. For example, in the study of the mechanism of circulatory collapse in severe infections not amenable to antibiotic therapy, the testing of a drug or, perhaps in the future, the trial of a mechanical heart booster could be interwoven and both studies completed at the same time. Such design assures the experimenter that he could benefit the human subjects of his experiments.

Modern design of human experiments opens up new vistas in the understanding of complex biological systems with immediate promise of human benefit. Experiments so designed should yield more knowledge at the same risk to the human subject—and this is an ethical benefit. But these more complex experiments also uncover new ethical problems demanding increasing vigilance in the protection of the human subject.

The Role of Mathematical Theory

When it is impossible for ethical reasons to perform a given experiment to test a particular hypothesis, it may be useful to turn to the mathematician for the deduction of an alternative hypothesis which could be tested by experiment. As W. G. Cochran has pointed out:

A fruitful mathematical theory will predict the results of experiments not yet carried out—in some cases impossible to carry out. In the intensive studies of the Rhesus factor during the 1940's, Mendelian analysis predicted the existence of two genes not then discovered and the seriologic properties of two new antibodies. Epidemic theory can indicate by how much the probability of a major epidemic will be reduced by immunization of any given proportion of the susceptible population in a public-health program. In evolution and the study of inbreeding, the consequences of forces acting over many generations can be worked out.[8]

The increasing role of mathematics in the medical sciences should make this approach more and more feasible.

If we can agree that scientific medical research can continue to serve ethically as the basis for medical progress, there is an immediate need to re-examine the design of human experiments from both the scientific and ethical points of view; to reshape the design of human experiments and take advantage of new technology; to increase, improve, make more relevant the data collected in human experiments, and yet, at the same time, strengthen the ethical principles of medical research.

REFERENCES

1. Rheumatic Fever Working Party of the Medical Research Council of Great Britain and the Sub-committee of Principal Investigators of the American Council on Rheumatic Fever and Congenital Heart Disease, American Heart Association, "A Joint Report: The Treatment of Acute Rheumatic Fever in Children. A Cooperative Clinical Trial of ACTH, Cortisone, and Aspirin," *Circulation,* Vol. 11 (1955), pp. 343-77; *British Medical Journal,* Vol. 1 (1955), pp. 555-74.

2. Since this manuscript was presented and submitted, it has been learned that two control studies are now under way in the United Kingdom.

3. H. K. Beecher, "Surgery as Placebo—A Quantitative Study of Bias," *Journal of the American Medical Association,* Vol. 176 (1961), pp. 1102-1107.

4. A. B. Hill, J. Marshall, and D. A. Shaw, "A Controlled Clinical Trial of Long-Term Anticoagulant Therapy in Cerebrovascular Disease," *Quarterly Journal of Medicine,* Vol. 29, New Series (1960), pp. 597-609.

5. D. D. Rutstein, R. B. Stebbins, R. T. Cathcart, and R. M. Harvey, "The Absorption and Excretion of the Streptomycin in Human Chronic Typhoid Carriers," *Journal of Clinical Investigation,* Vol. 24 (1945), pp. 898-909.

6. Such an agreement should not be confused with the rumored surreptitious drug testing said to be conducted at times by a few United States drug manufacturers in countries not having standards so rigid as those of the Food and Drug Administration in the United States.

7. Rheumatic Fever Working Party of the Medical Research Council of Great Britain and the Sub-committee of Principal Investigators of the American Council on Rheumatic Fever and Congenital Heart Disease, American Heart Association, A Joint Report Prepared by D. D. Rutstein and E. Densen, "The Natural History of Rheumatic Fever and Rheumatic Heart Disease: Ten-Year Report of a Cooperative Clinical Trial of ACTH, Cortisone, and Aspirin," *Circulation*, Vol. 32, pp. 457-76; *British Medical Journal*, Vol. 2, pp. 607-615; *Canadian Medical Association Journal*, Vol. 93 (1965), pp. 519-31.

8. W. G. Cochran, "The Role of Mathematics in the Medical Sciences," *New England Journal of Medicine*, Vol. 265 (1961), p. 176.

WILLIAM J. CURRAN

Governmental Regulation of the Use of Human Subjects in
Medical Research: The Approach of Two Federal Agencies

MEDICAL AND scientific research in the United States concerning the
health and illnesses of man has become of such steadily growing
magnitude—from $161 million in 1950 to $2.5 billion in 1968[1]—that
it was perhaps inevitable that public concern for the protection of
human subjects would lead to public regulation of the use of humans in clinical medical investigation. On the federal level, action
to adopt administrative controls took place in the two major federal
agencies concerned with medical research at approximately similar
times in the 1960's: the Food and Drug Administration (FDA) and
the United States Public Health Service, particularly the National
Institutes of Health (NIH), both units of the Department of
Health, Education and Welfare. The responsibilities of these agencies are quite different. The FDA is the national government's
largest regulatory agency protecting consumers in the use of foods,
drugs, and cosmetics. The NIH, on the other hand, is the federal
government's primary agency supporting (through research grants
and contracts, and demonstration, construction, and training grants)
and conducting (through its own scientific and clinical facilities)
medical research. The background that led these agencies to install
programs in this field is significantly different.

Pre-1960 American Law Concerning Medical Research

In the years prior to the current decade, there was little "law"
in the United States concerning medical research. There were no
specific federal or state statutes purporting to regulate research organizations or investigators in their research methods, their areas
of research, or the use of subjects or patients in such work. There
were also no reported court actions involving liability issues or

criminal action against research organizations or personnel. Among the few scientific writers or legal scholars interested in the field, the hypotheses of the law—the predictions of what American courts would do if confronted with a need to determine legal principles applicable to this field—were drawn from a small number of appellate court decisions in the United States and Great Britain involving common law actions of medical malpractice.[2] From this meager collection, the general conclusion was drawn that investigators might well be "experimenting" at their own personal risk of a liability suit should any harm come to the patient. This principle was expressed as early as the late 1890's in a summary of the law concerning the skill and care demanded of physicians and surgeons.[3] In a book that went through three popular editions and was considered a "bible" of medical malpractice law by many physicians in this country, the statement was made flatly: "In the treatment of the patient, there must be no experimentation."[4] There seems, however, to have been an assumption in these legal decisions that the experimentation was unauthorized and violative of the basic understanding between the patient and the doctor who had undertaken to treat him. This assumption was based on two factors: (1) that the doctor was bound to act within the accepted methods of medical practice applicable to the practitioner's field of medicine; and (2) that the doctor had not sought or received the permission of the patient to deviate from these methods. In the early cases,[5] and even as late as 1934 in *Brown* v. *Hughes*,[6] the courts did not look kindly upon experimentation and equated it with rash action on the part of the clinician-defendant who was responsible for the care of the patient. *Fortner* v. *Koch*,[7] an important decision by a respected state Supreme Court in 1935, however, seemed to sanction clinical investigation and to recognize the need of medicine to engage in it. The Michigan Supreme Court authorized such investigation as a part of medical practice without subjecting the researcher to strict liability (without fault) for any injury, so long as the patient knew of the experiment and consented to it, and so long as the experiment did not "vary too radically from the accepted methods of procedure."[8] This Michigan decision could be viewed as an important step forward. First of all, it removed experimentation in a clinical situation from the "outlaw" category. Up to this time, experimentation in medical practice was considered an intentional transgression on the person of the patient. It would be the tort of battery. It was treated in theory as imposing strict liability for any harm incurred and was closely akin to the famous 1868 English case of *Rylands* v. *Fletcher*[9] and its progeny where unusually dangerous or inappropriate use of property (a use that is not thought socially valuable to the court) subjects the user to strict, non-fault liability.

The *Fortner* case also brought into the open the two assumptions underlying most of the earlier decisions—the matters of patient consent and accepted standards of practice. The court's application of the first assumption would seem to be quite proper under past and current common law. Though the requirements of consent are still far from clear, it would currently seem to be accepted as obligatory among responsible medical investigators. This cannot be said, however, for the court's treatment of the second assumption. The court imposes an obligation on the investigator-clinician not to deviate "too radically" from accepted methods even though he is conducting an investigation and even though he has informed the patient and received his consent to the investigational procedure. This restriction would seem clearly unacceptable to research interests, at least in many instances. Almost by definition, clinical investigation must deviate from the normal or traditional in some *significant* degree. As Renée Fox has said: "Human experimentation, like all research, is to some extent a voyage into the unknown."[10] This voyage cannot be undertaken on fully charted seas, at least not if the voyager wishes to discover something new.

Legal commentators have tried to explain this limitation in the *Fortner* case.[11] It means, they assert, that the physician can choose between "more than one accepted method of procedure" according to his own "best judgment."[12] They suggest that physicians do this when they perform exploratory operations or when they try one drug after another until they find "a remedy that works."[13] The authors conclude that this mode of practice is both experimental medicine and accepted procedure. They go on to say: "The physician cannot experiment rashly, of course; that is what is meant by saying he 'must not vary too radically from the accepted method of practice.' "[14] It seems to me that this was an unfortunate choice of words by Shartel and Plant. To accept this interpretation would be to read *Fortner* as making no break with the past. It would again equate experimentation (if a significant deviation from accepted practice) with "rashness," the very word used in the earlier cases. This does not seem to me a necessary interpretation. The earlier cases rejected experimentation; *Fortner* does not. The Michigan Court said: "We recognize the fact that if the general practice of medicine and surgery is to progress, there must be a certain amount of experimentation carried on."[15] The Court accepted that experimentation is necessary not merely to treat the individual patient, but also to help medicine to progress—that is, that the object of experimentation is the production of new general knowledge, the discovery of new procedures and methods. This cannot be achieved solely by trying out a series of already recognized treatment methods on a particular patient. No progress in medicine and surgery could result from this concentration on accepted regimen.

What, then, did the Michigan Court mean by its restrictive language? I submit that it can only mean to contain experimentation within the bounds of reasonableness as judged by other colleagues engaged in similar practice involving clinical research. In research, acceptable standards would be determined by examining the practice and procedure followed by reputable and qualified clinical investigators. Today, even more than in 1935 when *Fortner* v. *Koch* was decided, a "researcher's test" of reasonableness should be applied to clinical medical investigation. It is generally said that since at least 1950 the more traditional avenues of clinical therapy have been thoroughly explored and basic research has indicated entirely new routes to be tracked out. Exploration of quite novel approaches in medicine, chemotherapy, and surgery has been the order of the day in clinical investigation during the decades of the 1950's and 1960's.

Viewed in its most favorable interpretation, therefore, the law concerning human experimentation could be expected to develop on a case-by-case basis in traditional common law fashion. The courts would look to expert witnesses drawn from the research field to testify as to common, accepted practices in clinical research. On this hypothesis, it would be in the best interest of the research community to foster the development of identifiable, articulated, acceptable standards of care in research—standards that would also foster productive and imaginative progress in research results.

Early Research on Standards of Care in Clinical Investigation

The need to identify and to develop acceptable standards of care as an aid to the courts (admittedly in defense against arbitrary establishment of rules of conduct by the courts) began to receive limited but respectable support in the clinical research community in the late 1950's and early 1960's. Reaction to the need tended to take either or both of two forms: (1) a movement to develop a code or set of guidelines or principles to govern the use of humans in research; and (2) an effort to study existing practices in reputable research organizations.

Discussion about codes focused on the ten principles of the so-called *Nuremberg Code*.[16] A National Conference on the Legal Environment of Medical Science held in Chicago in 1958 spent most of its deliberations in the area of medical experimentation on producing a commentary on the Nuremberg decalogue.[17] One of the most important new developments in these years was the formulation of a Draft Code of Ethics on Human Experimentation by the World Medical Association in Geneva in September 1961.[18]

The first effort in the area of research into actual practices of clinical researchers was a questionnaire survey by Dr. Louis G. Welt of the University of North Carolina.[19] Dr. Welt questioned medical school departments of medicine concerning whether or not they had a "procedural document" dealing with human experimentation and asking them also about their views concerning the principles that should guide the clinical investigator. He also asked whether they thought a committee of disinterested faculty should review the experimental design to assure appropriate attention to moral and ethical problems. Responses were received from sixty-six departments. The results were quite significant. Only eight departments had a procedural document, and only twenty-four had or favored the establishment of a committee to review research proposals.

In response to the interest provoked by the National Conference mentioned earlier, the National Institutes of Health approved and funded a research project[20] at the newly established Law-Medicine Research Institute at Boston University.[21] The objectives of the project were to study and to report on actual practices of medical researchers and research organizations throughout the United States regarding ethical and moral problems in the use of human subjects and related medico-legal matters. The report of the project and its various publications produced useful findings and recommendations, some of which foreshadowed developments later in the 1960's.

The research into actual practices in the Institute study utilized two general methods: the survey questionnaire and a series of invitational work conferences that were made up of researchers and concentrated upon specialized topics. Of significance was a questionnaire survey in 1962 which followed up in greater detail Dr. Welt's earlier survey.[22] This survey of eighty-six departments of medicine produced fifty-two responses (60.5 per cent). This time the replies were no more encouraging, if one were seeking evidence of a movement toward establishing guidelines or procedures concerning research. Nine institutions were found to have procedural documents, and five more institutions indicated either that they were in the process of developing such a document or that they favored developing one for their institution. When the "procedural documents" were examined by the research project staff, however, it was revealed that only two of the nine could be said to be general guidelines covering all clinical research. Four documents covered only clinical drug trials, two pertained only to the use of normal volunteers, and one was a set of guidelines for the procedures of a review committee.

Some departments answering "no" to the question of whether they had adopted procedural documents nevertheless indicated in answer to other questions that they did apply some informal ethical guidelines on the use of human subjects in research. A small group of respondents consistently replied to all questions that they preferred to leave such matters in the hands of the clinical investigator. Ten departments replied that the department head routinely reviewed all research proposals and monitored the research activities of his staff. On the question of review committees, the results of the Institute survey closely paralleled Dr. Welt's earlier effort. Twenty-two departments replied that they had review committees that examined questions concerning the use of human subjects. The committees reviewed research protocols and were usually advisory only. Some covered only the particular department of medicine replying to the questionnaire, but most seemed to apply to the entire medical school or hospital involved. The committees were concerned with such matters as general research design, qualifications of the investigator, safety of the subject, and financial support of the study. All respondents indicated that the matter of selection and recruitment of research subjects was solely the responsibility of the investigator.

The survey also contained questions about legal precautions. Twenty-three respondents indicated that either or both the institutions and investigators were covered by liability insurance. (Twelve covered both; in eleven only the investigator was covered by his own insurance.) The other answers to this question were either unclear or in the negative. When asked if the departments or institutions provided indemnification for injury to a research subject, no respondent answered positively. Eleven answered "no," while the remainder either did not answer or gave unclear responses, indicating they did not understand the question. The departments were asked if they used special consent forms for research. Only sixteen answered positively. Two additional departments indicated that they used standard patient consent forms. One of the institutions replying "yes"—that it did have a special consent form—gratuitously added "but it is seldom if ever used."

The other predominant method used to collect data and opinions was a series of invitational work conferences of leading researchers drawn from all over the country to discuss informally the issues involved in the study. This format was selected after the project staff experienced some difficulties with communication in questionnaires and interviews early in the project. Many investigators and institutional officials expressed the view that the information sought was sensitive and confidential. The invitational work conferences were designed to avoid invasions of confidentiality and privacy and to provide an informal atmosphere away from the home base of the participant-researchers. It was hoped that the more relaxed format (the meetings were always chaired by one of the participant-researchers, not the project staff) would enable the participants, stimulated by their colleagues, to provide basic information and opinions that could not otherwise be obtained within the confines of the project's time-span, finances, and manpower. Four useful conferences were held concerning pediatric research, the concept of subject consent, the use of prisoners, and the conduct of clinical drug trials.

The field research by Dr. Welt and the Law-Medicine Institute as well as the efforts to encourage the development of professional and institutional guidelines were, of course, almost entirely "pre-Thalidomide" and pre-Estes Kefauver and his congressional investigations into the drug industry.

It is apparent that in the medical research community, prior to 1962, there was a general skepticism toward the development of ethical guidelines, codes, or sets of procedures concerning the conduct of research. On the legal side, it was assumed that any legal principles applicable to the field would be built slowly and deliberately on a case-by-case basis as a result of the small numbers of personal liability suits that might inevitably be expected. There was little, if any, discussion in the literature of the possibility of regulation of medical research by the federal government. It was the posture of both the FDA and the NIH to allow and to encourage clinical investigators to use a high level of imagination and freedom in the pursuit of their research objectives. They were to be guided by their own professional judgment and controlled by their own ethical standards as well as those of their institution.

THE FDA PROGRAM

The First Reaction: Congressional Hearings and Thalidomide

Direct action to regulate clinical investigation took place in the Food and Drug Administration more than two years before the first official action at NIH and the Public Health Service concerning extramural research programs. Of course, congressional action, not administrative initiative at FDA, caused the first significant governmental regulation of the conduct of medical research by that agency. Extended congressional investigation was followed by statutory enactment in the Drug Amendments Act of 1962.[23] The direct precursors to the law were the long and often heated investigational hearings of Senator Kefauver's Subcommittee on Antitrust and Monopoly that began on December 7, 1959.[24] The Drug Law of 1962 was a great personal triumph for Estes Kefauver, perhaps the most significant of his distinguished career. The law probably would never have been enacted, however, without the vast public outcry for stronger drug-control laws that resulted from the terrible outbreak of infantile deformity (phocomelia) caused in Western Europe in 1961 and 1962 by the drug Thalidomide. The drug, developed in West Germany, never got a foothold in the United States due largely to one medical officer, Dr. Frances O. Kelsey, in the FDA's Bureau of Medicine. Dr. Kelsey withheld approval of a new drug application for the drug by one of its American sponsors, the William S. Merrell Company.

Ironically, Dr. Kelsey was not called before Kefauver's Subcommittee to testify about Thalidomide after the story of her work was broken in the *Washington Post* by a leading drug reporter, Morton Mintz.[25] The FDA-Thalidomide story was heard before Senator Hubert H. Humphrey's Subcommittee on Reorganization and International Organization. FDA Commissioner George P. Lar-

409

rick and Dr. Kelsey testified. Senator Humphrey "stuck to the subject," as Richard Harris tells it,[26] but Senators Karl Mundt and Jacob Javits kept insisting on a review of the general subject of clinical investigational use of new and unapproved drugs. Mundt drew the concession from Larrick that the FDA was engaged very little in the control of clinical testing, that it did not know what drugs were being tested, how many doctors were involved in testing, or upon whom the drugs were being tried out. Senator Mundt said: "Well, now, in simple talk it seems to me this is a loophole in the law through which you could drive a South Dakota wagonload of hay."[27]

The South Dakota Senator thought that "ordinary prudence" should dictate that limited, controlled testing of a small quantity of the drugs ought to be tried out on human beings (whom he called "the world's most expensive variety of guinea pig") before the drug was "spread out over an unlimited number."

After this incident, the Senate continued its interest not only in a stronger drug-control bill, but in controls over the investigational use of drugs. And Senator Javits offered the "patient consent" amendment to the Kefauver-Harris Bill in its last stages before enactment.

Drug Investigation Controls Prior to 1962

Senator Mundt was basically correct in his conclusions about the absence of FDA regulation of the clinical testing of drugs prior to 1962. This is not to say that the FDA did not have the statutory authority to regulate investigational use of drugs under the 1938 law. On the contrary, it most probably did, but the agency did not exercise this power. Under the 1938 law, the FDA merely required the drug manufacturer to seek to receive an investigational-use exemption from the law that would otherwise have kept the untried drug out of interstate commerce. Upon receiving the exemption, the manufacturer was free to distribute the drug so long as it carried the label: "Caution—New Drug—Limited by federal [or United States] law to investigational use." The FDA did not require notice of actual shipments of the drug, or information on the research protocol or on the qualifications, number, or location of investigators using the drug. The Thalidomide incident brought out the great and sobering reality of this program's weakness. After Merrell withdrew its new drug application for Thalidomide on March 8,

1962, the company and the FDA undertook to notify all investigators and to recall all supplies. At first the FDA had been under the impression that only forty to fifty doctors in the United States were involved in Thalidomide testing. By August 7, however, the FDA had found and been in touch with 1,248 investigators, 410 of whom had not even tried to communicate with patients for whom they had prescribed the drug. By August 21, 1962, the FDA discovered that over two and a half million tablets had been distributed to 1,267 doctors who had prescribed the drug to 19,822 patients, including 3,760 women of child-bearing age.[28] John Lear of *Saturday Review* was never satisfied with the figures about Thalidomide use in the United States.[29] We will probably never know how much the drug was used, or by whom, or how much of the stuff is still in family medicine cabinets all over the country. In defense of the FDA, it should be noted that the agency concentrated its meager staff in the ethical drug field upon review of the new drug applications themselves. At this point, the drug could make its breakthrough into the general market where it could do the greatest damage,[30] and Dr. Kelsey stopped Thalidomide at this stage. As a result, the United States has certainly not experienced the thousands of phocomelia births that occurred in Europe.

Prior to the 1938 law, there was no control of any kind over new drugs entering the market, and the dangers were far greater then. A thoughtful industry lawyer has pointed out that even in the 1938 legislation it took a similar tragedy concerning elixir-sulfanilamide to move Congress to insert requirements of testing before marketing.[31] Jurow asserts that "at no time during the five-year period of gestation through which the 1938 legislation had passed did anyone suggest such a requirement."[32]

The Drug Amendments of 1962

The Kefauver-Harris Bill, known as the Drug Amendments of 1962, was passed by Congress and signed by President John F. Kennedy on October 10, 1962. The Act makes fundamental changes in the basic laws regulating the ethical drug industry. Of particular importance to academic medicine and to clinical investigators, however, were the following requirements: that there be proof of therapeutic efficacy for drugs as well as the earlier requirement of safety; that drug advertising be controlled more effectively and the labeling of drugs fully disclose contraindications, precautions, and

411

harmful side effects; that the requirements for new drug applications be strengthened and automatic approval of an application after a passage of time be eliminated; that the FDA impose comprehensive regulations on the clinical testing of new drugs.

As may well be imagined, there was opposition to the requirement that manufacturers prove the efficacy of their drugs. This meant a fundamental change in the philosophy of public regulation of the drug industry. From a policeman of safety, the FDA was transformed into an arbiter of value, quality, and success in scientific achievement.

The efficacy requirement had significant effects on the need for and the scope of government controls over clinical investigation. Prior to the 1962 law, the clinical trials needed only to prove the safety of the drugs. The importance of clinical trials under the new law is well brought out in the statutory definition of "substantial evidence" of efficacy:

"Substantial evidence" means evidence consisting of adequate and well-controlled investigations, including clinical investigations, by experts qualified by scientific training and experience to evaluate the effectiveness of the drug involved, on the basis of which it could fairly and responsibly be concluded by such experts that the drug will have the effect it purports or is represented to have under the conditions of use prescribed, recommended, or suggested in the labeling or proposed labeling thereof.[33]

After 1962, effort would have to be made—and supported by Congress—to strengthen the FDA as a scientific organization. The point was made well in the Report of the Commission on Drug Safety. The Commission concluded:

[T]he FDA must be brought into the mainstream of science. As an aid to recruiting and retaining qualified scientists, a constant effort must be made to enhance the scientific stature of the agency.[34]

FDA Regulation of Clinical Testing: First Efforts

The first move at FDA to regulate clinical investigation came just two months to the day before the President signed the Drug Amendments Act of 1962. In response to the Thalidomide incident, Commissioner Larrick issued on August 10, 1962, a set of regulations and solicited comment thereon. These regulations were issued under the authority of the 1938 Act—clearly answering the question for the FDA, at least, that authority had existed all along for such action. With the passage of the new law and its added requirements, the regulations were revised and their final form was published in the Federal Register of January 8, 1963, to become effective on February 7, 1963.

The 1962 Act removed any ambiguity about FDA authority to regulate the testing of new drugs. The new law *requires* (the 1938 Act was permissive) the Secretary of Health, Education and Welfare (and by delegation the FDA) to promulgate regulations for exemption for investigational use. Three types of conditions were suggested in the Act that could, in the discretion of the Secretary, form the basis for such regulations "relating to the protection of the public health."[35] Briefly, the three suggested statutory conditions are (1) submission to the FDA before any clinical testing is done of reports of preclinical tests, including animal tests adequate to justify the proposed clinical testing; (2) signed agreements from investigators that patients to whom the drug will be administered will be under their personal supervision or the supervision of investigators responsible to them, and that drugs supplied to them will not be distributed to anyone else; and (3) the establishment and maintenance of adequate records to enable the FDA to evaluate the investigations.

The requirement regarding patient consent was not in the bill that went before the Congress for vote; it was added to the above section by amendment on the floor of the Congress. As first suggested by Senator Javits, it would have required that patients be "appropriately advised that such drug had not been determined to be safe in use for human beings."[36] No exceptions were allowed. In cooperation with Senator Carroll, however, Senator Javits later modified the amendment to make it permissive at the discretion of the Secretary and subject to such exceptions as the Secretary might by regulation prescribe. Senator Javits said that the amendment was necessary because the matter could not be left to state law. He produced a legal research memorandum from the Library of Congress which concluded that not a single state had any statute which "covered the use of an experimental drug and required the physician to inform the patient of such use."[37] This was a strong argument in a Senate still discussing the Thalidomide tragedies. The lack of "law" in the field of clinical investigation was now a serious issue, as the commentators had warned all during the 1950's.

The final version of the "consent provision" of the 1962 law as it came out of the Senate-House Conference Committee was

413

stronger than the Senate version and closer to the House provision.

It made consent of the subject mandatory and gave the FDA no discretion in its application. It also spelled out two exceptions to the requirement that could be applied by the clinical investigator himself in his own professional judgment, rather than vesting the power to determine exceptions by regulation in the FDA. The FDA was required, however, to enforce the entire section of the law by further regulations. As finally adopted, the provision reads as follows:

Such regulations [on exempt use for investigational purposes] shall provide that such exemption shall be conditioned upon the manufacturer, or the sponsor of the investigation, requiring that experts using such drugs for investigational purposes certify to such manufacturer or sponsor that they will inform any human beings to whom such drugs, or any controls used in connection therewith, are being administered, or their representatives, that such drugs are being used for investigational purposes and will obtain the consent of such human beings or their representatives, except where they deem it not feasible or, in their professional judgment, contrary to the best interests of such human beings. Nothing in this subsection shall be construed to require any clinical investigator to submit directly to the Secretary reports on the investigational use of drugs.[38]

After passage of the new law, the FDA set about preparing regulations in regard to all of the new provisions. As indicated earlier, the FDA had begun preparation of investigational new drug (IND) regulations before the passage of the Act. With this head start, these regulations were the first issued under the new law, becoming effective on February 7, 1963. The remaining major regulations, including those on new drug applications (NDA), were not issued until June 20, 1963.

The regulations concerning investigational use of new drugs were extensive.[39] Since the 1962 Act did not provide details on the procedure for the IND, as it did for the NDA, the leeway for action by the regulatory agency was much greater. The first requirement under the 1963 regulations is for notification to the FDA by the sponsor prior to any interstate shipment of investigational drugs. According to the 1963 Annual Report of the FDA, about 2,680 investigational drugs were reported as being under clinical trial on humans on or after August 10, 1962, when the regulations were first issued.[40] By June 30, 1963, some 1,039 "notices" had been filed under the new regulations for interstate shipment of investigational drugs. About 1,143 drugs were reported as discontinued from clinical evaluation. FDA officials can stop the shipments of investigational drugs on the basis of the notice alone if they conclude that the preclinical investigation does not support the safety of the drug for clinical testing.

In addition to the required information on preclinical testing, the regulations require information on what are described as the three phases of investigations. These phases are grouped in two categories: (1) *clinical pharmacology*, which includes Phases I and II; and (2) *clinical trial*, which applies to Phase III. The description of the phases conforms basically to scientific usage. During Phases I and II, the experimental design may be modified on the basis of experience without notifying the FDA; the changes can be reported in later progress reports. The regulations also specifically allow these phases to overlap. No significant changes can be made or investigators added in Phase III without FDA approval.

There are specific requirements in the regulations concerning all three phases of clinical investigation. Extensive information is required on investigators concerning their training and experience generally and as it relates to the planned drug trial, in particular. A summary of the research design for each phase must be provided. For Phases I and II, a general outline must be submitted identifying the investigator or investigators, the hospital or research facilities where the clinical pharmacology will be undertaken, any expert committees or panels to be utilized, the maximum number of subjects involved, and the estimated duration of these phases of the study.

Though not directed primarily at ethical problems, it should be apparent that these regulations provide the framework for excellent procedural safeguards for the protection of research subjects. Some commentators have pointed out that the quality of a research design is itself an ethical question—that a poor research design is inherently unethical since it cannot achieve the scientific results being sought. From this point of view, the regulations of the FDA concerning the adequacy of the research design and the qualifications of the investigators deal with ethical as well as scientific issues. In addition, it should be noted that the regulations specifically mention the use of expert committees or panels at the research institution that may be involved in reviewing research proposals. This would be similar, in principle, to the review committees required under the PHS-NIH program discussed later in this paper.

In Phase III, the sponsor is required to submit a "reasonable protocol" developed on the basis of the earlier phases of the investigation. The regulations go on to outline various requirements for Phase III testing. The plan must contain data concerning the specific nature of the investigation to be conducted, together with information or case-report forms to show the scope and detail of the planned clinical observations and the clinical laboratory tests made and reported, the names and addresses of investigators, the approximate number of subjects, and the estimated duration of the clinical trial. In order to be considered adequate, the research plan must ordinarily contain, among other things, provision for the utilization of more than one independent investigator, each of whom must keep adequate records designed to permit evaluation of all discernible effects attributable to the drug in each subject treated. Individual records are required on each subject relating to his involvement in the study and also containing information on any other treatment given as well as a "full statement" of any adverse effects and useful results observed, together with a statement of an opinion as to whether such effects or results are attributable to the drug under study.

Periodic progress reports are required, and reports of adverse effects caused by or probably caused by the drug must be reported by the investigator to the sponsor "promptly." If the adverse effect is "alarming," it must be reported immediately. The sponsor must report to the FDA when any investigation is discontinued with the reasons therefore. He must also notify each investigator if a trial is discontinued and also whether a new drug application has been approved on the drug.

The regulations further provide that the sponsor shall not unduly prolong distribution of the drugs for investigational use (as had often been the case prior to the 1962 law). The sponsor is required either to discontinue the investigation and withdraw the drug, or to file a new drug application. The NDA must be filed within sixty days after receipt of a notice from the FDA requiring such a filing, or the drug must be withdrawn. This requirement can be avoided for so-called "service drugs" that have little market value and yet high utility for a small number of patients.

The Consent Requirement: Early Inaction

As can be seen from the above description, the FDA could not be described as dragging its feet on bringing the new law into effect with regulations on investigational drug trials. The only major area where clarification of the law was not provided in the new regulations was in regard to the subject-consent provision. The new regulations merely repeated the language of the law exactly as it appeared in the Act.

One may well ask why the FDA took no action to clarify the ambiguous language of the 1962 law regarding a safeguard in the law considered so important by the Congress. What was meant in the exceptions by the terms "not feasible" and "not in the best interests" of the subjects? To leave these terms undefined was to invite wide variation in the application of the law.

Some speculation on this inaction can be offered. First, the "new" regulations of 1963 were largely the same as the regulations on clinical investigation issued in August 1962, before the Congress had added the consent requirement. The FDA and its enforcement and legal staffs were heavily occupied with preparing the many other regulations required to carry the new legislation into effect. In addition, because of the lateness of Congress in adding this particular amendment to the law, there was no legislative-hearing material to help the FDA and only sparse floor debate on the meaning of the terms. The FDA may also have hesitated because the law implied that the clinical investigators were not directly responsible to the FDA on the consent requirement, but reported only to the drug sponsor.

Among the few authoritative pronouncements on the consent provisions in these early years was a special contribution of Dr. Kelsey to a publication of papers on the moral, ethical, and legal implications of clinical research, edited and published by the Law-Medicine Research Institute.[41] Dr. Kelsey was then Chief of the FDA's newly established Investigational Drug Branch, Division of New Drugs. Dr. Kelsey denied that the exclusions in the law could be applied in circumstances where "the investigator feels that informed consent would interfere with the design of the experiment or would disturb the 'doctor-patient' relationship."[42] Dr. Kelsey's opinion would seem to have closed a large gap in the consent requirement. Many investigators had thought that "not feasible" could mean not convenient to the research design they had in mind, such as the use of some form of deception of the subjects.

Dr. Kelsey also noted that the debates in the House and Senate prior to passage of the bill indicated that the exceptions to obtaining consent would apply to situations where the patient was unconscious, where the subject was a child in an emergency and the parents could not be reached, in the case of a mentally incompetent patient with no known relatives, or where the patient was suffering from an incurable disease and the doctor felt that imparting knowledge of the disease would be detrimental to the patient's welfare.

Dr. Kelsey made it clear that the consent requirement applied to all human subjects of clinical investigation, whether patients or normal subjects, such as medical students, prisoners, laboratory personnel, or volunteer religious groups. This latter reference had a particular significance for such research groups as those at the NIH Clinical Center that utilized as normal subjects religious pacifists (conscientious objectors to military service) in some of their clinical investigations.

The paper also attempted to settle certain other difficult questions that had been raised since the law's passage. Dr. Kelsey wrote that the consent requirement would not bar either "blind" or "double-blind" studies. She asserted that the law does not require that the subject be informed as to which preparation he receives—either the investigational drug, a placebo, or a drug of established activity (the latter two being used as controls)—so long as he is told that he is engaged in an experiment involving an experimental drug. Though she did not spell it out, apparently this means that the subject could be told that he "might" get any one of the three. On this basis, the investigation would meet the requirements of the 1962 law and regulations.

Pronouncements such as Dr. Kelsey's may not have gone so far as some investigators might have wanted in mitigating the rigors of the consent requirement, but it certainly could not be considered aggressively strict.

Commissioner Larrick, up to his retirement, refused to clarify the legal provisions on patient consent. He reiterated his stand in a letter to Dr. Henry K. Beecher of the Harvard Medical School and the Massachusetts General Hospital on September 20, 1965, with copies being sent to Dr. Kelsey, Dr. Sadusk, and Mr. Goodrich.[43] In part, the letter reads as follows:

Dr. Joseph F. Sadusk, Jr., our Medical Director, has made me acquainted with the series of letters which have passed between both of you since your original letter to me of December 22, 1964 in which you asked for an interpretation of the patient consent provisions of the Kefauver-Harris Drug Admendments of 1962. . . . Your letter was specifically directed to a quotation of Dr. Frances Kelsey, which appears to have been taken from the article entitled, "Patient Consent Provisions of the Federal Food, Drug and Cosmetic Act" which appeared in the book, "Clinical Investigation in Medicine: Legal, Ethical and Moral Aspects" (Boston University Law-Medicine Research Institute, 1963). This article was cleared by the Food and Drug Administration prior to publication.

. . . In the final analysis the law is clear in that the basic rule is that patient consent must be obtained except where a conscientious professional judgment is made that this is not feasible or is contrary to the best interests of the patient. It is my present opinion that it is not possible to go beyond this generalization at this time and that individual cases of alleged violation of consent provisions, when charges are made will have to be decided upon the facts in that particular case.

Rule-Making at the FDA in 1966

In late 1965, FDA Commissioner George P. Larrick and a number of other senior staff members retired. On January 17, 1966, Dr. James Lee Goddard, then head of the Public Health Service's Communicable Disease Center in Atlanta, took office as Commissioner of Food and Drugs, the first physician to head the agency in forty-five years. Dr. Goddard was no stranger to assignments outside the uniformed service of PHS. He had formerly served as the first Civil Air Surgeon at the then newly created Federal Aviation Agency. Dr. Goddard set about with accustomed vigor to reorganize and revitalize the FDA.[44]

Among the most serious problems facing Dr. Goddard in the drug field when he arrived at the agency, according to Assistant General Counsel William W. Goodrich,[45] were a long-standing and growing backlog of NDA's, a failure even to begin the review of therapeutic effectiveness of the new drugs marketed from 1938 to 1962, and a "problem of serious proportions" with the kinds of scientific data being presented to the FDA in the IND's. Goodrich reported that an administrative review of the IND problems in preparation for testimony before Congress had revealed that the FDA needed to require stricter adherence to the rules promulgated in 1963. He pointed to widespread industry deviations from required practices, including the submission of "wholly fictitious" data. He also said: "Patient consent, as required by law, was not being obtained in too many instances."[46]

The new administration set about correcting these deficiencies.

The NDA regulations were revised to provide a more effective format for the applications. Dr. Goddard arranged with the Public Health Service to detail seventy physicians and pharmacists to his agency to help in clearing up the backlog of NDA's. By the end of June 1967, the backlog was eliminated. In order to undertake the efficacy review of the three to four thousand drugs approved during the 1938-1962 period, the new Commissioner negotiated a contract with the National Academy of Sciences-National Research Council to conduct the review under the highest standards, utilizing the services of the country's leading scientists. With these actions, Dr. Goddard moved effectively to make the FDA a fully participating member of the scientific community.

In the area of the IND's, Dr. Goddard, Assistant General Counsel Goodrich, and the new director of the Bureau of Medicine, Dr. Herbert L. Ley, Jr., and their respective offices worked together to produce the first interpretive rulings at the FDA concerning patient consent. The *Statement of Policy Concerning Consent for Use of Investigational New Drugs on Humans* was published in the Federal Register on August 30, 1966.

The forces leading up to this action at the FDA, the first in four years of administering the Drug Amendments of 1962 and the first in over twenty-five years of basic legal authority concerning clinical drug investigation, are fairly clear: (1) the change in administration at the FDA; and (2) the growing indications of failure to obtain subject consent in many investigations. One unfortunate incident in the field seems, however, to have been of particular importance: the cancer-cell implant case at the Jewish Chronic Disease Hospital in Brooklyn, New York.[47] Elderly patients at the hospital had been used as subjects in a study of rejection of live cancer cells. There was apparently no foreseeable danger to the patients, and they were told of the experimental nature of the implants. The consent of the subjects was obtained, but they were not told that the cells were cancerous. Though no new drugs were under investigation in the project, one of the attorneys involved in the case wrote to Senator Javits and Congressman Rogers protesting against the consent provisions of the 1962 law as legalizing the use of humans as guinea pigs without their consent whenever the investigators should consider it in the best interests of science. Congressman Rogers questioned the HEW General Counsel, Allanson Willcox, about the matter,[48] and was kept informed during the period when the new *Statement of Policy* was being formulated.

Congressman Rogers made some suggestions concerning the *Statement* that were accepted during the drafting stage.[49]

The Patient-Consent Regulations of 1966

It may be helpful to provide a description of the basic thrust and philosophy of the consent regulations before examining them in detail.

1. The regulations are clearly a substantive attempt to provide comprehensive rules regarding patient consent in clinical drug trials.

2. They do purport to define all of the significant terms in the patient-consent provisions of the 1962 law.

3. They use the *Declaration of Helsinki* of the World Medical Association and the *Nuremberg Code* as guidelines for the regulations.

4. The regulations distinguish between therapeutic and non-therapeutic investigations. They allow no exception from the consent requirement in non-therapeutic studies.

5. They allow the use of controls and "blind" and "double-blind" studies so long as the subject is told he may receive a placebo or otherwise be used as a control.

6. The regulations adopt the term "consent" or "informed consent" as the statutory requirement, using a combination of *Helsinki* and *Nuremberg* to define the term, rather than adopting any standard derived from the recent common law medical malpractice cases involving the same term.

7. The regulations define the key words and phrases of the statutory exception, "not feasible" and "contrary to the best interests of such human beings," and in so doing follow closely the explanations of these exceptions as offered in the congressional debates by the sponsors of the consent amendment.

The above list is my own. Others, including the FDA, may describe the regulations differently and feature other aspects of the agency action. I believe, however, that this list highlights the basic intentions behind the regulations.

By adopting the *Declaration of Helsinki*[50] as a primary source of guidance on ethical standards, the agency was able to adopt principles already approved by the medical profession on a world-wide basis. The American Society for Clinical Investigation, The American Federation for Clinical Research, and other medical research groups had already given their endorsement to the World Medical Association's *Declaration*.

In the first of seven sections in the regulations interpreting the statutory consent requirement, the FDA adopted the *Helsinki Declaration's* distinction between therapeutic and non-therapeutic clinical research, though these terms were not used. In non-therapeutic cases (where investigational drugs are administered "primarily for the accumulation of scientific knowledge, for such purposes as studying the drug behavior, body processes, or the course of a disease"), consent of the subject must be obtained in all instances. In therapeutic situations ("patients under treatment"), the regulation requires that consent be obtained "in all but exceptional cases."[51] The "exceptional cases" are defined in Subsection (d) as the two exceptions contained in the 1962 law. The regulations then go on to define the two exceptions. The term "not feasible" is defined as being limited to those cases where the investigator cannot obtain consent because of inability to communicate with the patient or his representative—for example, when the patient is in coma or "otherwise incapable" of giving consent, his representative cannot be reached, and it is imperative to administer the drug without delay.[52] This definition follows closely the Senate discussion. Senators Carroll and Kefauver mentioned the patient-in-coma type of case in the Senate debates.[53] Both Senators also mentioned emergency cases involving children. Senator Kefauver referred to these as cases "requiring emergency administration of medicine" to children.[54]

The exception for cases "contrary to the best interests of such human beings" are defined in Subsection (g) as applying "when the communication of information to obtain consent would seriously affect the patient's disease status and the physician has exercised a professional judgment that under the particular circumstances of this patient's case, the patient's best interests would suffer if consent were sought." Again, this definition follows the Senate debate and adds little if anything to it. Most particularly it refers to Senator Carroll's example of the patient with cancer who has not been told the nature of his disease.[55]

The last Subsection of the regulations provides a definition of consent. It reads as follows:

(h) "Consent" or "informed consent" means that the person involved has legal capacity to give consent, is so situated as to be able to exercise free power of choice, and is provided with a fair explanation of all material information concerning the administration of the investigational drug, or his possible use as a control, as to enable him to make an understanding decision as to his willingness to receive said investigational drug. This latter element requires that before the acceptance of an affirmative decision by such person the investigator should make known to him the nature, duration, and purpose of the administration of said investigational drug; the method and means by which it is to be administered; all inconveniences and hazards reasonably to be expected, including the fact, where applicable, that the person may be used as a control; the existence of alternative forms of therapy, if any; and the effects upon his health or person that may possibly come from the administration of the investigational drug. Said patient's consent shall be obtained in writing by the investigator.

As indicated earlier, this definition is adapted after the requirements for patient and subject consent in the *Helsinki Declaration* and the *Nuremberg Code.* In public pronouncements, the FDA usually identifies the consent regulations with the *Helsinki Declaration;* but in the definition of consent, which is the most extensive borrowing of language from any other codification in the entire regulations, the great bulk of the borrowing is from *Nuremberg* rather than *Helsinki.* A comparison of the provisions will point this out. The first principle of the *Nuremberg Code* reads as follows:

1. The voluntary consent of the human subject is absolutely essential.

This means that the person involved should have legal capacity to give consent; should be so situated as to be able to exercise free power of choice, without the intervention of any element of force, fraud, deceit, duress, over-reaching, or other ulterior form of constraint or coercion; and should have sufficient knowledge and comprehension of the elements of the subject matter involved as to enable him to make an understanding and enlightened decision. This latter element requires that before the acceptance of an affirmative decision by the experimental subject there should be made known to him the nature, duration, and purpose of the experiment; the method and means by which it is to be conducted; all inconveniences and hazards reasonably to be expected; and the effects upon his health or person which may possibly come from his participation in the experiment.

The duty and responsibility for ascertaining the quality of the consent rests upon each individual who initiates, directs, or engages in the experiment. It is a personal duty and responsibility which may not be delegated to another with impunity.

The arrangement of the substance of the FDA definition of consent as well as the language follow *Nuremberg* closely; actually, no specific wording is taken from *Helsinki*. The *Helsinki* pronouncement, however, shares characteristics with both *Nuremberg* and the FDA definition. For example, all three use the concept of "free choice" or "free consent." All three emphasize informing the subject of the nature of the research and the risks involved. *Nuremberg* and FDA add the requirement that the subject be told the *duration* of the research or administration of the investigational drug to the subject. Two aspects of the FDA regulation are closer to *Helsinki* than to *Nuremberg*. One is the requirement that the subject be given "a fair explanation of all material information concerning the application of the investigational drug." There is no such language in the *Nuremberg* first principle, but the *Helsinki Declaration*, in reference to therapeutic research, requires "a full explanation."[56]

The other FDA requirement in the 1966 regulations that is closer to *Helsinki* than *Nuremberg* is the demand for written consent from all subjects. *Nuremberg* makes no reference to method of recording consent. The *Helsinki Declaration* mentions it only in regard to non-therapeutic clinical research where it says: "Consent should, as a rule, be obtained in writing."[57] The written consent requirement has since been modified by the FDA.

The only significant requirements in the FDA regulation that were not drawn from either of the two codifications are (1) the reference to informing subjects that they may be used as controls; and (2) the requirement that the subject be informed of "the existence of alternative forms of therapy, if any." The first of these requirements is drawn directly from the statute. The second is original with FDA, and we cannot attribute this phraseology to any previously published official source. The withholding of otherwise-known effective treatment was, however, the first classification of serious violations of ethical requirements in the use of human subjects in the famous paper Dr. Henry K. Beecher published on June 16, 1966.[58] In all probability, the Beecher paper influenced the FDA action, at least in the latter stages of its preparation. The *Ethical Guidelines for Clinical Research,* adopted by the American Medical Association on November 30, 1966 (after publication of the FDA regulations in August), do contain a requirement that the patient-subject involved in "clinical investigation primarily for treatment" be informed of "alternative drugs or procedures that may be available." The FDA may well have had available earlier drafts of the AMA guidelines, since they were quite liberally distributed by the AMA for comment.

After the publication of the consent requirements, many comments were received by the FDA, and the regulations were discussed at scientific meetings. As a result, some modifications were made in the regulations by amendments issued on March 9, 1967.[59] The preamble to the amended consent regulations specifically identifies them as "in consonance with" the *Helsinki Declaration* and the new *Ethical Guidelines for Clinical Investigation* of the AMA. The FDA thus underscores the endorsement of the medical profession, American and international, behind the basic principles of the FDA code. That the medical principles are called "guidelines" and "ethical" considerations while the FDA code has the binding effect of law is not discussed. Also, the FDA does not mention the extensive borrowing from the *Nuremberg Code* in the FDA regulations. Apparently it was thought more important to identify the regulations with more recent pronouncements. Reference to the twenty-year-old *Nuremberg* decalogue would not serve this purpose.

The most significant modification of the former regulations in the 1967 amendments was the removal of the requirement of written consent for Phase III studies. Oral consent may be substituted where "taking into consideration the physical and mental state" of the patient-subject, the investigator deems it is "necessary or preferable to obtain consent in other than written form." A record of the obtaining of oral consent must be placed in the medical history of the patient-subject receiving the drug.

The new regulations also make some changes in the definition of consent as a result of questions and comments concerning this important requirement. The unnecessary and possibly confusing reference to "informed consent" as an alternative term for "consent" was dropped entirely. The FDA thus makes it clear that the regulatory definition is controlling and that attorneys should *not* look to the growing case law on "informed consent" in medical malpractice cases where research is not involved for definition of the term. The phrase "fair explanation of all material information" referred to earlier was changed to "fair explanation of *pertinent* information." The most extensive clarifications came in the second full sentence of the definition. (It is reprinted herein with the added words italicized. The words in parentheses are those stricken out of the earlier definition.)

This latter element means that before the acceptance of an affirmative decision by such person the investigator should *carefully consider and* make known to him (taking into consideration such person's well-being and his ability to understand) the nature, *expected* duration, and purpose of the administration of said investigational drug; the method and means by which it is to be administered; (all inconveniences and) *the* hazards involved; the existence of alternative forms of therapy, if any; and the *beneficial* effects upon his health or person that may possibly come from the administration of the investigational drug.

This amendment allows the investigator to take into account the patient-subject's well-being as well as his ability to understand and eliminates the requirement that the patient-subject be told about all inconveniences of becoming involved in the study. The first of these could become a serious weakening of the consent requirement. Protection of the "well-being" of the patient (not the healthy volunteer who does not need it) is covered by the statutory exceptions, or at least this was the intention of Congress. It would seem unnecessary to refer to it again at this point unless it could be used to broaden the investigator's opportunity to abbreviate his explanation of the nature of the research and the hazards involved so as not to "upset" the patient's "well-being." Prior to the regulations, this rationalization was the most common of all used to excuse seeking a meaningful consent of patient-subjects. The second consideration—that of the ability of the subject to understand—is, on the other hand, a useful clarification. It goes along well with the dropping of the term "informed" consent. As has been pointed out frequently by clinical investigators, it is hardly possible to inform any non-physician, non-scientist subject of all aspects of the research. Actually, it is not possible for any subject, since some aspects of the problem and some of its hazards are not fully understood even by the investigator. The clarification here by the FDA should allow the investigator to tailor his explanation to the intelligence and experience of the patient-subject. It is not so much the essential content of the explanation that will be altered, but the method and language used to achieve basic understanding. If the subject's intelligence, education, or experience renders him incapable of achieving the basic understanding required in the definition, he should be eliminated as a subject, or if his participation is essential, a representative (or guardian or conservator) must be appointed to protect his interests and to consent on his behalf.

Most investigators will greet the elimination of the requirement that the subject be told of *all inconveniences* in the study with approval. It is not at all simple to determine what an "inconvenience" is in a given case. To attempt to go over these issues at the time of seeking consent may overly prolong the explanation and confuse the subject as to which are "hazards," which he must weigh seriously, and which are "inconveniences." As the experiment proceeds, the inconveniences will be revealed. They will be no secret to the subject. (They might entail such things as being awakened twice each night for added laboratory tests, or being interviewed twice each day as to how he "feels.") If these inconveniences are too much for the subject, he can protest and have them changed, or he can withdraw from the investigation.

The consent regulations of the FDA are a considerable accomplishment from the legal viewpoint, if one accepts the purpose behind them. They do not cover all aspects of patient-subject protection, since they are limited by congressional authority to a concern with the matter of consent to the administration of investigational drugs. There are other areas where protection could be provided for research subjects, but the FDA does not, under these regulations, have authority to take further action.

If these regulations can be faulted on major issues of ethical consideration, it is in regard to the interpretation of the two statutory exceptions to obtaining consent. The first exception, "not feasible," is said to apply where it is not possible to communicate with the patient or his representative, and it is imperative that the drug be administered without delay. The "example" given of such a situation is a patient in coma. Admittedly, as pointed out earlier, this interpretation is drawn from the congressional debates. Nevertheless, it raises ethical problems. I doubt that any patient in coma should be admitted to an experimental trial utilizing an investigational drug without any consent or communication, even with the patient's "representative." The justification offered is that the drug must be given without delay. This would assume that no other recourse was available in the treatment of the patient. The regulation seems to assume that the patient would die or suffer other irreversible, substantial harm if the drug were not given. We would also have to assume that the investigator and the attending treating doctor were reasonably confident of the efficacy as well as the safety of the drug in this emergency situation. If this is the case, I submit that the drug is *not* being administered as a part of a research study; rather, it is being administered in a clinical situation.

The rules of clinical practice and medical malpractice apply to this case, not solely the rules of experimental medicine. In order to act, the physician taking care of the patient would be required to decide whether or not the drug should be administered in an effort to save the patient. The matter of consent here would be covered by the general-treatment consent obtained by the attending physician when the patient first entered treatment. In any other situation, I submit, comatose patients or patients in full coma should not be admitted to a research study. The only time such patients could be used, it seems to me, is when they have already been admitted to the study with proper consent at an earlier stage when they were conscious and able to understand and exercise a reasonable judgment. In such cases, the administration of the drug might still be continued after the patient had become too ill to communicate. The decision to continue or to stop administration of the drug, or to break the code of a "blind" or "double-blind" study to determine what the patient was receiving when he has lapsed into coma, would have to be the responsibility of the physician-investigator and the patient's attending physician.

It may be argued that patients in coma "or otherwise incapable of giving consent," as the regulation says, could be admitted to an investigational drug trial as long as the consent of a "representative" is obtained. I submit, however, that this would be ethically and legally doubtful unless, as in the discussion above, the drug's potential efficacy had already reached quite a high degree of proof, and there was no other accepted method of treatment. If this were not the case, the seriously ill patient in coma or otherwise out of communication could not reasonably be expected to benefit from the administration of the drug. Without potential benefit, the "representative" might well have no legal grounds for giving his consent on behalf of the patient.[60] The FDA regulations themselves would, of course, entirely rule out the application of the exception to non-therapeutic situations. The potential degree of direct therapeutic benefit would, however, have to be quite high in these exceptional cases, since they are justified by the regulation only where administration of the drug without delay is essential. But in such situations the reason for administering the investigational drug is not part of an experimental design. It is intended as an emergency therapeutic measure in a desperate effort to save the patient. As such, all of the rules of accepted medical practice must be followed. Read in this context, even though the drug is still labeled "investigational," this categorization would not bar its use in an emergency clinical situation (not investigational) where consent was not possible, but it was believed on good clinical grounds that the drug was the last reasonable hope to save the patient.

The regulatory interpretation of the other statutory exception—"contrary to the best interest of such human beings"—presents similar ethical problems. The regulation here is much vaguer than that concerning feasibility, and no examples of its application are given. The language, however, suggests the example given in the Senate debates of the patient who might be seriously or terminally ill with cancer, but might not know it. To obtain consent to administer the investigational drug, it is assumed, might require that he be told the truth about his condition. Even if we accept this justification, it does not seem to me to require eliminating entirely the obligation to obtain some form of consent from the patient. The patient can be told that he is receiving some new medication, and the explanation can be fitted into the particular situation to the extent of the patient's awareness, even if the prevarications are continued and, perhaps, reinforced. In addition, if the possible hazards of the drug are significant, these might well be explained to the patient's family or representatives, if they know the truth about the patient's condition.

The regulation also allows the investigator to dispense with consent on the essentially clinical grounds of the "best interests" of the patient. The investigator is thus allowed to wear two hats—that of investigator and that of physician for the patient. There are situations where this is the case. Where it is not, however, it can be hoped that the investigator will consult the patient's physician before making any decision to dispense with consent. If the attending physician does not approve, the investigator should not proceed without consent. Difficult questions arise in situations where there is no attending physician other than the investigator. Some might advocate that the patient in such circumstances be furnished with independent medical consultation for the legal protection of both the patient and the investigator. Proposals of a similar nature in the field of organ transplants can be found in the Uniform Anatomical Gift Act[61] and the Statement on the Ethics of Human Transplantation of the National Academy of Sciences.[62] The Uniform Act requires that the certification of the death of the donor of an organ be made by a physician not participating in the transplant operation. The NAS Statement suggests the utilization of independent medical judgment on a number of issues concerning the transplant procedure itself.

The last point one might note in regard to both of these regulations is that they may be taken to sanction "experimentation" on seriously ill and terminally ill patients, even those in coma and close to death. This subject would in itself require many pages to explore thoroughly. It can be noted that one of the most complete ethical codes—that of the Public Health Council of the Netherlands, published in 1955—flatly disapproves of experiments on dying patients under any circumstances. This type of flat prohibition presents difficulties in any practical application, and it has not been adopted in any of the later codifications or ethical guidelines. But clarification regarding the involvement of terminal patients in clinical research in the United States may be necessary in future years.

An understanding of the philosophy behind the FDA regulations requires a realization of the public responsibility of the Food and Drug Administration to protect consumers of foods, drugs, and cosmetics in the United States and to regulate the industries that produce these goods on a competitive basis. The FDA is a regulatory agency. Its comparative emphasis upon firm administrative controls and upon cooperative support of the better practices of the industry may vary from time to time, but policing the industry in the interests of the consumer remains its primary responsibility. It should be expected that the FDA would eventually be forced, because of its essential mission, to take action in the field of clinical testing of drugs and in the regulation of the conduct of clinical investigators. The degree to which it attempts controls and the freedom of choice it leaves to the industry and to clinical investigators in the conduct of research are the root issues. The approach of the FDA in addressing this problem can best be explored, it seems to me, by contrasting the present FDA position with the approach taken by the other major federal agency active in the field—the National Institutes of Health.

THE PHS—NIH PROGRAM

General Background

The national medical research institute program of the federal Congress can be dated from the establishment of the National Cancer Institute in 1937. With the creation of this first institute came also the first extramural research grants awarded on a competitive basis to medical researchers in the United States. Major growth and proliferation of the categorical institute programs occurred after World War II. The Division of Research Grants was established in 1946; the National Heart Institute was authorized in 1948; and the regrouping of other laboratories in 1948 resulted in the formation of the Experimental Biology and Medicine Institute and the National Institute of Dental Research. In 1949, the National Institute of Mental Health was established, merging with it the Mental Hygiene Program of the Public Health Service. In 1950, omnibus legislation established the National Institute of Neurological Disease and Blindness and the National Institute of Arthritis and Metabolic Diseases, the latter absorbing the Experimental Biology and Medicine Institute. The Clinical Center of NIH, incorporating most of its intramural clinical research activities, was opened in 1953 on the Bethesda, Maryland, campus. The Division of General Medical Sciences, a non-categorical research grant program, was authorized and established in 1958 and became the National Institute of General Medical Sciences in 1963. The National Institute of Child Health and Human Development also began operation in 1963. In 1968 legislation authorized the establishment of a National Eye Institute, and the John E. Fogarty International Center for Advanced Study was put into operation. The above is not an exhaustive list of the NIH's far-flung activities. The recent reorganization of the Public Health Service further strengthens the NIH in the over-all structure of the Department of Health, Education and Welfare.

The expansion of research activities and grant support by NIH over these years is an even more dramatic story. In round-dollar figures, the NIH medical research budget went from $17 million in the 1948 fiscal year to $803 million in 1967 and an estimated $873 million in 1968.[63] The total magnitude of all NIH programs in 1968 is in the order of $1.2 billion, a twelvefold increase since 1956.

The NIH is a different type of organization than FDA. It is not a regulatory agency, and its responsibilities relate mainly to the support of a national program of health science research. In this capacity, the NIH, under congressional policy, makes research grants to other responsible research institutions and investigators, contracts for specified research studies, and conducts its own intramural research program in its own facilities. This paper will be concerned with the first of these activities, the extramural research project grants program, and particularly with the ethical guidelines for the use of human subjects in clinical investigation.

The first contrast between the FDA program and that of NIH in the above area is one of magnitude. The FDA is concerned with controls over a huge industry spending millions on research and the production of new drugs. During 1967, the FDA received a total of 671 Notices of Claimed Investigational Exemption for the testing of new drugs. Over the past four years (including 1967), the FDA processed approximately 4,100 such notices.[64] These impressive figures may, however, be contrasted with considerably larger numbers of applications processed yearly by NIH. In 1967, NIH (not including the National Institute of Mental Health) awarded over 21,000 grants for research, training, demonstrations, and construction.[65] Some 13,937 of these were research grants. In addition, the NIMH made nearly 5,000 awards, of which 1,707 were research grants. All of these grants represent only those funded from a much larger number of applications. An impression of the total number of applications may be gathered from the 55.4 per cent approval rate for research grant applications in fiscal 1967.[66]

To cope effectively and fairly with this great volume of applications, the NIH has over the years developed a quite elaborate and complex system of review. First of all, it must be realized that the NIH research support program is primarily a *project* system— that is, the NIH supports an idea, a proposal for research. This proposal must be fully developed and must stand on its own merit as being scientifically significant and potentially beneficial to science and mankind. Any scientist may make a proposal and join the competition on the relative merits of his ideas and his ability to spell them out in accordance with the rigorous high-level requirements of scientific research design. This system may be contrasted with a policy of supporting the man or the institution rather than the project. The project-support system is more openly competitive than selection based upon the competence or prominence of the investigator or institution. Selection based upon competence or potential competence tends to become quite conservative with the use of limited objective criteria such as age, place of training, and experience in the case of investigators, and facilities, equipment, staff, and research resources in the case of institutions. Of course, it cannot be denied that the NIH project-review system weighs heavily the background and relative competence of the investigator and the place where the research is to be conducted. But these cannot be the sole bases of awards or priority.

A research-project application first receives an administrative review by the Division of Research Grants staff to assure basic compliance with NIH requirements. The grants are then reviewed by study-section panels composed primarily of leading scientists not employed by the government and drawn from leading research institutions and universities throughout the country. The panels are rotated in membership frequently. Of course, because institutions significantly involved in important medical and scientific research are clustered in certain areas of the country, membership may not be evenly distributed among the states.

Procedures have been developed to avoid conflict-of-interest and favoritism in the review of research projects. When an application is received from a particular institution, it cannot be reviewed by a consultant from the same institution, and study-section members from the applicant institution cannot participate in the discussion or vote on the application. Procedures have also been instituted to provide review of a study-section member's own applications in study sections other than the one on which he is serving. The study sections review grant proposals on the basis of scientific merit. To aid in the funding process, however, they also collectively rate the projects on a relative priority scale.

After examination and rating by the study sections, the proposals go before the Advisory Councils of the respective Institutes. These statutory bodies are composed of leading scientists and also of non-scientists who have shown an interest and concern for research and have backgrounds that can bring important and different points of view on national goals to the Councils. Procedural rules are also imposed at this level to avoid conflict-of-interest in the review of proposals. In determinations of the National Advisory Councils, collective judgment is influenced mainly by the relevance and importance of the proposals to advance the program objectives of the Institute rather than relative scientific merit. Scientific merit is expected to have been assured in the study-section review.

The Academic Freedoms of NIH

The NIH is staffed in all major levels of the organization by well-trained, experienced scientists and research administrators. It will be recalled that one of the criticisms that was made of FDA before Dr. Goddard took office was its lack of high-level scientific competence. This criticism certainly cannot be made of NIH. The NIH is a part of the research and academic community. Its values are in most part the values of academic medicine in the United States. The heavy participation of university faculty in the decision-making process at NIH reinforces this relationship. In his Godkin Lectures at Harvard in 1963, Clark Kerr, then President of the University of California, complained: "[S]ome faculty members tend to shift their identification and loyalty from their university to the [research-grant] agency in Washington."[67] Dr. Kerr did not mention any particular federal agency in this statement, and most university faculty (as distinguished from administrators) would probably not agree with the statement in any case. Loyalty to an institution, be it the university at which he is serving or a particular research organization which may from time to time support his work, is significant to the scholar and scientist in a relative manner as a part of his general responsibility to his discipline, to teaching, and to research in the acquisition of knowledge. The faculty member's freedom to pursue these objectives as he sees fit is probably the value he places highest and guards most tenaciously. NIH has traditionally respected this attitude on the part of university researchers. The agency has applied the philosophy of academic freedom to the administration of the scientific aspects of its extramural project-grants program. Institutional policies govern regarding faculty and staff salaries and terms of employment. Decisions on publication of research findings are left in the hands of the principal investigator. A great deal of freedom is allowed principal investigators in changing the research design in order to take advantage of new leads in the research not discovered until the research has begun. Such freedom of movement is essential, of course, to assure success in research.

Research Involving Humans: Development of Policy

Given this background, it is not surprising that NIH did not impose regulations or guidelines concerning the use of human subjects in its extramural project-grants program during its early years. Ultimate responsibility in these matters was determined to rest with the universities and other research institutions and with the principal investigators. This is not to say that the NIH staff, study sections, and Advisory Councils were unconcerned with ethical considerations or with protecting research subjects from hazards revealed or suspected as a result of project application review, site visits, or progress reports. Informal action was taking place constantly, and advice was being given to investigators and institutions. There were discussions of ethical considerations in the National Advisory Councils from time to time over these years.

Perhaps the best evidence of the genuineness of the NIH's concern for ethical principles and the protection of research subjects can be gathered from an examination of its own practices in clinical investigation in its own clinical research facilities. The Clinical Center at Bethesda has, since its inception in 1953, acted under a well-developed set of principles and procedures for the protection of patients and subjects involved in studies at the Center. As pointed out by Dr. Stuart M. Sessoms, then Assistant Director of the Center,[68] no study about which ethical questions might have been raised could be initiated until approved by a medical review committee composed of representatives of each research Institute and Center staff.

Dr. Sessoms also stated:

The patient or subject of clinical study is considered a member of the research team and is afforded an understanding suited to his comprehension of the investigation contemplated, particularly any potential danger to him.[69]

This acceptance of the subject as "a member of the research team" is one of the earliest expressions of the concept of medical research as encompassing the subjects as well as the investigators as colleagues in a cooperative enterprise.

The policy of the Clinical Center also indicates that where any unusual hazard may be involved for patients or subjects, the written consent of the subject is required and a statement must be entered in the patient's chart or in a separate memorandum indicating the patient's understanding of the procedure and its purpose, including potential hazards to him, and his willingness to participate.

As noted earlier, the National Advisory Health Council had sporadically discussed the advisability of applying particular guidelines concerning ethical matters to the extramural grants program. But in late 1963 NIH began to study the subject in greater depth. In July 1964, a meeting was held involving the NIH Director, staff assistants from the Office of Program Planning, and a small group of outside advisers. The Director, Dr. James A. Shannon, forwarded the report of the group to the Surgeon General on January 7, 1965.[70] The *ad hoc* committee made four recommendations that may be summarized as follows:

1. That an appropriate inter-professional group should be encouraged to formulate a statement of principles relating to moral and ethical aspects of clinical investigation.

2. That there is a need for factual information concerning actual research procedures and activities.

3. That NIH should consider providing advice, at the request of grantees, concerning ethical problems and risk-reducing practices in clinical research.

4. That research grant documentation relating to the use of human subjects in clinical investigation should be identified for special consideration throughout the NIH-PHS review process.

Dr. Shannon, in his memorandum of transmittal of the document, endorsed all four statements in principle, but urged that the highest priority be given to "the rapid accomplishment of the objectives" of the first and fourth recommendations.

The NIH Guidelines on Clinical Investigation

The result of the study and recommendations of NIH concerning moral and ethical issues in clinical research was the resolution of the National Advisory Health Council adopted on December 3, 1965. It reads as follows:

Be it resolved that the National Advisory Health Council believes that Public Health Service support of clinical research and investigation involving human beings should be provided only if the judgment of the investigator is subject to prior review by his institutional associates to assure an independent determination of the protection of the rights and welfare of the individual or individuals involved, of the appropriateness of the methods used to secure informed consent, and of the risks and potential medical benefits of the investigation.

Surgeon General Stewart accepted the recommendation of the Council and promulgated the following policy statement on February 8, 1966:

No new, renewal, or continuation research or research training grant in support of clinical research and investigation involving human beings shall be awarded by the Public Health Service unless the grantee has indicated in the application the manner in which the grantee institution will provide prior review of the judgment of the principal investigator or program director by a committee of his institutional associates. This review should assure an independent determination: (1) of the rights and welfare of the individual or individuals involved, (2) of the appropriateness of the methods used to secure informed consent, and (3) of the risks and potential medical benefits of the investigation. A description of the committee of the associates who will provide the review shall be included in the application.

The policy at first applied only to research and research training grants. Assurances of compliance and apparently the prior review and approval of each grant application by the institutional review committee were required with each separate grant application. This was a time-consuming operation and meant increased "paper work" for each principal investigator applying.

On July 1, 1966, the Surgeon General issued a revision of the *Policy Statement* extending the requirements of "prior review of research involving human beings" to all PHS grants. He also revoked the requirement of individual assurances of compliance accompanying each grant application and provided instead for an institution-wide assurance that could be filed once to cover all subsequent grant proposals. The institutions were required to file an assurance or agreement of compliance (an example of an acceptable assurance was supplied with the revision) along with evidence of compliance with the requirements set forth in the assurance. The institutions were also required to furnish a description of the review committee or committees to be utilized at the institution and an indication of the methods to be used by the institution to assure that the advice of the review committee or committees would be followed.

The grantee institutions were also required to report any changes in their policies and procedures or in the composition of their review committees.

In December 1966, the Surgeon General issued a further clarifying statement relating mainly to behavioral and social science research. It was asserted that the grantee institution is responsible for assuring that investigations are "in accordance with the laws of the community in which the investigations are conducted and for giving due consideration to pertinent ethical issues."

437

Scope of the NIH-PHS Guidelines

Again, as in regard to the FDA consent requirements discussed earlier, it may be helpful to summarize briefly the major thrust of the guidelines.

1. The *Policy Statement,* as revised, sets up what is primarily a self-regulatory system in the research institutions and universities funded by the PHS and NIH. This does not mean, of course, any abdication of responsibility on the part of the Public Health Service and NIH. The agency staff, consultants, study sections, and Advisory Councils will still continue to identify concern with ethical matters and the welfare of subjects and will continue to question applications if the gravity of risks to subjects so indicates.

2. Broad guidelines for action, rather than detailed, substantive regulations, are provided.

3. The guidelines are three in number:

   a. protection of the rights and welfare of subjects

   b. the obtaining of "informed consent"

   c. assessment of the risks and potential benefits of the investigation.

4. At the institutional level, the assessment and surveillance of these guidelines are vested in a review panel of the peers of the investigator at his own institution. The review committees can include not only clinical researchers with competence to review the scientific content of the projects, but such other members as clergy, lawyers, philosophers, and laymen from the community. The members cannot, however, have a vested interest in any particular project in whose review they participate.

5. The action by the institutional review committee is not an independent review of the guidelines for the protection of the research subjects; it is a review of the "judgment" of the principal investigator. In other words, the committee must give weight to the decision of the investigator concerning his methods for complying with the guidelines.

6. By the revision of July 1966, PHS added an institutional responsibility to assure that the procedural aspects of the *Policy* would be complied with throughout the institution. The revision also requests copies of any general principles adopted by the institution as ethical guidelines in clinical research. These can be original with the institution, or endorsements of such pronouncements as the *Declaration of Helsinki* or the *AMA Guidelines*. The institution is not specifically required to adopt any substantive ethical principles, however, so long as their methods and procedures otherwise comply with the Policy and the institutional assurance and protect the rights and welfare of the subjects.

The guidelines now in operation are consistent with the traditional NIH philosophy of reliance on decentralized institutional controls over many aspects of the scientific research it supports. The policy avoids extremes in the exercise of federal responsibility and leaves a great deal of flexibility for the exercise of local judgment.[71]

The Guidelines in Operation

As of May 28, 1968, the NIH had received 1,485 institutional assurances of compliance with the guidelines and required procedures. Of these, 1,312 have been approved and accepted by NIH. The remainder had either been inactivated or are still under review.

An evaluation of the effectiveness of the guidelines and the institutional review system over so short a period of time would be quite difficult. Some comparison can be offered at the NIH level, however, in regard to so-called "problem projects." These are proposals presenting possible hazards to subjects. The hazards may be medical, psychological, or sociological in nature.[72] Estimates at the study-section level over a period of years from about 1960 onward placed these problem projects at about 2 to 3 per cent per year. Firm figures have been collected since 1966. They indicate a steady decline in the problem projects coming before the National Advisory Councils—from 93 to 21—between the June meetings in 1966 and those in 1968. The decline in the percentage of problem projects among the total projects involving human subjects is even more dramatic. The percentage in 1966 was 7.4, but had dropped to 1.7 in 1968. The projects coming before the June, 1966, meetings were submitted to NIH before the ethical guidelines went into operation.

439

During this same period, the spread of problem projects among the study sections was surveyed. Thirty-two separate study sections reviewed at least one application that presented a problem of hazards to research subjects. On the Council level, the problem projects were fairly evenly distributed among Arthritis (30), Child Health (28), and Heart (25), with the remaining 36 applications scattered over the remaining Institutes and Divisions. It is difficult to assess the effect of this characterization of "problem projects" on the approval rate for the projects. Certain projects were approved and funded in view of counterbalancing benefits to the research subjects; in other cases, the possible hazard to subjects was limited to future years of the project and could be reviewed subsequently by NIH and the institutional review committees.

Further Analysis of the Guidelines

Some comment should be made on the three key guidelines selected by the National Advisory Health Council to form the basis of the *Policy Statement*. The first—protection of the rights and welfare of the subject—is a universal admonition and should provide the basis for a broad, working philosophy for principal investigators and institutional review committees. It is quite common to rest the general development of policy upon such a universal goal. The second guideline is also broad in nature, requiring the obtaining of the subject's informed consent. There is no doubt but that subject consent is the most important single requirement in all of the ethical codes concerned with the use of humans in clinical research. The earlier detailed examination of the FDA regulations illustrates the complexity of the issue. The lack of further definition of the term can present difficulties. The use of "informed consent" rather than "consent" can lead to confusion as to whether NIH and PHS intend to apply the term in the sense in which it has been used in medical malpractice cases not specifically involving medical research. As noted earlier, the FDA dropped the term "informed consent" in its 1967 revision in an effort to avoid such a connotation and to insure a uniform interpretation of the term nationally. By retaining the term and not defining it, it can be assumed that NIH and PHS are willing to have the application of the consent requirement differ from state to state according to local law. This is a justifiable policy—one consistent with the traditions of NIH and its effort to allow a significant degree of local judgment to be exercised concerning the ethical guidelines. It may, however, be necessary to clarify the consent requirement in some respects in such areas as the use of mentally incompetent persons, children, and prisoners. It is also not clear whether any exceptions are allowed to the consent requirement, though exceptions can be read into the term "informed consent" as it has been applied in common law medical malpractice cases in some jurisdictions.

The last of the three guidelines is the most complex from the point of view of legal and ethical interpretation. It has no direct counterpart in the FDA regulations, but is close to two of the Basic Principles of the *Declaration of Helsinki*.[73] The guideline also recalls the sixth principle of the *Nuremberg Code*.[74]

The difference between the FDA regulations and this guideline is that the FDA requires a consideration of risks and benefits as a part of the consent issue. The subject weighs the risks or hazards to him against the benefits he may derive from the investigational drug. In the PHS-NIH guideline, risk-benefit is separately considered, apparently by the investigator and the review committee. Of course, we would assume that the subject also has the opportunity to weigh the risks and benefits in giving his consent to participation in the study.

Under this guideline, it would seem that the review committee must, in order to review the judgment of the principal investigator on this issue, assess the merits of the research study. There would be no other way to estimate the study's potential medical and scientific benefits. If the research design is poor or other aspects of the study are not acceptable scientifically, any significant risk to the subjects would be without justification.

The assessment of risks and benefits by the review committee should provide a further safeguard for the welfare of subjects. There could be cases where the subject has consented to assume risks that on reflection the review committee finds too grave, despite the potential benefits. The committee, by refusing approval, would be protecting the subject even against his own willingness to take the risk. On this ground, the guideline is highly commendable in its effort to protect the subject's welfare. But some scientists and philosophers might be heard to object that the subject ought to have the right to take heroic risks for his own potential benefit, or for the sake of others, or for medical science generally.

From a legal view, the problem with this guideline is the fact that it adds to the responsibility of the review committee in a diffi-

441

cult area for the exercise of scientific judgment. Courts and juries may second-guess this balancing of interests in risk and benefit at some future time after the fact and in a case situation where harm actually did come to the subject. (The courts, after all, will not be reviewing cases where nothing went wrong.) At this stage, hindsight can be applied not only to the harm actually occurring to the subject, but to the benefits—the actual success or failure of the project, rather than the potential benefits that the review committee was required to consider. The court and jury may be admonished not to apply hindsight, but they can be tempted to do so in an effort to provide compensation for an injured plaintiff. This guideline does, it seems to me, open up a question of the justification of the research. The question, once opened, can be subject to constant reassessment after the fact, based upon very inadequate means of weighing the separate values under consideration—that is, the individual welfare of research subjects and the eventual good of science, medicine, and mankind.

The Review Committee System

From a legal viewpoint, one of the most interesting features of the PHS-NIH policy is the establishment of institutional review committees. This system is the heart of the self-regulation allowed to the research community itself under this government policy. The establishment of these committees cannot help but have a profound effect upon these institutions in their approaches and attitudes concerning research practices. It will be recalled that in the Welt and Law-Medicine Institute surveys prior to the installation of the PHS-NIH Policy, only a small number of institutions had adopted ethical guidelines or established review committees.[75] With review committees set up for PHS-NIH grant applications, it can be expected that many, if not most, of the institutions will extend the responsibility for review to all research projects involving human subjects throughout the organization. It will be difficult not to do so. The connotation of second-class citizens could be said to attach to the subjects in research projects not having the protective review of the committee. Also, researchers may wish equally to have the support of the committee in endorsing their judgments that no significant hazards are involved in their non-NIH research studies.

At present there is little data available concerning the functioning of the review committees.[76] A 10 per cent sample of approved institutional programs was, however, analyzed by NIH in 1968 in regard to panel membership. In a total of 142 institutions, the great majority (104, or 73 per cent) of the committees are limited in membership to immediate peer groups; thus, they represent only professional groups of scientists or physicians without the addition of theological, legal, philosophical, or lay members. Broad inter-disciplinary groups in which the applicant investigator's co-professionals are in a minority were found in only 11 institutions. The remaining 26 institutions utilize some associates from other professional or lay backgrounds, but these members are in the minority. Among this group of committees, 18 include lawyers on the panels, 16 include lay associates, and 1 includes both lawyers and clergy. Committee size is highly variable. Some large institutions use more than one group. Some of the largest research organizations use several panels with one central group acting as an appeals board and policy coordinator. A few institutions employ a large panel from which a smaller group (typically three in number) is formed on an *ad hoc* basis to review individual projects. This is a good system with built-in flexibility for coping with problems of conflict-of-interest and with gathering a panel on short notice from among busy—and often absent—faculty and staff associates. It is not entirely clear in this category whether an appeal lies to the full panel if the three-man initial review finds problems with the application. In all probability, such an appeal should be available. Otherwise, the full panel has little real function, and the smaller *ad hoc* groups carry heavy responsibility.

It may be that in the future NIH should further encourage the institutions to widen the membership of their review committees. At present, if this sample is at all representative, the great majority of the panels seem quite parochial in nature. It must be admitted, however, that not much is known about committees of this type and what the function of non-scientists or non-medical members should be on the panels. The role of lawyers either as members or as advisers to the panel is perhaps the simplest to describe. Lawyers can advise on the procedures and methods of the panels in carrying out their functions as reviewers and decision-makers. They can also advise on local law applicable to particular situations. Physicians are generally more apt to be aware of the lawyer's utility in the latter area than in the former. It may be necessary to educate the clinical members to appreciate the lawyer's interest, skills, and knowledge in procedural matters and the methods of decision-making. Care must be taken, however, to avoid legal members dominating the discussion and decision of certain aspects of the issues before the committees.

The function of theologians and philosophers on the panels may also be fairly clear. Their interest will be in ethical issues and human values. The philosopher will probably be an academician. (Our society seems to support such thinkers in few other places.) He is apt to be interested in the ethical issues before the committee in a relatively abstract way. The theologian, on the other hand, may come from a more varied background. He may be a university faculty member like his philosopher colleague, but he is perhaps more likely to be associated with a local church, parish, or synagogue. He may be a hospital chaplain or a pastoral counselor. As such, he is interested not only in general ethical principles but in particular religious beliefs, personal attitudes, and the welfare of individuals. As such, he can be a valuable member of the review committee. The question of religious participation in the review committees attached to religiously affiliated hospitals, however, can present special problems.

The role of other professionals, businessmen, and laymen from the community is not so easily related to the particular knowledge, understanding, or skills useful to the review committees in their deliberations. Perhaps the most important function these members will perform will be in forcing the professionals to interpret their deliberations and decisions to these general community representatives. Lay members will thus tend to transform the committees from closed associations of like-minded professionals who "understand" one another into a more open forum of community responsibility. If this can occur, it will be all to the good, it seems to me.

Lay members can also be considered "consumers" in the sense now being applied in some other areas of community decision-making, such as the anti-poverty programs, model cities projects, and comprehensive health planning. Whether these consumers should include research subjects is another question that might be asked. When adding lay members, the institutions would also have the opportunity to exercise greater flexibility in such matters as age, sex, ethnic and racial background, and geographic distribution than can be applied in selecting professional members.

To a lawyer, the most significant aspect of the institutional review committee system is that it allows for the building of a body of general principles over a period of time on a case-by-case basis.

Most lawyers in the United States brought up lovingly in the common law tradition will experience an automatic, positive reaction to this method of regulation. I am certainly among them. The use of review committees is a common law approach. These committees will be building the law as they go along. This seems to me a wise approach to a field where the subject matter itself, clinical investigation, is still developing dynamically. Specific rules can become obsolete quickly in such a field. This is not to say that general guidelines are not useful and significant in addition to the common law principles that may be developed by the committees. On the contrary, the committees will need general principles, such as the PHS-NIH guidelines, upon which to build the application to specific cases. General principles are needed in regard to such matters as subject consent and research design so that investigators can work within some basic framework.

The reference to the common law should be examined carefully, however. Lawyers are apt to seize upon tort law (the law of personal liability) as the obviously similar field. Here the courts are concerned with assessing fault and with redressing personal injuries or wrongs, such as in automobile accidents or medical malpractice. But the institutional review committees are not considering issues such as these at all. If I were to analogize the review committee system to any legal area, it would be to licensing hearings rather than to liability suits. The committees are concerned with authorizing, or preventing, an investigator from carrying on a particular activity—a research project. They are seeking to prevent harm from being done to research subjects, rather than to redress harm already done. The review committees can probably learn a great deal from the procedures and practices of administrative law regarding licensing adjudication.

In these early years, the leeway allowed to local institutional committees may produce substantial variation in the operation of the review panels. The variation may result as much from lack of background, sophistication, and interest on the part of the panel members as from differences in local law or institutional organization. In the beginning, there will be few settled principles of procedure or substance that can be easily adopted and followed. Nevertheless, principles will grow if the panels take their work seriously, record their deliberations and decisions, and attempt to generalize their conclusions. The guidelines do require that the committees keep records of their deliberations. These records, if well organized and intelligently developed, can be the basis for building a local common law of committee review.

It has been suggested that efforts should be made, perhaps by NIH itself, to publish the decisions of these institutional review committees so that general principles can be developed across the country concerning the ethics of clinical investigation. This is an interesting idea, again analogous to the common law system in American courts. It has much to commend it, but there are serious problems in adopting it. Again, the suggestion tends to assume that these committees are like courts deciding appeals in tort liability suits. The problems here are much more complex than this. First, one would have a huge volume of uninteresting and unimportant cases (for this purpose) if one reported every project reviewed by every review committee. It would also be difficult to select the projects which, among those approved, presented serious ethical issues. One could not select for publication only the applications denied either, since many close decisions might be missed this way. The criteria for selecting the cases to be reported would be difficult to develop. Futhermore, as a practical matter, many committees probably operate in such a way that few applications are clearly and unequivocally turned down. The research protocol is probably returned for further explanation and revision until the problems are ironed out to the satisfaction of the investigator and the review committee. At the end of all this, what would be reported? If an impasse should result, the investigator might well be allowed to withdraw the application rather than have it stamped "disapproved."

All of these practical considerations militate against simply publishing review committee "decisions" as such. Any publication system raises problems relating to confidentiality and privacy and to the reputation and integrity of the researchers, subjects, and review panels involved. It may be more advisable at this time to encourage some competent legal and social-science research into the workings of selected institutional review committees from which useful generalizations can be made rather than to move into some common law-like decisional reporting system.

The Responsibility of NIH

It was noted earlier that the adoption of these guidelines and the placing of important responsibility for self-regulation in the institutions did not remove responsibility from NIH staff, consultants, study sections, and Advisory Councils in identifying and reviewing applications and taking action to safeguard subjects in PHS-NIH supported research projects. The attention given in these earlier pages to institutional procedures is in no way intended to denigrate the importance of this federal responsibility. It would seem important, therefore, to examine this aspect of the total program at this point.

As noted earlier, the NIH staff and study sections have always given attention to ethical issues in project applications, both before and after adoption of the 1966 guidelines. Much of the action in this regard has been informal, involving inquiries to the principal investigator or site visits. Discussions would also take place in study-section review of applications. Often the issue would be inextricably woven into the general issue of the merits of the application. A project that seemed to present undue hazard to subjects would often be questionable on other scientific grounds. If such a project received a low rating indicating almost certain rejection, it would be difficult to assign weight to the significance of the ethical problem.

The effect of the 1966 policy upon this system at NIH is difficult to assess at this time. Earlier it was noted that the number of "problem projects" involving possible hazards to subjects has declined sharply since 1966, the year just before adoption of the ethical guidelines. This decline may be due to the institutional review committees intercepting and rejecting or modifying the projects before they get to NIH. Under the guidelines, however, the institutional committees are not required to review projects before submission to NIH. They can review them after processing at NIH as long as they examine them before the research actually begins. It is not clear what actual practice is at present. In the 10 per cent sample of approved institutional assurances examined earlier, 60 per cent of the institutions review projects before submission to NIH. In 4 per cent, it is clearly stated that review will take place only after approval by NIH. In the remaining 36 per cent, the review was either optional before or after submission to NIH, or it was unclear what method was utilized. Under these conditions, the responsibilities of the NIH staff, consultants, and review system have themselves remained flexible. It would seem advisable to clarify these matters.

The first step in the clarification of areas of responsibility might

447

be to require all institutional committees to review applications prior to submission to NIH. The Bethesda staff, consultants, and study sections could then act under the assumption that a responsible group had found the projects acceptable on ethical grounds. It would also be clear that unless NIH and its review system should stop a project, it would go into operation on the basis on which it was submitted. The NIH could make no assumption that a later review would correct problems not discovered or corrected by the NIH review system. From this point forward, responsibility would rest with NIH. If problems should then arise on ethical grounds, NIH staff, consultants, study sections, and Advisory Councils should be specifically obliged to raise these issues, and they should have the authority to reject an application solely on the basis of ethical questions.

It would seem advisable also to encourage more extensive communication between NIH staff and the institutional review committees after project applications are filed and questions of an ethical nature are raised. They may be the same questions examined by the committee and answered to their satisfaction. Such communication may clear up the doubts of the NIH staff or consultants. Whenever NIH determines to turn down a project on ethical grounds, it would seem that this decision and the reasons for it should be communicated to the institutional review committee. Such communication would not be for the purpose of allowing the committee to protest or to appeal to NIH for any reconsideration, but as an informational feedback to help to educate the institutional committees. Such an exchange would enable the committees to evaluate their own collective assessment of the projects under their review. It would help the two systems, one local and one national, to work in harmony toward similar goals.

Conclusion

In these pages I have attempted to analyze the approaches of two federal agencies in regard to the public regulation of certain aspects of medical research involving human subjects. The particular focus has been upon ethical considerations and safeguards to protect the rights and welfare of the research subjects.

The difference in approach between the two agencies can be explained largely on the basis of their character and responsibilities. The Food and Drug Administration is an administrative, regulatory agency concerned with protecting the consuming public. Its program in the field of clinical drug testing is regulatory in nature and applies to all phases of clinical investigation and to research design. Its action regarding the ethics of drug testing is in the same vein. It is concentrated upon assuring that investigators obtain the consent of patients and subjects to whom investigational drugs are given in the course of clinical trials. Exceptions to this requirement are allowed only in accordance with statutorily established conditions. The FDA program of control is applied uniformly throughout the country.

The National Institutes of Health, on the other hand, is a research organization supporting and conducting an extensive national program of medical and scientific research. In its extramural project grants program, it applies a philosophy of encouraging academic freedom and imagination in the research it supports in the interest of achieving the best possible scientific results. Instead of a substantive, regulatory program uniformly applied across the nation, it has installed a system of decentralized, institutional review committees and generalized ethical guidelines to protect patients and subjects in the projects it supports. It also takes direct responsibility for the protection of research subjects under its own system of national review of project applications. The review committee structure is an interesting and imaginative approach to lawmaking. The FDA, as well as the NIH, makes provision for use of such self-governing, common law-producing mechanisms. This institutional review system cannot help but have a profound effect on the medical research community.

Most of this paper has concentrated on providing a background concerning the philosophy of the agencies against which the particular programs could be viewed and on giving a rather detailed examination of the separate operation of the two programs. Much of the interpretation of the effects of the programs and a large part of the actual comparison of approaches on specific issues in juxtaposition one to the other must necessarily be left to the reader.[77]

REFERENCES

1. These are estimated figures. It might also be noted that medical research has risen in this same period from 5.5 per cent of the total of all research and development expenditures to 10 per cent of the total. *Basic Data Relating to the National Institutes of Health—1968* (1968), p. 1.

2. For writings along this view, see particularly, Irving Ladimer, "Ethical and Legal Aspects of Medical Research on Human Beings," *Journal of Public Law*, No. 3 (1955); Elwyn L. Cady, Jr., "Medical Malpractice: What About Experimentation?," *Annals of Western Medicine and Surgery*, Vol. 6 (1952), pp. 164-70.

3. See Note, 37 L.R.A. 830, 836.

4. L. J. Regan, *Doctor and Patient and the Law* (2d ed., 1949), p. 381; (3d ed., 1956), p. 370. The author was a physician who also had received a law degree. The book was addressed to physicians and other medical personnel. After Dr. Regan's death, the book was totally rewritten under new authorship and was addressed more to legal readers. See C. J. Stetler and A. R. Moritz, *Doctor and Patient and the Law* (4th ed., 1962).

5. See particularly the earliest American decision, *Carpenter v. Blake*, 60 Barb. 488 (N.Y., 1871).

6. 94 Colo. 295, 30 P. 2d 259 (1934).

7. 272 Mich. 273; 261 N.W. 762 (1935).

8. *Idem*, at 282, and at 765.

9. L.R. 3 H.L. 330.

10. R. C. Fox, "Some Social and Cultural Factors in American Society Conducive to Medical Research on Human Subjects," *Clinical Pharmacology and Therapy*, No. 1 (1960), p. 423.

11. B. W. Shartel and M. L. Plant, *The Law of Medical Practice* (1959).

12. *Ibid.*, p. 38.

13. *Ibid.*

14. *Ibid.*

15. 272 Mich. 273; 261 N.W. 762 (1935).

16. The Code was developed for the Medical Case at the Nuremberg Trials. See *U.S. v. Karl Brandt, et al.*, Trials of War Criminals Before Nuremberg Military Tribunals Under Control Council Law No. 10, The Medical Case, Vol. 2 (1947), pp. 181-83. See also, Leo Alexander, "Limitations in Experimental Research on Human Being," *Lex et Scientia*, Vol. 3, No. 1 (January-March, 1966), pp. 65-73.

17. "Clinical Research: Legal and Ethical Aspects, Session III," *Report of the National Conference on the Legal Environment of Medical Science*. Published jointly by the National Society for Medical Research and the University of Chicago (paper, 1960).

18. *British Medical Journal*, No. 2 (1962), p. 1119.

19. L. G. Welt, "Reflections on the Problems of Human Experimentation," *Connecticut Medicine*, Vol. 25 (1961), pp. 75-79.

20. N.I.H. Research Grant No. 7039, January 1, 1960.

21. The Institute was established on February 1, 1958.

22. Final Report of the Project, Chapter IX (mimeographed), pp. 3-18. The first principal investigator on the project, from January 1, 1960, to May 31, 1962, was Irving Ladimer, S.J.D. The principal investigator from June 1, 1962, until the end of the project was Donald A. Kennedy, Ph.D. The author of this paper was Director of the Institute at this time.

23. P.L. 87-781, 21 U.S.C. 355.

24. The story of these hearings and of the legislative battle over the 1962 law is vividly told in R. Harris, *The Real Voice* (1964).

25. Mintz received a number of national awards for his reporting of the Thalidomide story. He later wrote a book about the drug industry. See M. Mintz, *The Therapeutic Nightmare* (1965).

26. Harris, *The Real Voice,* p. 191.

27. *Ibid.*

28. FDA Press Release, August 23, 1962.

29. The articles by Lear have been and still are among the best and most penetrating on the subject of drug use and clinical investigation. On Thalidomide, see particularly J. Lear, "The Unfinished Story of Thalidomide," *Saturday Review* (September 1, 1962), p. 38.

30. At times, even this assumption was invalidated, however, due to the lack of an effective time limit on the period allowed for exempt use for testing purposes. Some unscrupulous producers, particularly those in the fraudulent cancer-cure business, distributed their wares under the exemption for years.

31. I. H. Jurow, "Government and Consumer Protection—Drugs," *F.D.C. Law Journal,* Vol. 22 (1967), pp. 593-601.

32. *Ibid.,* p. 595.

33. Section 505(d), Federal Food, Drug and Cosmetic Act.

34. Report of the Commission on Drug Safety (1964), p. 21. The Commission could not be considered unduly biased in favor of the FDA. It was composed of drug industry investigators and administrators and academic investigators and was established under a grant from the Pharmaceutical Manufacturers Association. The Commission was formed to examine and to report on the new drug law of 1962 and the FDA regulations issued in 1962, 1963, and 1964.

35. Section 505(i), Federal Food, Drug and Cosmetic Act.

36. 108 *Congressional Record* 17391 (1962).

37. *Idem,* p. 17395.

38. Section 505(i), Federal Food, Drug and Cosmetic Act.

39. 21 C.F.R. § 130.3 (1963).

40. Annual Report of H.E.W., Food and Drug Administration, 1963, p. 313.

41. F. O. Kelsey, "Patient Consent Provisions of the Federal Food, Drug, and Cosmetic Act," in Ladimer and Newman (eds.), *Clinical Investigation in Medicine: Legal, Ethical and Moral Aspects* (1963).

42. *Ibid.*, p. 338.

43. A copy of the correspondence is contained in the official file on the IND regulations of William W. Goodrich, Assistant General Counsel for the FDA, Washington, D.C.

44. As Secretary Gardner put it in the HEW *Progress Report* of January 1968: "In 1965, attacks on FDA reached a peak in the press, in Congress, and even among reputable scientists. . . . When the new Commissioner, Dr. James Goddard, took over, he supplied a quality of leadership that ended the attacks and began the modernization of the agency to meet today's needs."

45. W. W. Goodrich, "Rule-Making as Viewed by the Commisioner, the Congress, and the Court," *F.D.C. Law Review*, Vol. 22 (pp. 613-19), p. 614.

46. *Ibid.*, p. 615.

47. For a useful summary of the incident and its legal aftermath in a medical licensure action before the New York Board of Regents, see Note, "Experimentation on Human Beings," *Stanford Law Review*, Vol. 20 (1967), pp. 99-117. For the decision in the courts concerning the hospital governing board's access to the patient records, see *Hyman* v. *Jewish Chronic Disease Hospital*, 15 N.Y. 2d 317; 206 N.E. 2d 338; 258 N.Y.S. 2d 397 (1965).

48. A copy of the letter of reply of Mr. Willcox of June 19, 1965, is contained in the official files concerning the IND regulations of Assistant General Counsel for the FDA, William W. Goodrich, Washington, D.C.

49. Memoranda of February 23, 1966, and July 21, 1966, from Mr. Goodrich to Dr. Goddard indicate the communication and exchange of views. Copies of the memoranda are contained in the official files concerning the IND regulations of Assistant General Counsel for the FDA, William W. Goodrich, Washington, D.C.

50. "Recommendations Guiding Doctors in Clinical Research," World Medical Association, 1964, reprinted in the *British Medical Journal*, No. 2 (1964), p. 177.

51. Subsection (b) of the Statement, 31 Fed. Reg. 11415 (1966).

52. Subsection (f).

53. 108 *Congressional Record* 17398-17399.

54. 108 *Congressional Record* 17399 (1962).

55. 108 *Congressional Record* 17398 (1962).

56. Section II, 1.

57. Section III, 3c.

58. H. K. Beecher, "Ethics and Clinical Research," *New England Journal of Medicine*, Vol. 274 (1966), pp. 1354-60.

59. 32 Federal Register 3994 (March 11, 1967).

60. The case law on consent for medical treatment by parents on behalf of children seems to require that the child benefit from the treatment. Nothing in the case law, statutes, or the literature of the field provides support for parental or other guardian or representative consent for admission to a research project without potential direct benefit to the incapacitated subject. See W. J. Curran, "A Problem of Consent: Kidney Transplantation in Minors," *New York University Law Review*, Vol. 34 (1959), pp. 891-98. None of the cases before the courts have presented the issue of indirect benefit or non-therapeutic clinical research.

61. Uniform Anatomical Gifts Act, § 4(c), National Conference of Commissioners of Uniform State Laws. Adopted July 26, 1968.

62. *Cardiac Transplantation in Man*, A Statement of the Board of Medicine, National Academy of Sciences, February 28, 1968.

63. *Basic Data Relating to the National Institutes of Health, 1968*, p. 6 (Published by the NIH, Division of Research Grants, March, 1968).

64. *Annual Report of the Department of HEW, Food and Drug Administration, 1967*, p. 208.

65. *Idem*, Public Health Service, Table 5, pp. 136-137.

66. *Basic Data Relating to the National Institutes of Health*, p. 31.

67. C. Kerr, *The Uses of the University* (New York, 1963), p. 59.

68. S. M. Sessoms, "Guiding Principles in Medical Research Involving Humans, National Institutes of Health," *Hospitals, Journal of American Hospital Association*, Vol. 32 (1958), pp. 44–64. These principles were not amended until 1966 when they were modified slightly to bring them into accordance with the extramural guidelines. See "Group Considerations and Informed Consent in Clinical Research at the National Institutes of Health," July 1, 1966.

69. *Idem*, at 59.

70. The letter of transmittal and memorandum are entitled, "Moral and Ethical Aspects of Clinical Investigations," January 7, 1963.

453

71. For a more complete and authoritative review of the PHS policy and the reasoning behind it, see E. A. Confrey, "PHS Grant-Supported Research with Human Subjects," *Public Health Reports,* Vol. 83 (1968), pp. 127-33.

72. D. T. Chalkley, "Intent and Experience in Implementation of Public Health Service Regulations Concerning Projects Involving Human Subjects," presented at the Annual Meeting, American Psychological Association, San Francisco, California, August 31, 1968.

73. *Op. cit. supra,* note 18. The principles read as follows:
    "(3) Clinical research cannot legitimately be carried out unless the importance of the objective is in proportion to the inherent risk to the subject.
    "(4) Every clinical research project should be preceded by careful assessment of the inherent risks in comparison to foreseeable benefits to the subject or to others."

74. *Op. cit. supra,* note 16. Principle Six reads as follows:
    "(6) The degree of risk to be taken should never exceed that determined by the humanitarian importance of the problem to be solved by the experiment."

75. See pages 546-48 of this article.

76. *Op. cit. supra,* note 72.

77. As an independent observer in both areas, I can only express my admiration for the work of the officials in each of the agencies and thank them for their cooperation in producing this commentary.

ADVISORY COMMITTEE

Notes on Contributors

HENRY K. BEECHER, born in 1904, is Dorr Professor of Research in Anaesthesia at the Harvard Medical School. He is the author of *Research and the Individual* (Boston, 1959), *Physiology of Anesthesia* (New York, 1938), and editor of *Disease and the Advancement of Basic Science* (Cambridge, 1960). Dr. Beecher served as chairman of the *Ad Hoc* Committee at Harvard Medical School to Examine the Definition of Brain Death.

HERRMAN L. BLUMGART, born in 1895, is professor of medicine, *emeritus*, at Harvard Medical School, physician-in-chief, *emeritus*, at Beth Israel Hospital in Boston, and consultant in medicine for the Harvard University Medical Area Health Service. Dr. Blumgart is the author of some one hundred and fifty articles dealing mainly with the cardiovascular system.

GUIDO CALABRESI, born in 1932, is professor of law at Yale University. Mr. Calabresi is the author of numerous articles in the field of accident law. He served as law clerk to the Hon. Hugo L. Black, U. S. Supreme Court.

DAVID F. CAVERS, born in 1902, is Fessenden Professor of Law at the Harvard Law School. He is the author of *The Choice-of-Law Process* (1965) and co-author of *Electric Power Regulation in Latin America* (1959). Since 1958, he has been president of the Walter E. Meyer Research Institute of Law.

WILLIAM J. CURRAN, born in 1925, is Frances Glessner Lee Professor of Legal Medicine at the Harvard Medical School and School of Public Health. He is also a lecturer on legal medicine at the Harvard Law School. Mr. Curran is the author of *The Doctor as a Witness* (Philadelphia, 1965), *Medical Proof in Litigation* (Boston, 1962), and *Law and Medicine* (Boston, 1960). He was a founder and former director of the Law-Medicine Research Institute of Boston University.

ARTHUR J. DYCK, born in 1932, is Mary B. Saltonstall Professor of Population Ethics at the Harvard School of Public Health and a member of the Harvard Center for Population Studies as well as the Harvard Divinity School Faculty. Mr. Dyck is the author of *Moral Evaluations and Reality* (in progress) and co-author of *An Ethical Analysis of Population Policies* (in progress).

GEOFFREY EDSALL, born in 1908, is Superintendent of the State Laboratory of the Massachusetts Department of Public Health and professor of applied microbiology at the Harvard School of Public Health. He is the author of numerous articles on applied immunology and the role of the laboratory in public health. Dr. Edsall has served as a consultant to the World Health Organization on immunization and related problems.

DONALD FLEMING, born in 1923, is professor of history at Harvard University. He is the author of *William H. Welch and the Rise of Modern Medicine* (Boston, 1954) and co-editor of *The Intellectual Migration* (Cambridge, 1969) and *Perspectives in American History.*

Renée C. Fox, born in 1928, is professor of sociology at the University of Pennsylvania, with a joint appointment to the Department of Sociology and to the Department of Psychiatry in the School of Medicine. Miss Fox is the author of *Experiment Perilous* (Glencoe, 1959) and co-author of *The Emerging Physician* (Stanford, 1968). She has also written numerous articles on the sociology of medicine. Miss Fox is an associate editor of *Social Science and Medicine*.

Paul A. Freund, born in 1908, is Carl M. Loeb University Professor at Harvard. He is the author of *On Law and Justice* (Cambridge, 1968) and *The Supreme Court of the United States* (New York, 1961). Mr. Freund was president of the American Academy of Arts and Sciences from 1964 until 1967.

Louis L. Jaffe, born in 1905, is Byrne Professor of Administrative Law at the Harvard Law School. He is the author of *Is the Great Judge Obsolete?* (New York, forthcoming), *Judicial Control of Administrative Action* (Boston, 1955), and *Judicial Aspects of Foreign Relations* (Cambridge, 1933). Mr. Jaffe is also the co-author of *Administrative Law* (3d edition, 1968).

Hans Jonas, born in 1903, is Alvin Johnson Professor of Philosophy in the Graduate Faculty of the New School for Social Research. His most recent books include *The Western Tradition and Technological Man* (in progress), *The Phenomenon of Life: Toward a Philosophical Biology* (New York, 1968), and *Zwischen Nichts und Ewigkeit* (Gottingen, 1963).

Jay Katz, born in 1922, is adjunct professor of law and psychiatry at Yale University. He is the co-author of *Psychoanalysis, Psychiatry, and Law* (Glencoe, 1967) and *The Family and the Law*. Dr. Katz also has written numerous articles on psychoanalysis and the law.

Irving Ladimer, born in 1916, is associate clinical professor of community medicine at Mt. Sinai School of Medicine and program consultant for the United Health Foundations, Inc. Mr. Ladimer is the author of some fifty professional papers on medicolegal issues in human experimentation, health education, and public welfare.

Louis Lasagna, born in 1923, is associate professor of medicine and associate professor of pharmacology and experimental therapeutics at the Johns Hopkins University School of Medicine. Dr. Lasagna is the author of *Life, Death, and the Doctor* (New York, 1968) and *The Doctor's Dilemmas* (New York, 1962), as well as many scientific articles on clinical pharmacology.

Walsh McDermott, born in 1909, is Livingston Farrand Professor of Public Health and Chairman of the Department at Cornell University Medical College. Dr. McDermott is the co-editor of the *Cecil-Loeb Textbook of Medicine* and author of numerous articles on the health problems of communities and the use of science and technology in socio-economic development.

MARGARET MEAD, born in 1901, is curator of ethnology at the American Museum of Natural History and adjunct professor of anthropology at Columbia University. Her publications include *Anthropology: A Human Science* (1964), *Continuities in Cultural Evolution* (1964), *New Lives for Old* (1956), and *Coming of Age in Samoa* (1928).

FRANCIS D. MOORE, born in 1913, is Moseley Professor of Surgery at the Harvard Medical School and surgeon-in-chief at the Peter Bent Brigham Hospital in Boston. Dr. Moore's most recent publications include *Give and Take: The Development of Tissue Transplantation* (New York, 1964), *Metabolic Care of the Surgical Patient* (Philadelphia, 1959), and, as co-author, *Carcinoma of the Breast* (Boston, 1968).

TALCOTT PARSONS, born in 1902, is professor of sociology at Harvard University. His publications include *Evolutionary and Comparative Perspectives* (1965), *Structure and Process in Modern Societies* (1959), *Family Socialization and Interaction Process* (1955), and *Toward a General Theory of Action* (1951). Mr. Parsons was co-editor, with Kenneth B. Clark, of the *Daedalus* Library volume *The Negro American*, and has served as President of the American Academy of Arts and Sciences since 1967.

DAVID D. RUTSTEIN, born in 1907, is Ridley Watts Professor of Preventive Medicine and head of the department at Harvard Medical School. Dr. Rutstein is the author of *The Coming Revolution in Medicine* (Cambridge, 1967), and of numerous scientific articles in the field of epidemiology and preventive medicine.

JUDITH P. SWAZEY, born in 1939, is a research associate in the Harvard University Program on Technology and Society. Mrs. Swazey is the author of *Reflexes and Motor Integration* (Cambridge, 1969). She is currently collaborating with Renée C. Fox on a study of the social aspects of organ transplantation and hemodialysis. This research will be published as a book in 1971. Mrs. Swazey is assistant editor of the *Journal of the History of Biology*.

469